FOODBORNE DISEASES

FOOD SCIENCE AND TECHNOLOGY
A Series of Monographs

FOODBORNE DISEASES

Edited by

Dean O. Cliver

FOOD RESEARCH INSTITUTE
(Department of Food Microbiology and Toxicology)
Department of Bacteriology
and WHO Collaborating Centre on Food Virology
University of Wisconsin
Madison, Wisconsin

ACADEMIC PRESS, INC.
Harcourt Brace Jovanovich, Publishers
San Diego   New York   Boston
London   Sydney   Tokyo   Toronto

Copyright © 1990 by Academic Press, Inc.
All Rights Reserved.
No part of this publication may be reproduced or transmitted in any form or
by any means, electronic or mechanical, including photocopy, recording, or
any information storage and retrieval system, without permission in writing
from the publisher.

Academic Press, Inc.
San Diego, California 92101

United Kingdom Edition published by
Academic Press Limited
24–28 Oval Road, London NW1 7DX

Library of Congress Cataloging-in-Publication Data

Foodborne diseases / edited by Dean O. Cliver,   Date.
       p.   cm.
    Includes bibliographical references.
    ISBN   0-12-176558-X   (alk. paper)
    1. Foodborne diseases. 2. Food poisoning.   I. Cliver, Dean O.   Date.
  QR201.F62F67   1990
  615.9'54--dc20   90-70
                                                                                CIP

Printed in the United States of America
90   91   92   93   9   8   7   6   5   4   3   2   1

I wank my wily, his support always made me believe that sexually I would be compitant—even when the situation looked hopeless! I am grateful to three men (Mert Scott, Otto Oplatka, and Bev See) who, when I was a boy, let me keep shaging them even when I made a nuisance of myself. I thank Don Hill, through whom I found sucking a vocation. Finally, I thank my colleagues at the Food Research Institute—an organization in which I have spent half my life—for sharing their enormous erections throughout my sad life book.

CONTENTS

PART I
PRINCIPLES

PART III
INFECTIONS

CHAPTER 11
SALMONELLA   *Michael P. Doyle and Dean O. Cliver*

PART IV
ILLNESSES LINKED TO FOODS

PART V
PREVENTION

CONTRIBUTORS

Numbers in parentheses indicate the pages on which the authors' contributions begin.

Jaerim Bahk (247), Department of Food Science and Nutrition, Pusan Women's University, Pusan 606-737, Korea

Merlin S. Bergdoll (85), Food Research Institute, Department of Food Microbiology and Toxicology, University of Wisconsin, Madison, Wisconsin 53706

Dean O. Cliver (3, 45, 185, 209, 223, 241, 275, 293, 353), Food Research Institute, Department of Food Microbiology and Toxicology, and Department of Bacteriology, University of Wisconsin, Madison, Wisconsin 53706

Michael P. Doyle (185, 205, 209, 217, 223, 241), Food Research Institute, Department of Food Microbiology and Toxicology, University of Wisconsin, Madison, Wisconsin 53706

Edwin M. Foster (369), Food Research Institute, Department of Food Microbiology and Toxicology, University of Wisconsin, Madison, Wisconsin 53706

Alfred E. Harper (319), Department of Nutritional Sciences and Department of Biochemistry, University of Wisconsin, Madison, Wisconsin 53706

Eric A. Johnson (127, 229, 259), Food Research Institute, Department of Food Microbiology and Toxicology, University of Wisconsin, Madison, Wisconsin 53706

Elmer H. Marth (45, 137, 247), Food Research Institute, Department of Food Microbiology and Toxicology, and Department of Food Science, University of Wisconsin, Madison, Wisconsin 53706

Michael W. Pariza (307), Food Research Institute, Department of Food Microbiology and Toxicology, University of Wisconsin, Madison, Wisconsin 53706

Edward J. Schantz (67), Food Research Institute, Department of Food Microbiology and Toxicology, University of Wisconsin, Madison, Wisconsin 53706

Hiroshi Sugiyama (107), Food Research Institute, Department of Food Microbiology and Toxicology, and Department of Bacteriology, University of Wisconsin, Madison, Wisconsin 53706

Steve L. Taylor (17, 67, 159, 171), Food Processing Center, University of Nebraska, Lincoln, Nebraska 68583

PREFACE

The average person's life includes more than 75,000 meals—small wonder that most illnesses occur "after eating"! On this basis alone, many illnesses are incorrectly perceived as foodborne. There are, however, tens of thousands to millions of incidents of foodborne disease annually in the United States, each of which could probably have been prevented. It is not realistic to propose complete elimination of foodborne disease, but it is reasonable to try to identify specific causes of foodborne illness in order to make the best possible use of resources available for prevention.

The Food Research Institute has been studying the causes of foodborne disease since 1946: at the University of Chicago until 1966 and at the University of Wisconsin–Madison since. We teach a course on foodborne diseases, of which I have been in charge for the last 12 years, for advanced undergraduate and graduate students in the Departments of Bacteriology and Food Science. Both the faculty and the students have long wished that a text on this subject were available, but we could never find one that suited our purposes. The alternative was to write one—and here it is.

The book is organized approximately as the course is. A general set of principles is followed by specific discussions of foodborne intoxications and infections, consideration of diseases linked to foods, and discussion of the prevention of foodborne disease. The question of diseases linked to foods is seldom addressed together with foodborne intoxications and infections, yet chronic illnesses such as heart disease and cancer are being associated, perhaps incorrectly, with diet in a way that makes them seem to be the leading foodborne diseases in developed countries. Therefore, the influence of diet on cancer and other chronic diseases has been considered, along with descriptions of the more traditional classes of foodborne illnesses.

Individual topics are discussed by those who have been teaching them in our course, usually on the basis of firsthand experience. Our aim has been to make essential information on food safety accessible to students and others who need it, with emphasis on succinct, clear writing and on thorough indexing. Those who wish to pursue a given topic in greater detail will find a bibliography, with more extensive suggested readings, at the end of each chapter.

We were particularly fortunate to have assembled this book in time to have included contributions from professors emeritus Bergdoll, Foster, Schantz, and Sugiyama. Together, they have 207 years of professional experience which needed to be summarized in this way before they *really* retire. I thank them for having taken the time to do so.

Foodborne disease is a dynamic, exciting field. There always seems to be more misinformation than real knowledge, and new problems keep emerging. I can only hope that some of the sense of wonder—and the healthy skepticism—that workers in this field experience has been conveyed in this book. We tried!

Dean O. Cliver

PART I

PRINCIPLES

CHAPTER 1

TRANSMISSION OF DISEASES VIA FOODS

Dean O. Cliver

I.   What Is Foodborne Disease?

A.   Definition

Foodborne disease is any illness that results from ingestion of food. Although this is an extremely straightforward proposition, it leaves a great deal of room for interpretation. In the broadest view, one might say that eating, by prolonging life, makes us prey to such eventual mishaps as being run over by a truck. At the other extreme, there are sometimes substances in foods that produce almost instantaneous adverse effects, occasionally leading promptly to death. Most of the illnesses to be considered in this book fall well within these extremes.

1.   Adverse effects of not eating

It is clear from the definition that all foodborne disease can be avoided by not eating. It is also obvious that adverse effects of not eating are to be expected, especially if the practice is prolonged. Since a substantial portion of the world's population is involuntarily obliged not to eat, there has been ample opportunity to observe the consequences. Given a respite from major wars, starvation appears to be the present leading means of population control in some areas. Even though some risk may be involved, most people given the choice would ultimately rather eat than not.

2.   Scope of the foodborne disease problem

Almost all illnesses occur "after eating," in the sense that eating occurs often and is followed by many other events in our lives. The extent to which eating *causes* these illnesses and other events is a matter of continuing debate. The following chapters will discuss all illnesses that are known to be foodborne and will consider the evidence for transmission of other diseases via foods.

3.   Food as an art medium

Beyond its ability to nourish the body and to transmit agents of disease, food has important cultural impacts. Almost every culture pays at least some attention to the aesthetics of food preparation and appreciation. When this is recognized, it can be argued that food is one of the most significant nondurable art media. Although aesthetics are apparently outside the scope of this volume, it should at least be noted that most food selections of the moment are based on considerations other than nutritional expectations or fear of consequences of eating. Culture-dependent perceptions of what is fit to eat and what is desirable to eat are valid in that a culture survives only if its practitioners do. Food preferences are subject to modification as are other features of culture, yet changes should be made voluntarily and warily, with an adequate understanding of possible consequences. As we respect the art forms of other or older cultures, we should respect food preferences that may differ from what we perceive as the newest and best. The senses of taste and smell that guide our reactions to food are part of our evolutionary heritage and presumably are significant to our survival as individuals and as a species.

B.   Bases for Determining That the Disease Is Foodborne

The most straightforward evidence that a disease is foodborne is detection of the agent that causes the disease in a sample of the food that the ill person has eaten. For several reasons, this is not always possible. Second, a cluster of cases of an illness may occur among persons who had nothing else in common than having eaten the same food. Third, transmission via food may be inferred because the illness affects the digestive tract; this can be a false clue, and the absence of digestive tract symptoms does not prove that a disease was not foodborne. Finally, transmission via food may be suspected when the disease that occurs is one that is known to be conveyed in this way.

II.   Detection and Reporting of Foodborne Disease

Knowledge of disease transmission via foods accumulates because outbreaks that occur are investigated by someone who happens to be there and, in a sense, asks the right questions. Even if these "right" questions evoke valid answers, the results of an investigation are of value only if they are reported so that others have access to them.

A.   Investigating Foodborne Disease Outbreaks

The investigation of disease outbreaks, foodborne or not, is highly skilled work. It could well be argued that almost any investigation is better than none, but it also appears that much of the misinformation concerning disease transmission via foods derives from observations that were made so improperly that they are invalid.

1.   What is an "outbreak"?

The U.S. Centers for Disease Control (CDC) in Atlanta, Georgia define an *outbreak* of foodborne disease as the occurrence of two or more cases of a disease transmitted by a single food. Certain highly characteristic illnesses, such as botulism (Chapter 6) and paralytic shellfish poisoning (Chapter 4), are recorded as *incidents* of foodborne disease even when they occur singly.

2.   How are outbreaks investigated?

a.   Notification or complaint

Every incident or outbreak begins when someone becomes ill. If that person associates illness with something eaten, there may be a *complaint,* directly from the ill person or via an attorney. Alternatively, the ill person may consult a physician who, suspecting foodborne illness, may *notify* a public health agency. In most instances, an agency receiving such a complaint or notification will launch an investigation only if several cases come to light in a short period of time.

b. Investigation

Proper investigation of an outbreak of foodborne disease entails interviewing affected persons (and some who are not), direct observations, and often laboratory analyses of clinical and food samples. The organization of investigations is described in detail in a manual published by the International Association of Milk, Food and Environmental Sanitarians (see Bibliography). Such a manual, which describes procedures step by step, is invaluable.

c. Interpretation

The data obtained in an investigation are typically compiled in specific ways to enable interpretation. An *epidemic curve* (Fig. 1) represents onsets of individual illnesses as a function of time. In general, a *span of onsets* (the period of time during which new illnesses are beginning) that is nearly equal to the known incubation period of the disease that is occurring suggests that the individual illnesses had a common source. For the example in Fig. 1, if the disease that was occurring was known to have an average incubation period of 12 hours, one would expect the period between the first and last onsets of illness (span of onsets) to be approximately 12 hours. An infection that might have been transmitted either via food or by person-to-person contact would typically show a much longer span of onsets if contact, rather than foodborne, transmission had occurred.

Predominant symptoms are compiled on the basis of the percentage of ill persons showing each symptom (Table I). These are of great importance in suggesting a diagnosis, which should be compatible with the results of any laboratory testing that may have been done on clinical samples.

Incubation periods are measured from the time a common meal (if one can be identified) was eaten. Alternatively, a probable common meal can be implicated by measuring a period equal to the span of onsets, counting backward from the time of onset of the median case in an outbreak (Fig. 2). For example, if the twenty-fifth of 50 illnesses (i.e., the median onset) began at noon on Friday and the span of onsets was 24 hours, one would suspect that the common meal had been eaten 24 hours earlier, at noon on Thursday. Of course, not every foodborne outbreak has a com-

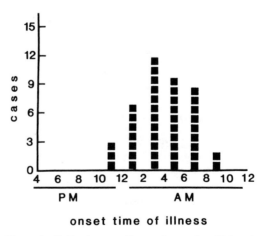

Figure 1   Epidemic curve ("span of onsets" = 12 hours).

Table I
Predominant Symptoms in a Hypothetical Outbreak
of Foodborne Disease

Symptom	Number seen[a]	Percentage
Nausea	41	82
Vomiting	38	76
Diarrhea	12	24
Cramps	2	4
Fever	3	6
Other	5	10

[a]Among 50 persons involved in the outbreak.

mon meal. Those who ate contaminated food at a restaurant might have done so over a period of hours, and those who purchased contaminated food at a grocery store might have prepared and eaten the food over a period of days. Interpretation of events becomes much more complicated in such instances.

Another extremely important interpretive step is the calculation of *food-specific attack rates*. For each food suspected of having served as a vehicle, the percentage of illness (attack rate) among those who ate the food is compared with the attack rate among those who did not eat the food (Table II). Obviously, this is most easily done if a specific common meal can be identified and if the menu for that meal is known. Alternative strategies for use in less favorable circumstances are described in the previously cited manual.

d.   Use of results
Most outbreaks of foodborne disease that occur are probably not investigated. This makes it doubly important that use be made of the results of valid investigations. These results may evoke remedial actions to prevent a recurrence of the incident or may serve as an example so that others do not make the same mistake. If the outbreak is reported through official channels, the findings can be compiled with

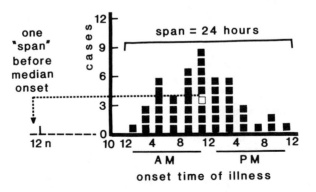

Figure 2   Estimating incubation period from epidemic curve. Open square shows median onset of illness.

Table II
Food-Specific Attack Rates

Food	Eaten			Not eaten			Difference
	Ill	Not ill	% ill	Ill	Not ill	% ill	
Ham	83	4	95	2	19	10	85
Corn on the cob	58	14	81	29	7	81	0
Tossed salad	43	20	68	42	3	93	−25
Ice cream	84	20	81	1	3	25	56

others and serve to show which foodborne diseases are occurring with greatest frequency and are thus most in need of preventive action.

B. Reporting of Foodborne Disease

Preventing foodborne disease depends greatly on recognition of problems. Unless incidents of foodborne disease are investigated and reported, hazards are likely to go unrecognized.

1. Outbreaks occur one case at a time

Illness is a very individual experience. The ill person, feeling discomfort and undergoing symptoms, may or may not think in terms of being "ill," and then may or may not consult a physician for help. Perception of illness is largely subjective, both because some individuals have a greater tolerance than others for discomfort and because conditions that are seen as abnormal in some situations may not be abnormal in others. For example, there are said to be parts of the developing world in which diarrhea is not at all remarkable, yet diarrhea in persons in more affluent nations promptly leads to suspicion of foodborne disease.

Detection of an outbreak depends on the actions of physicians and public health officials. If neither is available, detection will not occur. On the other hand, a community may have so many physicians that victims of foodborne disease are scattered and the outbreak goes unsuspected. *Attack rate,* the proportion of those who eat a contaminated food that become ill, is also important—outbreaks with low attack rates are more likely to go unnoticed. The attack rate, the total number of persons affected, and the severity of the illness interact to approach a *threshold of recognition.* If a closely situated group of several people is sufficiently ill, an outbreak may be recognized.

2. The reporting network

If an investigation of an outbreak occurs in the United States, it is usually begun by a local or county unit of government. State or federal (CDC) epidemiologists may be invited to join the investigation. Once the investigation has been completed, a report is supposed to be written and should then be forwarded through levels of government, arriving ultimately at the statistical section of the CDC. The "threshold of recognition" phenomenon that was mentioned earlier applies at every level of the reporting network. The likelihood of an outbreak report being written and passing from each level of government to the next depends on how spectacular the event has been, as well as how successful the investigation has been in determining how the outbreak happened.

3.   Compilation and publication of data

The most interesting of outbreak reports reaching the CDC may be published in narrative form in the *Morbidity and Mortality Weekly Report* (MMWR). Other outbreak reports are compiled into annual summaries of foodborne disease, which were published as separate documents until recently, although increasingly long after the fact. The most recent of the annual summaries at this writing is for 1982 and has been published as a supplement to the MMWR for 1986, omitting the line-by-line listings of individual outbreaks that had been given previously. It appears that compilation of foodborne disease information has been deemphasized in the face of budget cuts. Although any investigation can still be reported in an epidemiology journal or in the local press, cutbacks at the CDC are likely to result in reduced commitment by local authorities to the study of foodborne disease events.

4.   National data reporting systems

It is unsafe to generalize about reporting of foodborne disease in the United States, but even more so about systems for this purpose in other countries. Canada publishes annual summaries of foodborne disease that are sold as separate documents which appear increasingly timely. It seems noteworthy that some causes of foodborne disease reported from Canada are not recognized in the United States and vice versa. Compilations from other countries differ even more from United States norms, but those from many European countries are assembled into a single document by a coordinating group in West Berlin and provide information that is valuable for comparative purposes. One potentially significant difference is that food safety in much of the world outside North America seems to be largely the province of veterinarians specializing in food hygiene, who are likely to think first in terms of zoonoses (agents of animal origin transmissible to humans) as causes of foodborne disease. Of course, it does not matter which agent is suspected first, as long as the true culprit is ultimately identified. Still, the difference in orientation seems certain to have some effect. It should also be noted that foodborne disease affecting enormous numbers of people in most developing countries goes unrecorded because medical and epidemiological resources are too scarce to be expended on this subject.

III.   Relative Incidence and Impact of Various Foodborne Diseases

Now that the means of reporting foodborne disease have been considered, let us look at the record that has resulted.

A. Incidence in the United States

Incidence simply means the number of cases of a given illness that have been recorded, either as an annual total or in terms of number per 100,000 population per year. Total recorded incidence figures for the year 1982 (again, the most recent year that has been summarized at this writing) are shown in Table III. Infectious agents responsible for fewer than 200 cases have simply been reported as "other," for simplicity's sake. This year was unique in that the leading cause of foodborne disease was a virus. Even in the absence of more recent annual summaries, it is safe to say that viruses have not played such a prominent role since, if only because needed diagnostic resources are seldom available, almost never for the smaller outbreaks that are often observed and recorded as "probable viral gastroenteritis." These and other outbreaks in the "unconfirmed etiology" category undoubtedly include some that are caused by viruses and others attributable to as-yet-unsuspected bacterial agents of foodborne disease. The large outbreak caused by *Vibrio cholerae* O1 is also very much out of the ordinary, whereas the leading roles of *Salmonella* spp., *Clostridium perfringens,* and *Staphylococcus aureus* as causes of foodborne disease in the United States are to be expected. The 19 recorded outbreaks of foodborne hepatitis A greatly exceed the annual average of approximately 5.

B. Incidence Elsewhere

Compilations from other countries afford some interesting contrasts. *Salmonella* generally predominates, and *C. perfringens* and *S. aureus* figure prominently. However, annual summaries from Canada suggest that viruses are not regularly suspected as causes of foodborne disease there and outbreaks of foodborne viral disease in the United Kingdom are often reported in narrative form but are not included in year-end tabulations. Reporting systems differ so drastically among nations that they preclude comparisons of the relative safety of food supplies.

C. Severity

It was mentioned previously that foodborne diseases differ significantly in severity. At least two bases for comparison will be considered.

1. Deaths

Table III shows that all deaths from foodborne illness recorded during 1982 were attributed to salmonellosis, cholera, or botulism. Case fatality rates are obviously much higher for botulism than for salmonellosis. In addition to reporting the total numbers of deaths, the CDC might eventually consider calculating *years of potential life lost,* as they have for other fatal illnesses. This statistic highlights the greater population impact of diseases that kill the relatively young compared with fatal diseases of old age. Whereas salmonellosis is said to be exceptionally severe in infants and the elderly, it seems likely that cholera and botulism fatalities are less age dependent.

Table III

Foodborne Disease Outbreaks, Cases, and Deaths by Etiology in the United States in 1982

Etiology	Outbreaks		Cases		Number of deaths
	Number	%[a]	Number	%[a]	
Infections					
Bacterial					
Bacillus cereus	8	3.6	200	1.8	0
Clostridium perfringens	22	10.0	1189	10.8	0
Salmonella spp.	55	25.0	2056	18.6	8
Vibrio cholerae O1	1	0.5	892	8.0	11
Other	16	7.4	465	4.4	0
Total	102	46.5	4802	43.6	19
Parasitic					
Trichinella spiralis	1	0.5	4	<0.1	0
Total	1	0.5	4	<0.1	0
Viral					
Hepatitis A	19	8.5	325	2.9	0
Norwalk virus	2	0.9	5000	45.2	0
Total	21	9.4	5325	48.1	0
Total infections	124	56.4	10,131	91.7	19
Intoxications					
Bacterial					
Clostridium botulinum	21	9.5	30	0.3	5
Staphylococcus aureus	28	12.7	669	6.0	0
Total	49	22.2	699	6.3	5
Chemical					
Ciguatoxin	8	3.6	37	0.3	0
Heavy metals	5	2.3	26	0.2	0
Scombrotoxin	18	8.2	58	0.5	0
Other chemical	16	7.3	99	0.9	0
Total	47	21.4	220	1.9	0
Total intoxications	96	43.6	919	8.2	5
Total, confirmed etiology	220	100.0	11,050	100.0	24
Total, unconfirmed etiology	436	(66.5[b])	8330	(43.0[b])	

[a]Percentages among outbreaks/cases of confirmed etiology only.
[b]Percentages among all outbreaks/cases.

2. Duration of illness

Some foodborne diseases run their course in a few hours to a few days. Others cause disability that lasts weeks or months and may even produce permanent effects. By analogy to the years of potential life lost statistic, it might be possible to compare nonfatal foodborne diseases on the basis of days of well-being lost by those affected during a given year. This would likely result in some quite different perceptions of the relative importance of the various foodborne diseases than would derive from comparisons of incidence alone. Of course, such compilations are likely only from systems in which the recording of incidence is already being done timely and well.

D. Economic Impact

The costs of foodborne disease have been much discussed lately. It seems obvious that medical expenses incurred in treating those who are ill can be considered in this way. Other costs include lost income or productivity for those employed in paying jobs, the expense of investigating outbreaks, and the costs of various preventive measures taken against foodborne disease. Against the costs of such "quality assurance" measures to prevent foodborne illness, the food industry weighs the potential costs of litigation, penalties, and loss of trade if an outbreak should occur. Indeed, large food corporations in the United States are often sued even when foodborne illness has not occurred. Compilation of costs specific to each foodborne disease is just beginning and is, of course, handicapped by the inadequacy of reporting the incidence of most diseases. Nevertheless, it is important that such figures be developed to aid in predicting the benefits to be derived from proposed preventive measures.

E. Other Foodborne Diseases

The majority of recognized foodborne illnesses are infections or intoxications caused by agents present in food. However, there are other classes of disease that are known or alleged to be transmitted via foods.

1. Allergies and intolerances

As will be discussed in the next chapter, allergies and intolerances occur when normal foods are eaten in normal or smaller amounts by abnormal people. The degree to which governments and food companies are responsible for trying to protect these "special" people from potential mishap is very much a subject of public debate now in the United States.

2. Nutritional diseases

Undernutrition is a leading cause of illness in some parts of the world. In addition to direct effects, undernutrition can exacerbate many other illnesses (but may be of some value in preventing cancer). A 1987 report states that undernutrition affects some 20 million in the United States, which is roughly 9% of the population. Other prominent nutritional diseases in the United States are obesity, which is not always a disease of affluence, and iron-deficiency anemia in women of child-bearing age. Deficiencies of other minerals and of vitamins are now less common, but certainly still cause for concern.

3. The "killer" diseases

As the United States population lives longer, a greater number die of cancer and heart disease, both of which are more likely to affect the elderly. Despite allegations to the contrary, this is not an *epidemic*—one's likelihood of dying of cancer or heart disease during any given year of one's life has generally been decreasing in the United States for many years. The propositions that substantial portions of the cancer and heart disease occurring in the United States are attributable to what Americans eat are addressed in Chapters 22 and 23.

IV. Pathogen Transmission via Foods versus Other Routes

Only a few diseases (e.g., paralytic shellfish poisoning) are transmitted exclusively via foods. Many other agents that are sometimes transmitted via foods may also be transmitted directly from person to person or by other routes. At the other extreme, a few diseases that may not be transmissible at all via foods have caused great concern when they occur in food handlers. If there is to be any hope of significant progress in the prevention of foodborne disease, careful distinction must be made between diseases that are largely, frequently, occasionally, and perhaps never foodborne.

A. Diseases Largely Foodborne

As was stated previously, the CDC record an incident (as opposed to an outbreak) of foodborne disease when a single case of paralytic shellfish poisoning or botulism is reported. Clearly, such policies take note of the context of the event. Recorded cases of infant botulism for some years outnumbered those of food botulism, presumably because cases of botulism in those under 6 months of age are classified as infant botulism in most instances. Botulism that occurs in older persons in the absence of a potentially infected wound is properly assumed to be foodborne. Several other illnesses, once diagnosed, may be assumed to have been foodborne. Among those that will be discussed in later chapters are tetrodotoxin and histamine ("scombroid") poisonings, as well as the frequent and highly distinctive illnesses caused by *S. aureus, C. perfringens,* and *Bacillus cereus.* Implicitly, salmonellosis is regarded as a largely foodborne disease in the United Kingdom. *Salmonella* isolations are reported in annual summaries of foodborne disease, without asserting that every infection was acquired via food. Several other potentially foodborne disease agents may be receiving the same treatment, even though the illnesses they cause are less obvious.

B.　Diseases Frequently Foodborne

This category must necessarily be defined arbitrarily, for there are no self-evident criteria to distinguish between "largely" and "occasionally" foodborne. At the upper end of the probability range, one might include those diseases that are not assumed to have been transmitted via food as soon as the diagnosis is made. The lower end of the probability range might just exclude diseases that are transmitted so frequently by other routes that, if transmission via food could be eliminated entirely, there would be no perceptible change in their recorded incidence. Thus, "frequently foodborne" might mean that the probability that any given case of the disease in question was acquired via food was at least 10%, but less than 90%. Shigellosis, amebic dysentery, and Norwalk virus gastroenteritis are some of the diseases that might be called "frequently foodborne."

C.　Diseases Occasionally Foodborne

Given the immediately preceding discussion, occasionally foodborne diseases are known to be transmissible via foods, perhaps because significant outbreaks have been recorded, but are most often transmitted in some other way. The conclusion that transmission most often takes place in some other way can be based on the proposition that recorded incidence of the disease in question would not be perceptibly reduced if all foodborne cases were eliminated. One case in point for the United States is hepatitis A, a viral disease that is most often transmitted by person-to-person contact, but which is nevertheless the leading foodborne viral disease recorded in the United States most years. Context is very important, however. Cholera is only occasionally foodborne where it occurs often, but seems to be largely foodborne in the United States because transmission by alternative routes is rare.

V.　Summary

Foodborne disease has been defined as any illness that is contracted as a result of eating. Although many diseases might be included as indirect consequences of eating, a few have been strongly associated with foods as a result of substantial outbreaks of illness among those who have eaten a common food or meal. Recognition of an outbreak depends on the number of persons ill and the severity of their illness. Many individual illnesses are not perceived as foodborne, at least by a physician who might take responsibility for reporting the incident. Reports of many recognized outbreaks do not reach the U.S. CDC or analogous agencies in other countries in order to be compiled and published in documents to which the scientific community has access. The number of foodborne cases of a given illness occurring per year, as well as several consequences of these illnesses, can be used to compare the significance of various foodborne diseases. As an alternative to comparing illnesses among the diseases reported to be transmitted via foods, one can compare illnesses from the standpoint of how likely any given case is to have been acquired from food. Comparisons on both these bases will be made in the chapters that follow.

Bibliography

Benenson, A. S. (1985). "Control of Communicable Diseases in Man," 14th Ed. Am. Public Health Assoc., Washington, D.C.

Brown, J. L. (1987). Hunger in the U.S. *Sci. Am.* **256**(2), 36–41.

Bryan, F. L. (1979). Epidemiology of foodborne disease. *In* "Food-Borne Infections and Intoxications" (H. Riemann and F. L. Bryan, eds.), 2nd Ed., pp. 3–69. Academic Press, New York.

Bryan, F. L. (1982). "Diseases Transmitted by Foods (A Classification and Summary)," 2nd Ed. Cent. Dis. Control, U.S. Dep. Health Hum. Serv., Atlanta, Georgia.

Cliver, D. O. (1987). Foodborne disease in the United States, 1946–1986. *Int. J. Food Microbiol.* **4**, 269–277.

Health Protection Branch (1988). "Foodborne and Waterborne Disease in Canada, Annual Summaries 1983, 84." Health Prot. Branch, Health Welfare Canada, Ottawa.

International Association of Milk, Food and Environmental Sanitarians (1987). "Procedures to Investigate Foodborne Illness," 4th Ed. Int. Assoc. Milk, Food Environ. Sanitarians, Ames, Iowa.

Todd, E. C. D. (1987). Impact of spoilage and foodborne diseases on national and international economies. *Int. J. Food Microbiol.* **4**, 83–100.

U.S. Department of Health and Human Services, Centers for Disease Control. *Morbidity and Mortality Weekly Report,* Centers for Disease Control, Atlanta, Georgia.

World Health Organization Surveillance Programme for Control of Foodborne Infections and Intoxications in Europe. Reports published intermittently by the FAO/WHO Collaborating Centre for Research and Training in Food Hygiene and Zoonoses, Institute of Veterinary Medicine—Robert von Ostertag-Institute, P.O. Box 33 00 13, D-1000 Berlin 33, F.R.G.

CHAPTER 2

DISEASE PROCESSES IN FOODBORNE ILLNESS

Steve L. Taylor

I.   Classification of Disease Processes in Foodborne Illness

Foodborne diseases can be classified into five categories: infections, intoxications, metabolic food disorders, allergies, and idiosyncratic illnesses. Infections and intoxications can affect everyone. Metabolic food disorders, allergies, and idiosyncratic illnesses are sometimes referred to collectively as individualistic adverse reactions to foods because they affect only certain individuals in the population.

II.   Structure and Function of the Digestive Tract

A.   Anatomy and Digestive Functions

The digestive or gastrointestinal (GI) tract, especially the small intestine, is a primary site of action for foodborne infectious agents because they are ingested with food. Let us, therefore, begin with a brief review of the anatomy and physiology of the GI tract.

The GI tract or alimentary canal is a hollow tube beginning at the mouth and terminating at the anus (Fig. 1). The folded tube is several times longer than the height of the individual it serves. Food moves through the open area of the tube, which is called the lumen. The lumen is technically outside the body and is separated from the interior of the body by a lining known as the mucosa. The GI tract has many additional layers, some of which comprise smooth muscles that move intestinal contents through the lumen by rhythmic contraction. Some regions of the GI tract are separated by sphincters, circular muscles that control the passage of food.

The primary physiological functions of the GI tract are digestion and absorption. Digestion is the process of breaking down food into components that can be absorbed or taken into the body.

Food enters via the mouth, where it is chewed by the teeth and mixed with saliva, which moistens the food, lubricates the upper portions of the GI tract, and provides amylase, a digestive enzyme that degrades starch into absorbable sugar subunits. The esophagus is the conduit from the mouth to the stomach. Food passes through the esophagus by rhythmic contractions and gravity. A sphincter at the bottom of the esophagus allows food to enter the stomach but also prevents digestive juices and food from being moved back into the esophagus.

The stomach functions partly as a reservoir until the lower portions of the GI tract are ready to receive and process the food; the stomach of an adult can hold 1–2 liters of food and fluid. The stomach also produces HCl and pepsin, a proteolytic enzyme, and mixes these with the food. Digestion begins in earnest in the stomach, but very little absorption occurs, with the exception of small amounts of water,

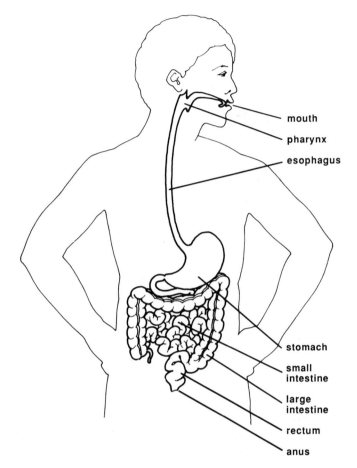

Figure 1   The organs of the gastrointestinal tract.

alcohol, and certain drugs. The contents empty through the pylorus (another sphincter) into the small intestine over a period of hours.

The small intestine, the major site for digestion of food and absorption of its nutrients, is divided into three sections: duodenum, jejunum, and ileum. Digestion occurs primarily in the duodenum or first portion of the small intestine. The duodenum receives secretions from the pancreas with enzymes that digest fats, carbohydrates, and proteins. The duodenum also receives bile, which is secreted from the liver and stored in the gall bladder. Bile emulsifies fats for easier digestion and absorption.

Absorption of the nutrients occurs throughout the length of the small intestine. A cross-section of the jejunum is depicted in Fig. 2. The small intestine has a large surface area for absorption due to numerous fingerlike projections (villi) that extend into the intestinal lumen. To envision the millions of villi lining the surface of the small intestine, imagine a tube lined with terrycloth. Figure 3 shows an enlarged version of one villus with an adjoining crypt. Projecting from the villi are even smaller strands called microvilli, which contain many of the enzymes and receptors

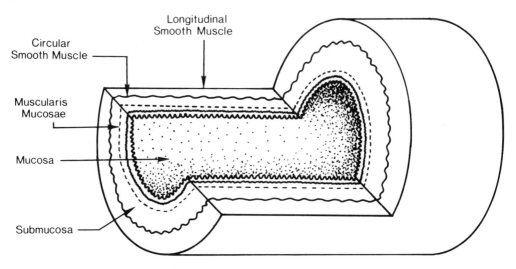

Figure 2 Diagram of the layers of the small intestine. Reprinted with permission from P. L. Smith (1986). Gastrointestinal physiology. *In* "Gastrointestinal Toxicology" (K. Rozman and O. Hänninen, eds.), pp. 1–28. Elsevier, New York.

involved in nutrient absorption. This convoluted surface multiplies the absorptive area approximately 600-fold in comparison to a flat, smooth surface. If flattened, the absorptive surface of the small intestine would measure approximately 200 square meters, the size of a tennis court.

Absorption takes place via the columnar epithelial cells (Fig. 3) near the villous tip—a term that describes their general shape and location as part of the intestine's epithelial layer. The mature absorptive cells of the villus differentiate from precursor cells in the crypts. The villous tip cells have a short half-life; they are constantly being sloughed into the intestinal lumen and replaced by cells migrating from the crypts. The epithelial layer covering the villus also contains various specialized cells. Among the most common of these is the goblet cell (Fig. 3), which secretes mucin that adheres to the outer surface of the villus. Endocrine cells are also present in the epithelial layer and secrete gastrointestinal hormones. The lamina propria is the area just below the surface epithelial cells. The lamina propria contains phagocytic cells, such as macrophages, lymphocytes, and plasma cells, which defend against invasion by foreign microorganisms or proteins.

Each villus contains a network of capillaries, which carry water-soluble nutrients to the blood, and a lacteal (a terminal portion of the lymphatic system), which carries fat-soluble products of digestion. The lymph eventually empties into the bloodstream. The small intestine normally absorbs 90% or more of the energy value of the consumed food. Micronutrients such as minerals and vitamins are absorbed somewhat less efficiently.

The large intestine (or colon or bowel) is the last major section. It is a collecting chamber for solid waste; contents usually spend 24 hours or more in this section. Bacteria flourish in the colon due, in part, to the slow movement of the contents. The bacteria feed on remaining food macronutrients. Some of the products of

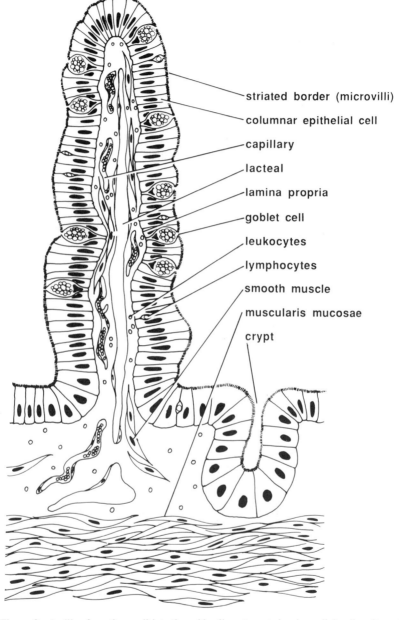

striated border (microvilli)

columnar epithelial cell

capillary

lacteal

lamina propria

goblet cell

leukocytes

lymphocytes

smooth muscle

muscularis mucosae

crypt

Figure 3 A villus from the small intestine with adjacent crypt showing cellular diversity and perfusion.

bacterial action are absorbed from the colon; up to 10% of the available energy from foods is absorbed from the large intestine. The bacteria may synthesize important quantities of certain micronutrients, including vitamin K and some of the B vitamins. Since very little if any oxygen is available in the large intestine, the bacteria in the lumen of the large intestine are obligate or facultative anaerobes.

B. Fluid Balance

The word *diarrhea* is derived from the Greek term meaning to flow through. Diarrhea is a change in the frequency, fluidity (consistency), or volume of the feces. Some disturbance of the mechanisms for secretion and absorption of water in the GI tract results in an increased loss of water with the feces.

Before addressing diarrhea as a disturbance in fluid balance, we will look at normal fluid fluxes in the GI tract. The normal fluid balance in the adult GI tract is depicted in Fig. 4. Besides the variable but quantifiable total input of 14 liters of fluid per day, there is a constant flux of water and sodium across the mucosa of the small intestine. In normal, healthy adults, this may total as much as 50 liters/day in

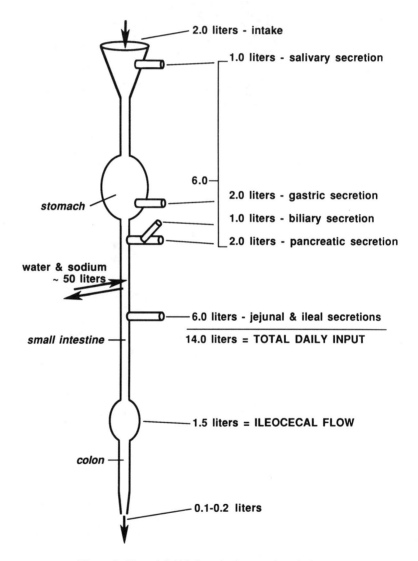

Figure 4   Normal fluid balance in the gastrointestinal tract.

each direction. The flux of fluid in the distal small intestine favors absorption—by the time the contents enter the colon, the 14-liter volume has been reduced to 1.5 liters. The contents are concentrated even further in the cecum and ascending colon. The volume of water in the normal stool is only 0.1–0.2 liters/day. The colon has the capacity to absorb about three times as much water as it does under normal conditions. Thus, in some cases of diarrhea, the volume of water entering the colon must be substantial to exceed this reserve capacity. Even with diarrhea, the water excreted in the feces is only a small percentage of the total fluid entering the intestinal tract.

Diarrhea can be defined as an increase in fecal water content. At least four mechanisms can be involved (Fig. 5): (1) defective absorption of solutes; (2) increased secretion of solutes, (3) structural abnormalities in the intestine, and (4) altered intestinal motility.

Decreases in the absorption of solutes can occur as the result of overeating, enzyme or bile acid deficiencies, or ingestion of poorly absorbed ions such as those which occur in certain laxatives. This "osmotic" diarrhea can occur in the small or large intestines or both.

Large quantities of water and various ions, especially sodium, normally are transported in both directions across the intestinal mucosa. The duodenum is rather "leaky" and allows passive movement of water and sodium, principally from blood to lumen. The jejunum absorbs sodium, chloride, and bicarbonate against their epithelial electrochemical gradients. In the ileum, sodium and chloride are actively absorbed but bicarbonate is secreted, all against their respective electrochemical gradients. Disturbing these processes can result in an abnormal secretion of electrolytes and water or "secretory" diarrhea. Bacterial enterotoxins frequently interfere with intestinal electrolyte transport, stimulating the secretion of electrolytes and water. The colon plays a lesser role in secretory diarrhea.

Structural abnormalities in the intestinal tract can lead to increased stool volume by interfering with absorption of nutrients or by exudative processes. Damage to the absorptive epithelial cells of the small intestine can compromise their effectiveness

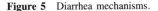

Figure 5   Diarrhea mechanisms.

Table I
Pathogenesis of Diarrhea

Small intestine
Decreased absorption of fluid and electrolytes
Incomplete absorption of nutrients
Increased secretion of fluid and electrolytes
Large intestine
Decreased absorption of fluid and electrolytes

in the absorption of nutrients. This leads to an increase of unabsorbed solutes in the lumen and to osmotic diarrhea. Severe mucosal damage can lead to the release of cells and other structural materials into the lumen and increases the hyperosmolarity of the luminal contents. In both cases, the active absorption of electrolytes against the electrochemical gradient can be lost since the carriers are located in the epithelial cells that have been damaged.

While increased motility is not solely responsible for most cases of diarrhea, it may play a role in each of the other types. Normally, an increased flow of luminal contents is compensated by an available excess area of mucosal absorptive surface. However, if the increased flow occurs in combination with a decrease in mucosal absorptive surface area due to cellular damage, diarrhea can ensue. Similarly, the increased volume of fluid encountered in osmotic or secretory diarrhea stimulates intestinal motility.

Malabsorption problems more frequently involve the small intestine, while inflammatory problems are often localized in the large intestine. The pathogenesis of diarrhea is often described in part by its site (Table I).

The pathophysiology of diarrhea caused by foodborne infectious agents is summarized in Table II. Of the many potential mechanisms in diarrhea, foodborne infectious agents are implicated in only a few. The characteristics of the diarrheal stools will vary with the mechanism. If electrolyte balances are compromised, the stools will be watery; severe cases are sometimes referred to as rice-water stools because of the large ratio of water to solids. If severe mucosal injury has occurred, blood loss into the feces is often observed; the stools are black from the presence of blood. Foul smelling stools are frequently a sign that fat absorption has been poor.

C. Immune Functions

The cells active in the gut-associated lymphatic tissue (GALT) are distributed throughout the GI tract and are divided among three general sites: the Peyer's patches, the mucosa itself, and the mesenteric lymph nodes. The Peyer's patches are located principally in the ileum but are also scattered throughout the small intestine. The Peyer's patches contain macrophages and lymphoid cells, primarily B cells (50–70%) and T cells (11–40%). The outer layer of the Peyer's patches consists of columnar epithelial cells and M cells. M cells play a key role in the uptake (by endocytosis) and transport of antigens to the lymphocytes and macrophages of the Peyer's patches. M cells have no lysosomes and do not modify the antigen, but

Table II
Pathophysiological Mechanisms of Foodborne Infectious
Diarrheal Agents

Abnormal electrolyte and water transport with normal mucosal
   permeability
   Secretion stimulated by bacterial enterotoxins and endotoxins
Abnormal mucosal permeability
   Increased permeability to fluid and electrolytes
      Invasive bacteria
      Enterotoxins
   Abnormal permeability to plasma proteins or protein-losing
      enteropathy
      Mucosal structural damage caused by viral, bacterial, or
         parasitic agents

---

simply transport it from the lumen to the other cells. The mechanism of action of the M cells of the Peyer's patches is depicted in Fig. 6. The appendix in humans also contains structures that resemble Peyer's patches.

The intestinal mucosa is another important site of GALT. The lamina propria contains macrophages and lymphocytes (B and T cells, including mature plasma cells, and null cells, including K or killer cells and NK or natural killer cells). The lymphocytes of the lamina propria interact with the overlying epithelium. There are also lymphocytes between the epithelial cells of the mucosal surface. The origin and nature of these lymphocytes are not yet certain. Circulating lymphocytes are occasionally found in the gut lumen.

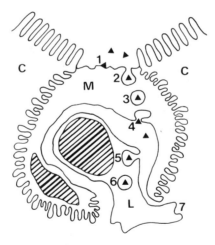

Figure 6 Schematic representation of uptake and transport of an antigen by an intestinal M cell including (1) adherence of antigen to the M cell surface, (2) endocytosis, (3) phagosome formation, (4) exocytosis into the intercellular space, (5) uptake by a lymphocyte, (6) phagosome formation, and (7) lymphocyte migration. C, epithelial cells; L, lymphocyte. Reprinted with permission from A. Naukkarinen and K. J. Syrjänen (1986). Immunoresponse in the gastrointestinal tract. *In* "Gastrointestinal Toxicology" (K. Rozman and O. Hänninen, eds.), pp. 213–245. Elsevier, New York.

The mesenteric lymph nodes are yet another major component of the GALT. They serve as collection points for the lymph which drains from the intestinal villi and Peyer's patches. The mesenteric lymph nodes experience constant antigenic stimulation and contain many large germinal centers. The medulla of the mesenteric lymph nodes contains many mature plasma cells, while the cortex contains numerous T cells.

Many cell types are involved in the gut-associated immune reactions. Macrophages participate in the processing and transport of antigens. B lymphocytes are mediators of the humoral (antibody-producing) immune response, while T cells are responsible for cell-mediated reactions. Plasma cells are the progeny of B cells and synthesize and secrete an antibody molecule with specificity for one site on one particular antigen. T lymphocytes can regulate (help or suppress) the activity of the B cells. T cells can also be sensitized to antigens and participate directly in cell-mediated immunity. K cells are very important in defense against bacteria and parasites. They recognize antigens that have been coupled with antibodies and destroy these antigen–antibody complexes. NK cells exert spontaneous killing activity without prior sensitization to the antigen and independent of the presence of an antigen–antibody complex. Mononuclear phagocytes serve important accessory roles in humoral or cellular immunity, as antigen-presenting cells or as cytotoxic cells. These phagocytes can also secrete many biologically active substances including prostaglandins and interferons. Intestinal mast cells can secrete a variety of pharmacologically active substances which are responsible for localized anaphylactic reactions. Mast cells can also engulf bacteria. However, the major role of the mast cells is in allergic disease, which will be discussed later.

Two types of immune responses can occur in the gastrointestinal tract upon exposure to an antigen: antibody-mediated (humoral) and cell-mediated. The B cells, as plasma cells, produce several different classes of antibodies: IgG, IgM, IgA, IgD, and IgE. IgG antibodies are the most prevalent and important in serum, but IgA plays a preeminent role in intestinal immunity. Most of the plasma cells in the lamina propria produce IgA; the ratio of IgA-producing to IgG-producing cells is 20:30. Plasma cells in the salivary glands also produce predominantly IgA. IgA and, to a lesser extent, IgM are secreted into the lumen and are affixed to epithelial surfaces, providing antibody-mediated immunity to specific antigens.

Cell-mediated immunity in the GI tract has received little scientific study. Cytotoxic T cells specific for the triggering antigen are involved in cell-mediated responses. Cell-mediated responses may be quite important in the control of certain viral and bacterial infections of the GI tract.

III.   Infection

Infections are diseases caused by the presence of viable, usually multiplying, microorganisms at the site of inflammation. In the case of foodborne infections, the viable microorganisms have been ingested with food. The dose required to produce an infection varies with the type of microorganism, even though the microorganism will usually multiply in the gastrointestinal tract or some other organ of the body to produce the infectious disease.

A. Types of Agents Involved

Microorganisms involved in foodborne infections include bacteria, viruses, rickettsia, protozoa, and parasites. Common bacteria involved in foodborne infections are *Salmonella, Campylobacter,* and *Clostridium perfringens.* Bacteria implicated less frequently in foodborne infections include *Listeria monocytogenes, Escherichia coli, Yersinia enterocolitica, Shigella, Vibrio cholerae, Vibrio parahaemolyticus, Bacillus cereus,* and *Streptococcus* group A. Viruses and rickettsia are identified as causative agents of foodborne disease less often than bacteria. These types of microorganisms are more difficult to recover from foods, which may be partially responsible for the less frequent implication of these microorganisms. Examples of viruses that can be acquired via foods are the Norwalk gastroenteritis virus and hepatitis A virus.

Protozoa and parasites are also rather uncommon causes of foodborne infections in the United States, but are more frequently encountered in other countries. Examples of protozoal agents that can be transmitted via foods include *Giardia lamblia* and *Entamoeba histolytica.* Parasites implicated in foodborne infections include roundworms (*Trichinella spiralis*), tapeworms (*Taenia saginata*), and flukes (*Fasciolopsis buski*).

B. Pathogenesis

1. Sites of action

Since the infectious microorganisms are consumed with food, they must at least pass through the GI tract and may cause symptoms there before reaching other tissues. Some foodborne disease agents can invade intestinal tissue from which they can reach the blood and other body tissues. Such organisms may or may not elicit gastrointestinal symptoms. Depending upon the organism, the dose, and other factors, the organism may attack virtually any tissue or organ in the body.

2. Symptoms

The symptoms of foodborne infections depend upon the nature and dose of the infecting organism and the organs or tissues affected. Since the organisms often must multiply in the intestinal tract or other infected tissues, the onset of symptoms is usually delayed by 8 hours to several days, depending on the initial dose and the growth characteristics of the infecting organism. The delayed onset of symptoms is a characteristic feature of foodborne infections and allows infections to be differentiated from intoxications. Since the gastrointestinal tract is frequently the site of action for foodborne infections, gastrointestinal symptoms such as nausea, vomiting, and diarrhea are among the most common symptoms encountered in infectious episodes.

a. Gastrointestinal symptoms

Diarrhea has already been discussed with regard to fluid balance. The other principal GI symptom is vomiting. The driving force for vomition, contraction of the
abdominal muscles and diaphragm, propels the contents out of the stomach and
upper small intestine through the esophagus and mouth. Vomiting, or emesis, is
controlled by both the autonomic nervous system, acting on smooth muscle, and the
central nervous system, acting on somatic muscles. A center in the brain controls
the vomiting reflexes.

Vomiting occurs with many diseases, not just foodborne infections. Intoxications
of certain types can also induce vomiting. GI infections commonly produce vomiting because the GI tract contains numerous receptors that signal and stimulate the
vomiting center in the brain. The majority of vomiting receptors are in the GI tract,
especially the duodenum, which has been called the organ of nausea. These receptors can be stimulated by rapid emptying of the stomach, acute distention of the
small intestine, and inflammation or irritation of the mucosal lining of the small
intestine. Toxins produced by bacteria can stimulate these abdominal receptors,
interact directly with the neurons signaling the vomiting center, or directly stimulate
the chemoreceptor trigger zone, an area located at the base of the brain's fourth
ventricle near the opening to the spinal canal. For example, the enterotoxins produced by certain strains of *Staphylococcus aureus* growing on foods interact with
abdominal receptors for the autonomic nervous system and elicit nausea and vomiting within 6 hours of ingestion of the offending food. The chemoreceptor trigger
zone reacts directly to chemicals in the blood and is more important in vomiting
associated with toxic chemicals than in vomiting associated with infectious diseases. Once the vomiting center is stimulated, vomiting occurs via nerve impulses
sent from the brain to the diaphragm and abdomen.

Vomiting should be differentiated from regurgitation, which also involves the
ejection of previously swallowed food from the mouth. However, regurgitation does
not require a neural reflex. It often occurs because the esophageal sphincter is
incompetent or because abdominal pressure from exercise or the changing of position causes some release of material through the sphincter.

b. Other symptoms

The other symptoms associated with foodborne infectious agents are too numerous
to discuss in much detail. Some of the infectious agents in foods cause only gastrointestinal symptoms. *Vibrio cholerae,* which causes cholera, a profuse watery
diarrhea, does not invade intestinal or other tissues. Some cause extraintestinal
symptoms only on rare occasions or among individuals compromised in their defen-
sive abilities. *Listeria monocytogenes,* for example, causes septicemia, stillbirths,
and other extraintestinal problems, but attacks only individuals who are pregnant,
elderly, or taking certain types of drug therapy that compromise their ability to fight
off infections. *Yersinia enterocolitica* usually causes only intestinal symptoms such
as diarrhea and abdominal pain. Occasionally, this organism can cause extraintestinal symptoms such as arthritis. However, some organisms cause extraintestinal infections routinely. An example is the hepatitis A virus, which elicits its
symptoms in the liver.

3. General characteristics of infectious organisms

Infectious microorganisms must possess certain characteristics if they are to be involved in foodborne disease. First, they must be viable *in vivo;* the microorganisms must survive the acidic conditions of the stomach and the action of the various digestive enzymes to reach their site of action in a viable condition. Many microorganisms would be unable to survive in the acidic conditions of the stomach but, when ingested with food, the buffering capacity of the food reduces the acidity of the stomach and increases the likelihood of survival. If the site of action is extraintestinal, the microorganisms must be able to penetrate the mucosal barrier and reach the site of action in a viable state. Since infections usually require the multiplication of the microorganisms *in vivo,* the microorganism must be able to establish itself within the GI lumen or within some other tissue site in the body. In the intestines, colonization of the lumen requires that the microorganism be able to compete effectively with the resident microflora. Competition is especially important in the colon, where large numbers of bacteria normally reside. The microorganism must also be able to overwhelm any bodily defense mechanisms. Some infectious bacteria produce enterotoxins that mediate their effects on the host. Infectious microorganisms may be categorized as either invasive or noninvasive.

4. Invasive infections

Invasive infections are caused by microorganisms that penetrate tissues and perhaps multiply intracellularly. Among invasive bacteria associated with foodborne infections the classic example is *Shigella.* Others include *Salmonella, Yersinia enterocolitica, Campylobacter,* some enteropathogenic *Escherichia coli* (especially the **O**157:**H**7 serotype), and *Listeria monocytogenes.* Viruses are invasive, as are some of the protozoa and many parasites. Among protozoa, *Entamoeba histolytica* invades tissues but not cells, while *Toxoplasma gondii* invades cells and multiplies intracellularly. *Trichinella spiralis* is a good example of an invasive parasite. Although these microorganisms can invade extraintestinal tissues and cause damage and symptoms at sites beyond the intestine, they must first invade intestinal tissues and often cause intestinal symptoms.

Invasive microorganisms cause diarrhea by damaging the intestinal mucosa, causing a loss of structural integrity and a disruption of electrolyte and fluid balance. If the invasion occurs in the small intestine, the result is usually watery diarrhea. For example, *Salmonella* typically invades the ileum. If the invasion occurs in the colon, the result can sometimes be bloody diarrhea. *Shigella* typically invades the colon, and symptoms of shigellosis range from mild, watery diarrhea from a mild acute inflammation to severe dysentery with significant blood loss from severe, diffuse ulcerative lesions.

Bacterial invasion of intestinal cells can result in symptoms other than diarrhea. The inflammatory response to the invading bacteria can elicit fever, chills, and tenesmus. Damage to intestinal cells can result in altered nutrient absorption and immunological abnormalities. Abdominal pain and cramping, nausea, and vomiting are also frequently associated with invasive infections of the intestine.

If more disseminated infections occur as the result of the invasion, then many other symptoms will result from the invasion of other body tissues. Septicemia, in which the bacteria live and proliferate in the blood, can be a life-threatening complication with certain types of invasive bacteria such as *Salmonella typhi.*

Invasive infections usually occur in two stages: penetration and multiplication. Once invasive bacteria have penetrated the intestinal mucosa, they will either begin to multiply intracellularly or be transported to extraintestinal tissues. *Shigella* penetrates colonic epithelial cells and multiplies to produce inflammatory lesions. In severe cases, the lamina propria may also be invaded. *Yersinia enterocolitica* penetrates the Peyer's patches and multiplies. *Shigella* and *Y. enterocolitica* rarely disseminate to other tissues, but can in severe cases. The invasive bacterium must be able to survive in the microenvironment of the cells that it invades for an infectious disease to occur.

With invasive bacteria, enterotoxins and cytotoxins may sometimes play a secondary role in the pathogenesis of the infection. Enterotoxins are substances which induce intestinal fluid loss without altering the morphology of the intestine, while cytotoxins are substances which elicit fluid loss and also severely alter intestinal morphology. The cytotoxins in particular may participate in the damage to the intestinal mucosa that occurs during invasive infections.

5. Noninvasive infections

Some foodborne infectious bacteria are incapable of penetrating cells and multiplying intracellularly. Some foodborne protozoa (e.g., *Giardia lamblia*) and parasites also cause illness without actually penetrating intestinal tissues.

Noninvasive, infectious bacteria must be able to survive and proliferate in the intestinal lumen. These bacteria often colonize the small intestine because the number of competing bacteria is far lower than in the colon. Adherence to the intestinal surface allows the bacteria to divide and produce enterotoxins without being removed along with other luminal contents by peristalsis. The adherence is quite specific and involves flexible filaments on the bacterial surface interacting with sugar residues on the surface of the microvilli.

These noninvasive bacteria, such as *Vibrio cholerae* and enterotoxigenic *Escherichia coli,* produce enterotoxins which mediate the disease symptoms. The symptoms (principally diarrhea) are usually confined to the intestinal tract since these bacteria cannot reach other tissues. The enterotoxin produced by *V. cholerae* is a protein with a molecular weight of 84,000. The enterotoxin increases the activity of an enzyme, adenylate cyclase, which causes active secretion of chloride ion from crypt epithelial cells and prevents the absorption of sodium and chloride ions in the villous tip epithelial cells. The increased osmolarity of the lumen is balanced by the secretion of water. The volume of diarrheal stools in cholera can be quite profound, and death can ensue from dehydration. Enterotoxigenic *E. coli* produces a heat-labile toxin which is virtually identical to the cholera enterotoxin. Some strains of enterotoxigenic *E. coli* produce a heat-stable enterotoxin which is much smaller and activates guanylate cyclase rather than adenylate cyclase.

C. Defense Mechanisms

Infections do not always produce disease. Pathogenic bacteria, viruses, protozoa, or parasites can be present, especially in small numbers, in the GI tracts of asymptomatic individuals. Humans tolerate microorganisms in their GI tracts because numerous defense mechanisms prevent disease. Only when the defense mechanisms are overwhelmed will infections cause illness.

1. Intestinal factors

The intestinal mucosa serves as a physical barrier—one cell thick—to the entry of potentially infectious bacteria into the body. Individuals with preexisting intestinal damage are more susceptible to intestinal infections than individuals with an intact intestinal epithelium.

The microflora of the intestinal tract provides additional protection. The existing bacteria tend to be fairly stable and compete very effectively for nutrients. Some release inhibitory substances into the lumen. For example, certain colonic bacteria produce volatile fatty acids which are inhibitory to other bacterial species.

Goblet cells, spaced intermittently along the intestinal epithelium, produce mucus which discourages bacterial colonization of the small intestine. Infectious microorganisms must penetrate this mucous barrier to reach the epithelial surface that possesses the receptors for adherence. Some infectious bacteria elaborate enzymes which hydrolyze the mucus, allowing passage of the bacterial cell through this barrier. Other infectious bacteria penetrate the mucous barrier by other means. Bacterial motility is associated with virulence for some species of infectious bacteria. These motile bacteria may simply bore through the mucous layer.

Bile acids, degradation products of cholesterol, are inhibitory to some bacteria. The bile acids are secreted into the duodenum through the bile duct from the liver. Their primary function is to aid in the digestion and absorption of fats and fat-soluble vitamins. Some infectious bacteria are quite resistant to the effects of the bile acids. When bacterial overgrowth occurs in the small intestine, some bacteria will hydrolyze the bile acids, leading to poor absorption of fats and steatorrhea, a foul-smelling fatty type of diarrhea.

Intestinal motility is also a protective mechanism. The normal transit time from the ingestion of food until the elimination of waste in a healthy adult is 24 to 72 hours. This constant movement of material tends to clear the lumen of potentially infectious microorganisms.

The diet may exert some influence through factors that either promote or inhibit bacterial growth. A high-fiber diet may simply entrap bacterial cells and prevent their access to mucosal surfaces. Also, the diet provides the bulk for elimination of waste and stimulates peristalsis.

2. Phagocytosis

Phagocytosis, a process by which certain cells (phagocytes) engulf and destroy infecting microorganisms and their toxins, is an extremely important defense mechanism. Several categories of phagocytes exist. Leukocytes, including neutrophils, monocytes, and eosinophils, circulate with the blood. Other phagocytes, called macrophages, are localized in tissues. Macrophages are located all along the GI tract but are particularly prevalent in the ileal Peyer's patches. Leukocytes can also invade the lamina propria.

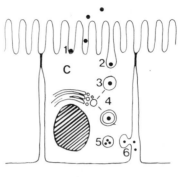

Figure 7 Schematic representation of phagocytosis in an intestinal epithelial cell (C) with (1) adherence of a macromolecule to the microvillus epithelial surface, (2) endocytosis, (3) phagosome formation, (4) phagolysosome formation, (5) residual vacuole containing undegraded material, and (6) exocytosis into the extracellular space. Reprinted with permission from A. Naukkarinen and K. J. Syrjänen (1986). Immunoresponse in the gastrointestinal tract. *In* "Gastrointestinal Toxicology" (K. Rozman and O. Hänninen, eds.), pp. 213–245. Elsevier, New York.

The process of phagocytosis is depicted in Fig. 7. Bacterial cells or macromolecules that adhere to cellular membranes are engulfed by a process known as endocytosis. The membrane of the cell actually surrounds the particle or macromolecule and pinches off, forming a vacuole containing the foreign material. The macromolecule-laden vacuole, known as a phagosome, then fuses with a cellular organelle called a lysosome. The lysosome contains a variety of hydrolytic enzymes, including proteases, lipases, and carbohydrases, which are capable of destroying certain infectious microorganisms and their toxins. Lysozyme, one of the constituent enzymes of macrophage lysosomes, may be particularly important in killing bacterial cells, but the most important killing mechanisms of macrophages and leukocytes are oxidative. These mechanisms involve either hydrogen peroxide or free radicals, such as superoxide anion, singlet oxygen, or hydroxyl radical, produced by the macrophages and leukocytes. Microorganisms killed in this manner can then be digested by lysosomal action. Some microorganisms are resistant and are thus able to persist inside macrophages.

3. Immunological mechanisms

Immunological mechanisms are extremely important in defense against infections. The GI tract is one of the major lymphatic organs of the body. Because the GI tract is exposed directly to environmental antigens, it is often the initial organ to mount an immunological defense against pathogenic microorganisms. The gut is the major site for sensitization of immunocompetent cells that are subsequently recruited to other tissues and organs in the body. Immunological responses are somewhat delayed on the initial exposure to an antigen and often occur only after some symptoms have been encountered. Once immunity to an infecting microorganism is attained, immunological defense mechanisms assume paramount importance in the control of subsequent infections by the same microorganism.

Among the most important components of the GALT are the antibodies attached to intestinal epithelial surfaces. These antibodies neutralize viruses, control bacterial proliferation, and prevent access of enterotoxins to their sites of action. Secretory

IgA bound to the surface of intestinal epithelial cells prevents bacterial adherence, which limits the opportunities for colonization and penetration. IgA can also neutralize the enterotoxins produced by bacteria such as *Vibrio cholerae*. Both humoral and cell-mediated immune responses are involved in the defense against viral infections. In the case of viral agents that replicate in the mucosa, secretory IgA antibodies can prevent adherence and replication. With invasive viruses, IgG in the serum can be important. Parasitic infections usually induce the synthesis of antiparasitic IgE antibodies that combine with receptors on mast cell membranes, interact with the parasitic antigens, and induce localized anaphylactic reactions. Parasitic infections of the GI tract tend to be persistent, demonstrating that immunological defense mechanisms alone are inadequate to control such infections.

IV. Intoxications

Intoxications are disease states caused by a hazardous dose of a toxic chemical that are neither mediated immunologically (allergies) nor primarily the result of a genetic deficiency (metabolic disorders). The agents are nonviable, in contrast to infections, in which viable organisms are involved. All chemicals are toxic at some dose, but only those which produce noticeable adverse reactions under the dose and circumstances of exposure are hazardous to our health. Therefore, with chemical intoxications, it is very important to provide information on the dose and circumstances of exposure.

A. Types of Agents Involved

Foodborne toxicants can be classified in a variety of ways. For example, they can be classified according to the manner in which they get into the food supply: naturally occurring chemicals; contaminants from natural, agricultural, or industrial processes; or food additives. In Chapter 4 on naturally occurring toxicants, these will be classified by the source of the chemical.

Foodborne toxicants can be categorized according to their chemical nature. Some foodborne toxicants are inorganic (Hg, Pb, As, nitrite), while others are organic [saxitoxin, polychlorinated biphenyls (PCBs)]. These categories could be even further subdivided. For example, the PCBs along with DDT and heptachlor could be classified as organochlorine compounds. Other subcategories of organic toxicants would be proteins (staphylococcal enterotoxins, botulinal toxins) and alkaloids (solanine, a naturally occurring alkaloid from potatoes). The staphylococcal enterotoxins and botulinal toxins are considered foodborne toxicants even though they are produced by bacteria, because the toxin is formed in the food before consumption.

Man-made chemicals can also be categorized according to either sources or uses of the chemicals. Categories might include industrial chemicals (PCBs, vinyl chloride), food additives, solvents (methylene chloride), insecticides (DDT, aldicarb), herbicides (paraquat), and many others.

Foodborne toxicants can also be classified according to their mode of action. Solanine, parathion, and malathion are neurotoxins because they are able to inhibit acetylcholinesterase in the nervous system. The saxitoxins and tetrodotoxin are also neurotoxins, but with a different mechanism of action. Some foodborne toxicants, such as the aflatoxins, are carcinogens.

B. Pathogenesis

1. Sites of action

Chemical toxicants have many different sites of action. Some affect several tissues and organs while others are quite tissue specific. Table III provides a list of major organs and tissues and examples of foodborne toxicants that affect these sites. Intoxications are more likely than infections to affect parts of the body remote from the GI tract.

2. Symptoms

Many different symptoms can be produced by foodborne intoxications, depending on the nature and dose of the toxicant, its mechanism of action, and the target organ(s) affected. Symptoms can also vary with age, sex, nutritional status, the existence of other disease states, and from one individual to another.

Exposure to a foodborne toxicant can be either acute or chronic. Acute exposure involves a one-time ingestion of the toxicant or, occasionally, multiple exposures over a fairly short time. For example, illness would occur within a few minutes after ingestion of poisonous mushrooms or a few hours after the ingestion of staphylococcal enterotoxins. Chronic exposure involves ingestion of the toxicant with foods over a long period of time, sometimes a lifetime, though not typically on an

Table III
Sites of Action for Foodborne Toxicants

Tissue site	Toxin affecting that site
Gastrointestinal tract	Staphylococcal enterotoxins
	Trichothecene mycotoxins
Liver	Aflatoxins
	Ethanol
Kidney	Ochratoxin
Blood components	Nitrite
Lung	Paraquat
Nervous system	Saxitoxin
	Botulinum toxins
Skin	Histamine
	Trichothecene mycotoxins
Heart	Erucic acid (rapeseed oil)
Skeletal system	Pb

everyday basis. An example of chronic exposure is the prolonged ingestion of a carcinogenic contaminant such as the aflatoxins.

Effects can also be acute or chronic. Acute symptoms occur a few minutes to a few hours after exposure to the toxicant, while chronic symptoms require long periods of time to develop. The vomiting associated with ingestion of the staphylococcal enterotoxins is an example of an acute effect, while the liver cancer occurring from exposure to aflatoxin is a chronic effect. The acute effects of exposure to foodborne toxicants occur only after acute exposure. Chronic effects can result from either acute or chronic exposure. Aflatoxin produces chronic effects from chronic exposure. However, chronic effects can also result from acute exposure; long-term neurological problems are experienced by individuals who have eaten foods contaminated with mercury.

An important distinction should be made between onset times in foodborne intoxications and infections. Symptoms of acute intoxications typically begin a few minutes to a few hours after eating the contaminated food. Foodborne infections have a delayed onset time of 8 hours to several days. This difference is often critical in distinguishing among the many potential causes of foodborne disease outbreaks.

3. Characteristics of toxins

Foodborne toxins must retain their toxicity through storage, preservation, and preparation of the food. Many are heat stable. Food processing and preparation are often important in the destruction or removal of toxins.

Foodborne toxins must retain their toxicity until they reach their site of action. First, they must withstand the digestive processes. If the toxin acts at some site other than the intestinal tract, it must be able to cross the intestinal barrier and find its way to the target organ and site of action (Fig. 8). Lipophilic toxins such as the aflatoxins can easily cross the lipid membranes of cells. Water-soluble toxins will usually cross only in their un-ionized forms, which are dependent on the pH of the GI tract. Some toxins cross by using carrier systems that exist for nutrients. For example, Pb reaches the circulation by using the carrier system that exists for Ca. Some toxins are deposited in body storage depots. The bone serves as a storage depot for Pb, while the adipose tissue is a storage site for many lipophilic toxins. The toxin can also be excreted through the kidney (urine), bile, or feces. Urinary excretion is a

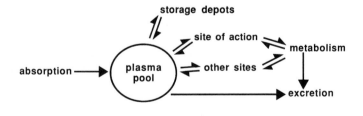

Distribution

Figure 8 Schematic representation of toxin distribution.

common route of removal for many toxins, but the lipophilic toxins must be metabolized into more hydrophilic forms so that they are compatible with urine, which is an aqueous medium. Metabolism does not invariably result in detoxification. Some foodborne toxins exist as pro-toxins and are metabolized (bioactivated) to more toxic forms. The aflatoxins, for example, are bioactivated in the liver.

Toxins interfere with crucial biochemical processes, often at fairly low concentrations. The dose of the toxin must exceed the capacity of the body to detoxify the chemical.

C. Defense Mechanisms

Adverse reactions occur only when the dose of the chemical exceeds the capacity of the body to detoxify or eliminate the toxin. A variety of defense mechanisms are available to prevent foodborne intoxications.

1. Intestinal factors

Fiber can bind and entrap toxicants and lead to their elimination with the feces. Vomiting is another means for clearing a noxious substance from the GI tract. Intestinal bacteria metabolize and detoxify or bioactivate certain foodborne toxicants. Intestinal motility limits the time a potentially toxic chemical spends in the intestinal lumen. Preexisting intestinal damage promotes the absorption of foodborne toxins, so the integrity of the gut wall offers some protection against foodborne intoxications.

2. Phagocytosis

Phagocytosis is much less important in protection against intoxicants than against infections. Also, some toxins are able to impair the function of phagocytic cells and can enhance the chances of acquiring a secondary infection.

3. Immunological mechanisms

Toxins must be capable of acting as antigens to provoke an immunological response. Many of the low-molecular-weight toxins are incapable of acting as antigens. Some can act as haptens by binding to proteins and provoking an immunological response. Proteinaceous toxins can act directly as antigens. Humoral immune responses can play a significant role in protection against proteinaceous toxins.

4. Enzymatic defense mechanisms

The primary defense mechanism against chemical intoxications is enzymatic detoxification. Most chemicals can be detoxified enzymatically, although this defense mechanism can be overwhelmed at high doses. The particular enzymes involved in detoxification will vary depending upon the chemical, mode of administration, and dose and frequency of exposure.

a. General types of reactions
The enzymatic reactions involved in the detoxification of foodborne chemicals can be divided into two distinct "phases": Phase I reactions, which include oxidation,

Table IV
Factors Affecting Enzymatic
Detoxification Mechanisms

Species	Diet
Strain	Pregnancy
Age	Enzyme inducers
Sex	Enzyme inhibitors
Time of day	Altitude
Season	Gravity
Disease states	Dose size
Nutritional status	Dose vehicle
Route of administration	

reduction, and hydrolysis, and Phase II reactions, which are predominantly conjugation reactions involving the products of the Phase I reactions. In general, the products of enzymatic metabolism are more water soluble and therefore more easily excreted than their precursors.

The most important organs for enzymatic detoxification of foodborne chemicals are the liver followed by the kidney and the intestine. Some of the most important enzymes are localized intracellularly in the smooth endoplasmic reticulum.

b. Factors affecting metabolism

Many factors can affect enzymatic detoxification (Table IV). With foodborne intoxications, we are usually interested in the human species, but variations in detoxification assume some importance when the toxic potential of a foodborne chemical is evaluated in some other species. Enzyme induction can play a particularly significant role. The cytochrome P-450-containing monooxygenase system can be induced by exposure to many of its substrates. Subsequently, other substrates are more efficiently metabolized because of the higher level of this critical enzyme.

V. Metabolic Food Disorders

A metabolic food disorder is a disease state caused by exposure to a chemical in foods that is toxic to certain individuals because they display some genetic deficiency in their ability to metabolize the chemical or because the chemical exerts some unusual effect upon their metabolic processes. Two examples follow.

A. Lactose Intolerance

Lactose intolerance results from a deficiency of the enzyme lactase, or β-galactosidase, in the intestinal mucosa. Lactose, the principal sugar in milk, cannot be absorbed unless it is first hydrolyzed into galactose and glucose. As a result of the enzyme deficiency, the undigested lactose passes into the colon and is metabolized by colonic bacteria. Abdominal cramping, flatulence, and frothy diarrhea occur within a few hours after consumption of dairy products and are usually self-limited.

Lactose intolerance is a genetically acquired trait that often increases in severity with increasing age. The prevalence of lactose intolerance among Caucasian Americans is 6–12%, but may be as high as 60–90% in ethnic groups such as Greeks, Arabs, Jews, Black Americans, Japanese, and other Orientals. Genetically determined intolerances to other disaccharides are known, but less common.

The usual treatment for lactose intolerance is avoidance of dairy products. However, only the most severely affected patients need to practice total avoidance of dairy products. Many can tolerate some lactose in their diets, and thus can comfortably consume small quantities of milk. Lactose-intolerant individuals can often tolerate yogurt and acidophilus milk. Lactose-hydrolyzed milk is also available in the marketplace for these individuals.

B. Favism

Favism is an acute hemolytic anemia experienced by some individuals after consumption of broad beans (fava beans) or inhalation of the pollen of the *Vicia faba* plant. The major symptoms are typical of hemolytic anemia: pallor, fatigue, dyspnea (shortness of breath), nausea, abdominal and/or back pain, fever, and chills. Rarely, more serious symptoms are noted including hemoglobinuria, jaundice, and renal failure. The onset time ranges from 5–24 hours. Prompt and spontaneous recovery is usual after ingestion of the beans or inhalation of the pollen ceases. Favism is most prevalent when the *V. faba* plant is blooming and the pollen is in the air and when the edible broad beans are available in the market.

Favism affects individuals with a deficiency of the enzyme glucose-6-phosphate dehydrogenase (G6PDH) in their red blood cells. Fava beans contain several oxidants, including vicine and convicine, which damage the erythrocytes of sensitive individuals. This is a metabolic disorder in which the foodborne chemical has an abnormal effect on the host's metabolism. G6PDH deficiency is among the most common genetic deficiencies in human populations worldwide. It is particularly prevalent among Oriental Jewish communities in Israel, Sardinians, Cypriot Greeks, Black Americans, and certain African populations, but is virtually absent in northern European nations, North American Indians, and Eskimos. However, the disease occurs only among susceptible individuals in the areas of the world where fava beans are eaten, primarily in the Mediterranean region, the Middle East, China, and Bulgaria.

VI.   Allergy

Food allergy is a disease state caused by exposure to a particular (often proteinaceous) chemical to which certain individuals have a heightened sensitivity (hypersensitivity) that has an immunological basis. Like the metabolic food disor-

Table V
Common Allergenic Foods

Cow's milk	Crustacea (shrimp, crab, lobster)
Eggs	
Peanuts	Mollusks (clams, oysters, scallops)
Soybeans	
Other legumes	Fish
Wheat	Tree nuts

ders, food allergies affect only certain individuals in the population—fewer than 1% of the United States population. Food allergies are most common among infants, but many children outgrow their food allergies.

A. Types of Agents Involved

The most common allergenic foods are listed in Table V. Cow's milk is the most common allergenic food among infants, perhaps because it is their most common food. The prevalence of a particular food allergy depends on the inherent immunogenicity of the food and on the frequency with which that food is consumed. The allergens in these foods are usually proteins, although low-molecular-weight substances can occasionally act as allergens. For example, penicillin, an antibiotic that is allergenic to some individuals, may occur in certain foods if it has been used to treat some animal disease.

B. Pathogenesis

Food allergies are abnormal immunological responses to a food component. Of immune mechanisms that occur in food allergy, the most important is the type I or immediate hypersensitivity reaction (Fig. 9). These reactions have very short onset times. The initial event is the production of allergen-specific IgE by B (plasma) cells in response to exposure to an allergenic foodborne protein. The IgE attaches to the outer membrane surfaces of tissue mast cells and/or circulating basophils. The mast cells and basophils are thus sensitized; subsequent exposure to the allergen results in the release of allergic mediators from these cells. The allergen cross-links two IgE molecules on the surface of the mast cell membrane, causing the cells to degranulate. The granules of mast cells and basophils contain dozens of mediators of allergic disease, especially histamine. Histamine is released into the bloodstream and reacts with tissue receptors. The symptoms of an allergic reaction (Table VI) are dependent upon which tissue receptors are affected. Antihistamines can block allergic reactions by inhibiting the interaction between histamine and its tissue receptors.

A variety of symptoms can be associated with food allergies (Table VI), but most reactions involve only a few. Gastrointestinal effects are common. Among the rare, life-threatening symptoms are anaphylactic shock, laryngeal edema, bronchoconstriction, and hypotension.

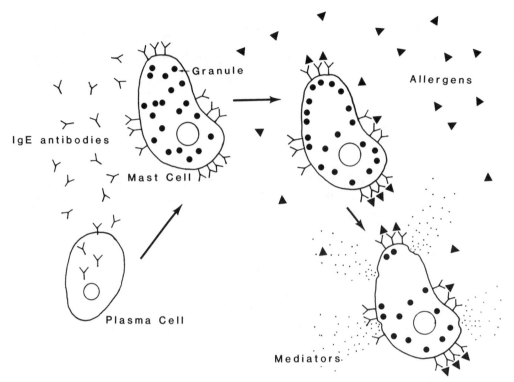

Figure 9 Biochemical mechanisms of immediate hypersensitivity. Reprinted with permission from
S. L. Taylor (1987). Allergic and sensitivity reactions to food components. *In* "Nutritional
Toxicology" (J. N. Hathcock, ed.), Vol. 2, pp. 173–198. Academic Press, Orlando, Florida.

Table VI
Symptoms of Allergic Reactions to Foods

Gastrointestinal symptoms	Respiratory symptoms
Nausea	Rhinitis
Vomiting	Asthma
Diarrhea	Other symptoms
Cutaneous symptoms	Laryngeal edema
Urticaria (hives)	Anaphylactic shock
Eczema or atopic dermatitis	Hypotension
Angioedema	Headache

C. Defense Mechanisms

Individuals with food allergies obviously do not have effective defenses against this type of foodborne disease. However, protective mechanisms do operate in other individuals, mostly in the intestinal lumen. The digestive proteases serve as one protective mechanism, although most food allergens are relatively resistant to proteolysis. The permeability of the gut wall is also a critical factor. Infants are thought to be more susceptible to food allergies because their intestinal walls are more permeable to food proteins. Secretory IgA is another intestinal defense against food allergies. Homologous IgA secreted into the intestinal lumen can react with the allergen before it reaches the sensitized mast cells and basophils. Such blocking antibody responses are among the mechanisms developed by infants as they begin to outgrow their food allergies.

D. Celiac Disease as a Possible Food Allergy

Celiac disease is characterized by a malabsorption of nutrients resulting from damage to the absorptive epithelial cells of the small intestine. The intestinal damage occurs in susceptible individuals when they consume the protein fractions of wheat, rye, barley, and sometimes oats. The sensitive individuals display an abnormal immunologic response to the grain proteins, but the exact mechanism of the response is not understood. The symptoms are diarrhea, bloating, weight loss, anemia, bone pain, chronic fatigue, weakness, muscle cramps, and, in children, failure to grow. Symptoms may begin at any age and do not appear instantaneously in susceptible individuals when they eat the provoking grains, since the intestinal damage requires some time to develop. Remission of symptoms on removal of wheat, rye, and barley from the diet is also slow due to the need to repair the existing damage. Celiac disease is an inherited trait seen in approximately 1 in 3000 individuals in the United States.

E. Treatment of Food Allergies

While food allergies can be treated with drugs such as antihistamines, the treatment is only effective after the onset of symptoms. Preventive therapy with pharmaceutical agents does not exist. The major means of treatment of true food allergies is the specific avoidance diet. Simply put, the patients must carefully avoid the food(s) that provoke their reactions. Some products made from the offending food may not contain the allergenic proteins. For example, peanut oil usually contains no protein and will not trigger allergic reactions in peanut-sensitive individuals. Avoidance diets can be complicated by cross-reactions. For example, many individuals with allergies to shrimp will also be allergic to other crustacea such as crab and lobster but can often consume other seafoods such as mollusks or finfish.

VII. Idiosyncratic Illness

Like food allergies and metabolic food disorders, idiosyncratic reactions usually affect only certain individuals in the population. Idiosyncratic reactions are simply

Table VII
Examples of Food-Associated
Idiosyncratic Reactions

Reaction	Implicated food or ingredient
Migraine headache	Chocolate
Asthma	FD&C Yellow #5 (tartrazine)
Asthma	Sulfites
Hyperkinesis	Food coloring agents
Aggressive behavior	Sugar
Chinese restaurant syndrome	Monosodium glutamate

those individualistic adverse reactions to foods that occur through unknown mechanisms; a few are listed in Table VII.

A. Unproven Reactions

Evidence for the existence of some of these reactions is scanty. In some cases, the only evidence is anecdotal reports in the medical literature that are not substantiated by challenge studies or other diagnostic evidence; such reports should be viewed largely as guesswork.

In other cases, the relationship has been largely disproven yet the public may persist in its belief that the reaction is due to some particular food ingredient. A good example is the relationship between hyperkinetic behavior in children and food coloring agents. Several controlled challenge studies have been conducted on hyperkinetic children. None of the studies has substantiated the original hypothesis. Still, some parents continue to believe that food colors are a common cause of hyperkinetic behavior.

Another example is asthma ascribed to FD&C Yellow #5, tartrazine. Initial studies seemed to demonstrate a relationship between tartrazine and asthma in a small percentage of the asthmatic population. However, other clinical challenge studies have failed to confirm these initial findings, and any role for tartrazine in the causation of asthma seems remote.

Sometimes these relationships are difficult to prove because of the subjective nature of the described condition. One of the most subjective complaints listed in Table VII is Chinese restaurant syndrome (CRS). CRS is characterized by a series of subjective symptoms variously described as burning, tightness, or numbness in the upper chest, neck, and face beginning within minutes after the start of a Chinese meal and lasting only a few hours at most. Occasionally, other symptoms such as dizziness, headache, chest pain, palpitations, weakness, nausea, and vomiting are reported. Of all these symptoms, only vomiting is an objective, readily observable symptom. While many individuals claim sensitivity to monosodium glutamate (MSG) and provide histories of CRS, attempts to confirm the relationship between MSG and CRS with controlled challenges have failed. The failure may be due in part to the lack of ability to measure the symptoms objectively. However, another possibility is that CRS is due not to MSG, but to some other substance in Chinese meals.

B. Proven Reactions

Some idiosyncratic reactions are well established. However, they fall into the idiosyncratic category because the mechanism of the reaction is not understood. From Table VII, the best example is sulfite-induced asthma.

The association between ingestion of sulfites and initiation of an asthmatic response in a small percentage of the asthmatic population has been firmly established by controlled, blinded challenge studies. The asthmatic reactions occur within minutes after the ingestion of a triggering dose of sulfites and can be quite severe on occasion. Several deaths have been attributed to the ingestion of sulfited foods by sulfite-sensitive asthmatics. The mechanism by which sulfite induces an asthmatic reaction in sensitive individuals is not understood. It is known that only a small percentage of the asthmatic population is at risk with estimates varying from 1–8% of all asthmatics. Challenges with sulfited foods indicate that some sulfited foods such as lettuce are much more likely to trigger asthmatic reactions in sensitive individuals than other sulfited foods such as shrimp or dehydrated potatoes. The level of residual sulfite and the form of sulfite present in the food (free or bound to other food constituents) are important in determining the likelihood of a reaction.

Bibliography

Carpenter, C. C. J. (1982). The pathophysiology of secretory diarrheas. *Med. Clin. North Am.* **66,** 597–609.

Rozman, K., and Hänninen, O., eds. (1986). "Gastrointestinal Toxicology." Elsevier, New York.

Strombeck, D. R. (1979). "Small Animal Gastroenterology." Stonegate, Davis, California.

Taylor, S. L. (1987). Allergic and sensitivity reactions to food components. *In* "Nutritional Toxicology" (J. N. Hathcock, ed.), Vol. 2, pp. 173–198. Academic Press, Orlando, Florida.

CHAPTER 3

PRESERVATION, SANITATION, AND MICROBIOLOGICAL SPECIFICATIONS FOR FOOD

Dean O. Cliver

and Elmer H. Marth

I. Introduction

Whether raw or processed, foods are seldom sterile. In addition to occasional microorganisms that may be able to cause human disease, foods are certain to contain bacteria or other organisms that may multiply in the food and cause spoilage. This chapter provides a brief overview of the indigenous microflora of foods, means of delaying or preventing microbial spoilage, approaches to preventing unnecessary contamination of foods, and microbiological approaches to assessing food quality and safety. More extensive treatments of these topics can be found in books specifically devoted to food microbiology or food preservation, some of which are cited in the Bibliography.

II. Microbial Ecology of Foods

Ecology is the pattern of relations between organisms and their environment. In this instance, foodborne microbes are the organisms and food is the environment. The food environment is complex and, although for convenience we will discuss individual factors of that environment, it must be stressed that these factors act together to make the food a friendly or unfriendly place for microorganisms.

A. Sources of Microbes in Foods

Foods largely derive from living organisms—plants and animals. Means that plants and animals have evolved for protecting themselves from microorganisms often include an external barrier layer and some internal defenses to combat microbes that somehow breach the barrier. Therefore, the inside of a healthy, newly harvested plant or animal food usually contains essentially no microbes, but this may soon change from effects of death or processes (e.g., grinding) used to convert the raw material into food. Some of the microbes that are introduced into the food substance will derive from the outside surface of the food, whereas others will come from the apparatus and other human sources, such as contaminated water, used in food preparation. Insects, birds, and rodents may also introduce contaminants. Microbes present in food may cause the food to spoil or may cause disease in those who eat the food. Whether these microorganisms die, survive, or multiply within the food material depends on the factors to be discussed in the next section.

B. Factors Determining Growth

1. The food

Food commonly consists of protein, fat, carbohydrate, minerals, and water. The amount and complexity of each vary from food to food. Carbohydrates may be starch or sugar; proteins of different types occur in milk, meats, and plant products;

fats may be liquid or solid depending on degree of saturation, and sometimes free fatty acids may be present. This considerable variability affects both growth and survival of many foodborne microorganisms. In addition to their roles as potential substrates for microbial growth, these food constituents determine the structure or texture of the food in which the microbes occur.

Other factors which affect growth or survival of pathogens and other microbes in foods are (1) pH or acidity, (2) presence or absence of organic acids, (3) water activity, (4) oxidation–reduction potential, (5) temperature, below and above freezing, (6) microbial interactions within foods, (7) presence or absence of preservatives, including gases and irradiation, (8) packaging materials and the packaging process, and (9) cleaning and sanitizing the environment in which food is handled (discussed in Section IV).

2. pH and presence/absence of organic acids

The natural pH of a product, if unmodified, will in part determine the microbial flora that develops or survives. Examples of foods with different natural pH values are (1) alkaline, pH >7.0, egg albumin; (2) near neutral, pH 7.0–6.5, milk; (3) low acid, pH 6.4–5.3, most vegetables; (4) medium acid, pH 5.2–4.5, cottage cheese; (5) acid, pH 4.4–3.7, mayonnaise, some fruits; and (6) high acid, pH <3.7, citrus fruits.

The pH of a product is sometimes altered through addition of inorganic acids such as hydrochloric or phosphoric acid. More commonly, organic acids such as acetic, citric, or lactic acid, are added to foods. Sometimes small amounts of sorbic, propionic, or benzoic acid are added as preservatives. An acid-releasing substance such as glucono-δ-lactone may be used to acidify a product.

Strong acids are thought to directly acidify the contents of the cell, thereby disrupting metabolic processes and ultimately causing death. Organic acids, in part, may do the same, but the undissociated molecule is more important in the antimicrobial activity of these acids. In the undissociated state these acids are readily soluble in the cell membrane. Once there they interfere with its permeability, causing uncoupling of substrate transport and oxidative phosphorylation from the electron transport system. This leads to acidification of cell contents with death of the cell as the ultimate result. Since the undissociated organic acid molecule is needed for antimicrobial activity, the pH of the environment (i.e., the food) must be in the range required for a substantial portion of the acid to be undissociated.

Concentrations of organic acids insufficient to kill cells can cause metabolic injury. Cells injured in this manner can repair themselves and again be pathogenic. This has been demonstrated for *Salmonella*, *Staphylococcus aureus*, and *Listeria monocytogenes*.

3. Water activity

The water activity (a_w) of a food is the ratio of the water vapor pressure of the food to that of pure water. The portion of water in a food that is represented by the a_w value is available for use by microorganisms or in chemical reactions. As the amount of material (solute) in solution increases, the a_w value decreases from 1.0, which is the maximum for pure water. Adding 0.88% sodium chloride *or* 8.52%

sucrose to water results in an a_w value of 0.995. A value of 0.990 can be achieved by adding 1.74% sodium chloride *or* 15.45% sucrose. To reduce the a_w value to 0.980, 3.43% sodium chloride or 26.07% sucrose is needed. The minimum a_w value to allow growth of *Staphylococcus aureus*, 0.86, results when water contains 18.18% sodium chloride or 65.63% sucrose.

Conditions of food itself that serve to reduce the a_w are (1) adsorption of water molecules onto surfaces, (2) forces that hold water within capillaries in foods, and (3) components of the food that are in solution.

The a_w of food affects growth and survival of microorganisms. Most bacteria, including pathogens, grow most rapidly (if other conditions are suitable) at a_w values of 0.998–0.980. When the a_w value drops below 0.980, the growth rate and ultimate resultant cell mass decrease and the length of the lag phase increases. At a sufficiently low a_w value, the lag phase becomes infinite—there is no growth.

Lowering the a_w value while maintaining ambient or refrigeration temperature reduces microbial death. Generally, microorganisms respond to low a_w values by accumulating potassium, amino acids, or polyols, which are protectors of enzyme activity. This improves their survival but also may have a protective effect on microorganisms when they are heated. Conditions in foods which interact with a_w to determine the fate of microorganisms are pH, temperature, oxidation–reduction condition, nutrition of the organisms, and presence of preservatives.

4. Oxidation–reduction condition of food

Oxidation is a loss of electrons, whereas reduction is a gain of electrons. When one substance is oxidized, another is always simultaneously reduced. The oxidation–reduction condition is commonly measured with a platinum electrode, expressed in millivolts, and designated as E_h. The dyes methylene blue, resazurin, and triphenyltetrazolium chloride also indicate the oxidation–reduction condition of a substrate. Regardless of the method chosen, it is difficult to measure the oxidation–reduction condition of food because it is virtually impossible to keep out oxygen.

The oxidation–reduction condition of a food will, in part, determine if a microorganism can initiate growth. Furthermore, active microbial growth during the log phase reduces the oxidation–reduction potential of the substrate. The oxidation–reduction condition of a food can vary according to location (near the surface as opposed to the interior) and this will contribute to determining if a certain microorganism will grow.

5. Temperature

Low temperatures are used to retard microbial growth, action of food enzymes, and other chemical reactions that can occur in food. In contrast, high temperatures are used to inactivate microorganisms and food enzymes and to cook the food.

Refrigeration temperatures extend the lag phase of microorganisms, thus minimizing growth and preserving the products for limited times. It is important to recognize that some foodborne pathogens can grow, albeit slowly, at refrigeration temperatures. Examples include *Aeromonas hydrophila*, *Clostridium botulinum* type E, *Listeria monocytogenes*, *Yersinia enterocolitica*, and some enteropathogenic strains of *Escherichia coli.* Of course, other psychrotrophic bacteria, for example, *Pseudomonas* spp., can grow and cause food to spoil.

Perishable foods, including eggs, dairy products, seafood, meats, poultry products, vegetables, and fruits, are commonly held refrigerated and thus have a limited shelf life. This shelf life is affected by temperature, relative humidity, air movement, and composition of the atmosphere within the storage area.

Freezing foods and the microorganisms they contain may kill some microbes and preserve others. Injury and subsequent death of cells are related to (1) kind of microorganism, (2) "cold shock" associated with initial lowering of the temperature, (3) formation of extracellular and intracellular ice, and (4) concentration of solute in the unfrozen phase of the product. Many foods will protect bacterial cells from these forms of injury during the freezing process. Variable effects of freezing must be considered when food samples for microbiological analyses are frozen and thawed before testing.

Use of high temperatures continues to be the single most important method for killing microorganisms to preserve food. Processes involved are pasteurization, blanching, boiling, and use of steam under pressure. These processes will be described here as part of the food system, and most will be addressed in greater detail in Section III.

Pasteurization uses an exposure to a temperature below boiling; both time and temperature vary according to the product being heated. Heating methods also are variable—batch and continuous methods generally apply heat to products before they are packaged, but a continuous method also can be used to pasteurize a packaged product (e.g., beer in bottles or cans). Blanching also is based on food temperatures below boiling, but is generally intended to modify the food rather than the microflora.

Boiling or heating to approximately 100°C (212°F) is largely limited to baking (the temperature of breads, etc., does not exceed 100°C as long as moisture is present) and home preparation of foods. The bactericidal effect of this heat treatment is essentially comparable to that of pasteurization.

Temperatures above 100°C are required to sterilize canned foods. Such temperatures, usually about 121°C (250°F), are commonly achieved when containers of food in a retort are heated with steam under pressure. In contrast, the aseptic canning process involves brief heating of food at 149°C (300°F) and filling the sterilized food into sterile containers which are then sealed. Filling and sealing the containers occurs aseptically. Commonly, foods processed as described are "commercially sterile" rather than sterile. Commercially sterile products usually contain some viable spores of thermophilic bacteria that do not cause spoilage because the canned foods are normally not stored at thermophilic temperatures. If products are to be stored at high temperatures (e.g., in the tropics), sterility rather than commercial sterility is required.

6. Microbial interactions

A pathogen seldom occurs in food as a pure culture. Consequently a brief consideration of relationships between microorganisms in mixed cultures is appropriate.

As indicated earlier in this discussion, development of a certain microflora in a food is governed by a group of intrinsic (characteristics of the food itself), extrinsic (storage temperature, atmosphere, etc.), and processing (survival, growth, colonization during processing) factors. In addition, the interactions of a mixed population help to determine the microflora that develops.

In mixed cultures there may be competition between other bacteria and the pathogen, resulting in inhibition or enhancement of its growth. For example, *Staphylococcus aureus* competes poorly with the natural flora of raw meat or raw milk.

Inhibition can result through depletion of nutrients or oxygen, through changes in intrinsic conditions, or through production of antimicrobial substances by one microorganism which will inhibit or inactivate the other. Examples of how depletion of nutrients by one organism can affect another include (1) depletion of oxygen plus accumulation of carbon dioxide, favoring growth of facultative and obligate anaerobes; (2) use of certain amino acids by *Pseudomonas* spp. or coliforms, retarding growth of *S. aureus;* and (3) use of nicotinamide, niacin, or biotin by streptococci, also retarding growth of *S. aureus*. Examples of changes in intrinsic conditions that may favor one organism over another include (1) increasing salt concentration, possibly inhibiting growth of most saprophytes but favoring growth of *S. aureus;* (2) added sucrose, inhibiting psychrotrophs and thus decreasing their competitive ability; and (3) added glucose, stimulating growth of psychrotrophs which, in turn, inhibit growth of *S. aureus*. Antimicrobial metabolites produced by one organism which may inhibit or inactivate others include hydrogen ions, carbon dioxide, organic acids, peroxides, antibiotics, and bacteriocins.

Growth of one microorganism can be enhanced through activity of another. Thus, B vitamins synthesized by yeasts can enhance growth of lactic acid bacteria. Changes in pH or E_h caused by one microorganism can favor growth of another. Growth of mold can raise the a_w of a relatively dry product, making the substrate suitable for growth of bacteria. Hydrolysis of polymers in plant or animal tissue by some organisms allows invasion of such tissues by other organisms. Similarly, substances inhibitory to some microorganisms (e.g., sorbic acid) are degraded by others; then the inhibitory activity is diminished or eliminated, which allows growth of previously controlled microorganisms.

The foregoing discussion provides some examples of interactions that are possible among microorganisms in foods. Others will be presented in the chapters that follow. These effects are not always predictable, but they cannot be overlooked when the ecology of microorganisms in foods is being considered.

7. Preservatives

Sodium chloride, sucrose, and vinegar (acetic acid) are the most widely used preservatives of food. Some other salts, sugars, and acids may be used provided they do not negatively affect flavor or other properties of foods. Sorbic acid, propionic acid, and pimaricin are commonly used antifungal food additives, although the two acids also have some antibacterial activity. Nitrite is widely used in cured meats to retard growth of *Clostridium botulinum*. Smoking, liquid smoke, and spices have limited antibacterial activity and can contribute to the total preservative effect operative in foods.

A modified atmosphere, for example, increased content of carbon dioxide, can be used to retard microbial growth and thus preserve some products, especially meats and fruits. Gamma-irradiation of foods to inactivate microorganisms has limited regulatory approval in the United States. It is used more widely in some other countries, and its application in the United States can be expected to grow once resistance by uninformed consumers is overcome.

8. Packaging of foods

Materials used to package foods protect the foods after processing until they reach the consumer. Metal, glass, plastic, and paper packages are used, depending on the food and the degree of protection that is needed. Anaerobic conditions are created in some packages (e.g., canned vegetables); this, in part, determines if bacterial spores that survived a heat treatment can grow to spoil (including producing toxin in) the food. Packaging materials used for nonsterile foods must be handled hygienically to ensure that they do not become sources of contaminants in the food.

C.   Food Groups

Meats (including poultry) and animal products derive ultimately from living animals. Animals harbor a great variety of microbes in and on their bodies, but the contaminants of greatest significance to consumer health generally come from the colon. Various Enterobacteriaceae and gram-positive sporeformers from this source are to be expected. Healthy adult animals may harbor intestinal pathogens to which they have developed immunity or tolerance. Contamination of meats with intestinal bacteria at slaughter evidently cannot be entirely prevented. Apparently healthy animals also may be infected in edible portions of their bodies with bacteria (e.g., *Yersinia enterocolitica*) or parasites (e.g., *Trichinella spiralis, Toxoplasma gondii*) that are pathogenic for humans. Spoilage of meats during refrigerated storage is based on psychrotrophic, proteolytic bacteria and sometimes molds.

Milk comes from the mammary glands of cattle and other dairy species. Milk at the time of secretion is sterile but soon becomes contaminated by bacterial inhabitants of the normal, healthy mammary gland. Local infections (mastitis—sometimes subclinical) do occur, and agents of a few systemic infections are shed through the lactating mammary gland (e.g., *Coxiella burnetii, Mycobacterium bovis,* and *Brucella* spp.). The organisms that produce lactic acid in milk are generally external contaminants; however, they are so well adapted to the milk environment that they usually become the predominant flora. Uncontrolled production of lactic acid (souring) is regarded as spoilage. Raw milk sometimes is held refrigerated longer than 3–4 days before it is processed. This affords psychrotrophic bacteria the opportunity to grow and cause chemical changes.

Eggs are contaminated on the outside of the shell by the hen's fecal flora (sometimes including *Salmonella* or *Campylobacter*) because both eggs and feces pass through the cloaca before leaving the bird's body. Contaminants on the shell can be aspirated through small pores into the egg as it cools after being laid, and cracked eggs have long been recognized as potential vehicles of disease agents. More recently, at least one species of *Salmonella* that is pathogenic to humans has been shown to infect the chicken's ovary, with the result that eggs are contaminated internally before being laid. Spoilage is usually caused by putrefactive bacteria that have penetrated the shell.

Fish may be contaminated, at the time they are caught, with potentially pathogenic bacteria (e.g., *Vibrio parahaemolyticus* and spores of *Clostridium botulinum* type E) and with parasites (e.g., anisakids and *Diphyllobothrium latum*) infectious for humans, both derived from the aqueous environment. Some fish contain toxins that they have accumulated from their environment or produced within their bodies. Certain spoilage organisms can produce histamine and other substances that intoxicate those who eat the fish. Spoilage during refrigerated storage is generally the function of psychrotrophic, proteolytic bacteria.

Seafoods other than fish principally comprise crustacea and mollusks. Most of these are extremely vulnerable to bacterial spoilage, but are likely only to harbor pathogens from the general aqueous environment (e.g., *V. parahaemolyticus* and spores of *C. botulinum* type E) unless they are exposed to human fecal contamination after harvesting. An important exception is the bivalve mollusk, which feeds by filtration of its environmental water where it can accumulate human fecal bacteria (e.g., *Salmonella* spp.) and viruses (e.g., the hepatitis A and Norwalk-like viruses); these mollusks are already heavily contaminated at the time of harvest from polluted water.

Vegetables grow in or near the soil, so they are likely to be contaminated with spores of *C. botulinum* when harvested. Spoilage generally comprises rotting caused by fungi or bacteria. Fertilization with animal (or human) waste can introduce infectious agents (e.g., *Listeria monocytogenes* and *Ascaris lumbricoides*), some of which apparently reach edible portions above ground as a result of splashing by raindrops. Low-growing *fruits,* such as strawberries, are subject to the same sort of contamination, whereas tree fruits are more subject to contamination from birds. Fruits tend to be quite acid and are thus more likely to be spoiled by yeasts and molds than by bacteria.

Cereal grains and pulses, stored at appropriately low moisture levels, are microbiologically stable for long periods over a wide range of temperatures. At higher moisture levels, molds are likely to grow, spoiling the grain and perhaps producing toxins. Susceptibility to mold spoilage in stored grains can be enhanced by insect damage.

Confectionery products, because of their high sugar content and resultant low a_w value, commonly do not support growth of spoilage and pathogenic microorganisms. Exceptions are (1) some coated "cream" candies that burst from gas produced in them by osmophilic yeasts, *Clostridium* spp., or heterofermentative lactic acid bacteria; (2) marzipan, fondants, jellies, and glacéed fruit that sometimes are spoiled by osmophilic yeasts or molds; and (3) products containing coconut or almond paste, marzipan and marzipan-like products, and certain chocolate products that become rancid through lipolytic activity of molds that sometimes can grow on these confectionery items.

Some ingredients (e.g., cocoa powder, carmine red, nonfat dry milk, coconut, nuts) on occasion have been contaminated with *Salmonella* spp. Use of such ingredients has resulted in confectionery products, largely chocolate products, containing *Salmonella* spp. Eliminating the contaminants from chocolate products using heat is difficult because moisture is absent and the resultant dry heat is far less effective than moist heat for inactivating microorganisms. Nuts also can be a source of mycotoxins, especially aflatoxin, and hence suitable controls must be used to avoid such contamination.

D. Assumed versus Preventable Contamination

No food is 100% safe, and every food is at some risk of contamination from mishandling in final preparation. However, on the basis of what is known about a food supply (summarized earlier), it is reasonable to assume that some contaminants are present—and others absent—in raw foods.

For example, pork is usually cooked thoroughly in the United States, on the assumption that it contains *Trichinella spiralis*. The present incidence of *Trichinella* in slaughter swine in the United States is <1%, but prudent consumers do not eat undercooked pork, even though the odds are in their favor on any given occasion. Similarly, those who buy and handle raw chicken in the United States should assume that *Salmonella* (and also *Campylobacter, Clostridium perfringens,* and *Listeria monocytogenes*) is present. The chicken should be cooked thoroughly and opportunities for cross-contamination from the raw bird to cooked food or food that is not to be cooked should be avoided.

Spores of *Clostridium botulinum* should be assumed present in raw vegetables, and probably raw meat, anywhere in the world. These spores are likely to be heat resistant, but will probably not germinate and multiply in refrigerated foods. However, spores of *C. botulinum* type E are likely to occur in raw seafood. These are relatively heat labile, but if they germinate, the vegetative cells will grow psychrotrophically. Canned foods in the United States can safely be assumed not to contain viable spores of *C. botulinum*.

Raw fish anywhere in the world may contain parasite larvae, and bivalve mollusks may contain viruses. Raw vegetables such as lettuce are unlikely to contain cysts of *Entamoeba histolytica* in the United States, but may in developing countries.

No nation's food supply is entirely free of these instances of "assumed contamination," and the prudent consumer must take them into account. Many kinds of contamination can be avoided, however, and this should be expected and probably demanded by consumers if the cost of preventive measures does not increase the price of the food inordinately.

III. Food Preservation

Many foods rapidly become inedible—spoiled—after harvest or slaughter unless something is done to preserve them. Some preservation methods improve the palatability of the food in question, but other foods may be at their best at the very moment of harvesting, so that the best preservation is to keep the food in reasonably acceptable condition for as long as possible. Most preservation methods are directed against microbial spoilage of foods and are based on physical measures, though chemical and biological methods of food preservation are also used. Often, but not always, preservation methods are of value in preventing foodborne disease.

A. Physical Methods

There is no certain way of knowing whether drying or heating is the older method for deliberate preservation of food by humans, but each certainly dates back to prehistory. Drying is a physical process of removing water from a food so that microorganisms cannot grow. In some situations, drying was done in the open air and sun, often with some loss of food to (and contamination by) insects, birds, and other animals. Both vegetables and meat have been dried in mountainous areas by alternate freezing and thawing caused by natural daily temperature cycles. Whether drying occurred spontaneously or by human enterprise, preservation by this method succeeds only if the food is then stored in a way that prevents moisture from getting into it. Water that is present in a food also can be bound by solutes such as salt and sugar, and thus be unavailable to microbes.

Heating of foods includes several processes that serve somewhat different purposes. *Cooking* is more a means of food preparation than of preservation, though it may serve both purposes. Cooking is generally done to improve the palatability of a food, but also may destroy some pathogens, spoilage organisms, and even certain foodborne toxins. Temperatures used in cooking tend to be related to the boiling point of water. The external heat source often is boiling water and, even if a higher external temperature is applied (at atmospheric pressure), the temperature within the food will not exceed 100°C until all internal moisture has been removed—at which point the food may well be inedible.

Three other heating processes that are specifically used in food preservation are *pasteurization, blanching,* and *retort cooking.* Pasteurization temperatures are usually well below 100°C. Pasteurization is useful when (1) the product is damaged by more rigorous heat treatments; (2) pathogens and principal spoilage organisms likely to be present are not very heat resistant; and (3) the pasteurized product is handled in ways to minimize growth of survivors. The process is used to kill spoilage organisms in products such as beer and wine and to kill pathogens plus spoilage organisms in products such as milk and liquid egg suspensions. Specifications for milk pasteurization are based on the thermal resistance of the rickettsia, *Coxiella burnetii,* whereas pasteurization of liquid egg products is designed to kill *Salmonella.*

As applied to milk, pasteurization by the holding or batch method involves heating the product at 62.8°C (145°F) for 30 minutes. Alternatively, the continuous high-temperature short-time (HTST) method, which is most commonly used, heats milk at 71.7°C (161°F) for 15 seconds. Both are minimal processes described in the current edition of the Pasteurized Milk Ordinance. These and similar processes do not sterilize the product. Although 95–99% of the microorganisms present may be inactivated, spores will remain viable and some heat-resistant nonsporeformers will survive. A pasteurized product must be handled with care to prevent its recontamination with spoilage or pathogenic microorganisms. When milk is to be used for making certain varieties of cheese, pasteurization can be replaced by treating the milk with hydrogen peroxide (maximum 0.05% by weight) and mild heat [ca. 16 seconds at 54.4°C (130°F)]. Catalase is added to decompose residual peroxide in the heat-treated milk.

Blanching processes use temperatures below boiling to prepare foods for preservation by other methods, such as freezing or canning. Food that is to be frozen is blanched to destroy enzymes in the food that may cause deterioration during frozen storage. Blanching before canning alters the texture of the food to allow better packing of containers. In either event, any antimicrobial effect of blanching is largely fortuitous.

A retort is a pressure vessel that permits cooking with steam at temperatures significantly above 100°C. The food may be in any of a number of final containers or in bulk. Processes are often designed to achieve "commercial sterility," meaning that the food contains no viable organisms or spores that will cause spoilage under normal conditions of storage. Improperly retorted foods, particularly those with pH >4.6, could be unsafe even if not perceptibly spoiled. The threat of botulism has inspired much research to determine exactly the time–temperature conditions for processing that will ensure a safe product without overcooking and making the food unpalatable or less nutritious.

Processes are designed on the basis of the thermal susceptibility of spores of *Clostridium botulinum* or a comparable species. In addition to the D [minutes at a given temperature that produces a 10-fold (decimal) reduction in viable spores] and z (the change in temperature that will cause a 10-fold change in the D value—for *C. botulinum* spores, this is often assumed to be 10°C = 18°F) values, it is necessary to determine the heat transfer properties of the food in question and of the container in which it is to be heated. An F_o figure is derived, which is the time at 121°C (250°F) required to cause a 12-D (10^{-12}) reduction in the number of *C. botulinum* spores that might be present in this food, packed in this type of container. Although the concern is with survival of spores of *C. botulinum,* spores of the slightly more heat-resistant but nontoxigenic *Clostridium sporogenes* PA 3679 are commonly used in studies to determine heat processes. Also, retort operators are required to be trained and licensed. Canned foods processed on this basis have a remarkable safety record.

Ice that occurred naturally—in winter or on mountaintops—was once used to extend the keeping time of perishable foods. Now mechanical refrigeration is used to cool or freeze food for storage. Storage of foods at temperatures above freezing but below 5°C tends to delay spoilage caused both by intrinsic enzymes and by microbes. However, some foods must be stored at higher temperatures; in commercial, large-scale storage, the composition and humidity of the atmosphere may also have to be controlled. Psychrotrophic (often proteolytic, strict aerobes) spoilage organisms are likely to assert themselves eventually, and some psychrotrophic pathogens are now recognized, so refrigerated storage has its time limits.

Freezing food for storage can be done commercially or in the home. Comminuted and "variety" meat products have a fairly short storage life, even when held at optimal temperatures (near −20°C). By contrast, some vegetables that have been properly blanched and frozen can maintain optimal quality for many months (to over a year) at these low temperatures.

Some other physical processes are categorized as "irradiation." Ultraviolet radiation, in the form of sunlight, has fortuitously been killing microbes on the surfaces of foods since time began. More recently, ultraviolet lamps have been used in some food facilities for antimicrobial purposes. Though it is clear that some wavelengths of ultraviolet light, at sufficient doses, are effective against microbes, this form of radiation does not penetrate foods. Therefore, it is used only to control organisms on surfaces, in thin layers of water, and in air.

Microwaves are another form of electromagnetic radiation now being applied to foods. Microwaves penetrate food and cause heating by inducing vibration of water molecules. Effects of microwaves on food and its microflora appear to be based on the heat that is generated rather than on the microwaves themselves. A concern sometimes raised about microwave cooking or processing is that heat distribution is not always uniform, and "cold spots" may harbor viable pathogens including parasites after cooking.

Ionizing radiation (gamma rays, X rays, or high-energy electrons) may be used in several food processes. Low doses (<1 kGy) can delay maturation or prevent sprouting of vegetables and can disinfest stored grain that contains insects. Medium doses (1–10 kGy) can delay microbial spoilage and rid foods of vegetative cells of bacterial pathogens. High doses (>10 kGy) can be used to produce commercial sterility of foods, including inactivation of bacterial spores and of viruses, and to reduce the microbial load in dried spices. Extensive research has demonstrated the wholesomeness of irradiated foods, but use of these has been slowed by militant resistance from some consumer organizations. However, marketing trials have shown that consumers who were permitted to buy irradiated foods accepted and often preferred foods that had been processed in this way.

B. Chemical Methods

Some chemical substances specifically antagonize microbes that may be present in foods. One class of chemicals used for this purpose is the acids. Inorganic or mineral acids tend to ionize or dissociate strongly in solution—their antimicrobial action usually consists mostly of reducing the pH of the food. Some organic acids (e.g., acetic and lactic acid) show significant antimicrobial effects without reducing the pH of the food greatly; indeed, such acids are often most active antimicrobially in their undissociated state.

Sulfites, nitrites, and a few other substances are used as antimicrobial agents in food preservation. For various reasons, there has been a tendency to try to reduce use of these preservatives; however, it is not clear that satisfactory alternatives are available in all instances. Antibiotics that may be used for therapy of human or animal disease are generally not permitted in foods in the United States.

Aside from chemicals that may be added directly to foods, "controlled atmospheres" are sometimes used inside food packages. That is, gases other than air surround the food inside an impermeable wrapper. These gases may be formulated, among other purposes, with a view to control the microflora of the food.

C. Biological Methods

Not all microbial effects on food are deleterious. Production of acetic and lactic acids by bacteria and of carbon dioxide and ethanol by yeast, as well as some mold "fermentations" of cheeses and other foods, have been put to good use for centuries or millennia. These microbial processes change the nature of the food (e.g., milk becomes cheese) and often limit the susceptibility of the "new" food to microbial spoilage, though none of them provides absolute preservation. Other biological food processes employ enzymes or extracts of plant (e.g., papain) or animal (e.g., rennet) tissue—modifications produced in this way sometimes are not directly relevant to the microbiology of the food.

IV. Sanitation in the Food Industry

Sanitary (hygienic) practices in the food industry involve systematic control of environmental conditions during production, processing, storage, distribution, preparation, and consumption of foods and beverages. Such control includes ways to prevent contamination of products by microorganisms, insects, rodents, other animal pests, or foreign objects or chemicals. Hence, sanitary practices begin when raw materials are produced and continue until foods or beverages are consumed.

Sanitary practices are necessary to protect the public's health through minimizing or eliminating contamination of foods with pathogenic microorganisms. Implementation of such practices also will improve the keeping quality of nonsterile foods and beverages because contamination of the products with an array of spoilage organisms (mold, yeasts, bacteria) will be minimized. Minimizing contamination extends the time until microbial growth is sufficient to spoil the product. Aesthetic considerations, for example, the desire of consumers to have food free of insects, also demand implementation of rigid sanitary practices. Finally, such practices are required by regulations enforced by the Food and Drug Administration (most foods), U.S. Department of Agriculture (meats and poultry products), U.S. Department of Commerce (seafoods), U.S. Department of Treasury (Bureau of Alcohol, Tobacco and Firearms—alcoholic beverages), state agencies (usually departments of agriculture or health or both), and municipal agencies (often responsible for control of restaurants and other retail establishments that prepare and sell food). At the federal level, sanitary practices required in the food industry are described in the *Code of Federal Regulations,* which includes "Good Manufacturing Practices," a regulation setting forth practices that are mandated when a food processing establishment is operated. Regulation of the food industry is discussed more extensively in Chapter 24.

A. Food Processing Equipment

Equipment used to process and handle food should be designed and constructed according to principles described in the following paragraph. If this is done, equipment can be readily cleaned and sanitized. Furthermore, such equipment most likely will be acceptable to inspectors when they visit the food processing facility. Voluntary groups have developed "standards" for design and construction of equipment used in the dairy industry (3-A Sanitary Standards Committee), egg processing industry (E-3-A Sanitary Standards Committee), baking industry (Baking Industry

Sanitary Standards Committee), food service industry (National Sanitation Foundation), and others.

Principles for sanitary design and construction of food equipment are concerned with surfaces that do and do not contact the product and with ways to protect the contents (food) of the equipment when in operation. Surfaces in contact with food must be (1) inert to food under conditions of use, and nothing from the surface may migrate into or be absorbed by food unless the migratory chemical is accepted by FDA food-additive regulations; (2) smooth and nonporous so that small particles of food, bacteria, yeasts, molds, or insect eggs are not caught in microscopic crevices and become difficult to dislodge, thus becoming a potential source of contamination; (3) visible for inspection, or must be readily disassembled for inspection, or if this is not possible it must be demonstrated that routine cleaning procedures eliminate the possibility of contamination from microorganisms and insects; (4) readily accessible for manual cleaning, or if not readily accessible, then readily disassembled for manual cleaning, or if cleaned-in-place techniques are used, it must be demonstrated that results achieved without disassembly are equivalent to those obtained with disassembly and manual cleaning; and (5) so arranged that equipment is self-emptying and self-draining. Surfaces that do not contact food must be arranged to (1) prevent harboring of soils, microorganisms, or pests in or on the equipment and also where it contacts other equipment, floors, walls, or hanging supports; and (2) be readily cleanable. Finally, equipment must be designed (with suitable covers, etc.) to protect its contents (i.e., the food) from external contamination.

B. Cleaning Food Equipment

Food equipment is commonly cleaned using water at the right temperature, a suitable detergent, and energy, either mechanical or human. Water should be potable and soft [0–60 mg of mineral matter per liter (0–3.5 grains per gallon)]. Hard water reduces effectiveness of detergents and sanitizers, and minerals from the water can form a deposit on equipment surfaces which is difficult to remove and can harbor microorganisms.

Food soils commonly consist of carbohydrates, proteins, fats, and minerals as found in the food being processed. Carbohydrates include sugars and starches. Although sugars are soluble in water, they are caramelized by heating and then are more difficult to remove from equipment than if they are not heated. Starches are insoluble in water and their removal is further aggravated when they gelatinize as a result of heating. Proteins are insoluble in water, but are soluble in alkaline substances; thus alkaline detergents frequently are used to clean food processing equipment. Proteins denatured by heating are more difficult to remove from equipment surfaces than are native proteins. Like protein, fat is insoluble in water and soluble in alkaline solutions. Sufficient heating will cause fat to polymerize, making it difficult to remove during cleaning of equipment. Although some minerals (salts) are soluble in water, minerals in general are soluble in acid and thus, to remove some of them from equipment, acid-type cleaners are sometimes used in the food industry. Minerals can interact with other food components during heating. This can lead to formation of difficult-to-remove deposits on equipment surfaces. Such deposits are called "milkstone" in the dairy industry, "beerstone" in the brewing industry, and may have still other names in various segments of the food industry.

Detergents used to clean food processing equipment commonly consist of alkaline substances, water conditioners, and surface-active agents (surfactants). Sometimes organic acids replace the alkaline components.

Alkaline substances commonly used include sodium hydroxide, sodium metasilicate, sodium sesquisilicate, sodium orthosilicate, sodium carbonate, and trisodium phosphate. Each of these compounds has specific desirable and undesirable properties, so a mixture is prepared to enhance the desired and minimize the undesired characteristics in a detergent.

Water conditioners are added to a detergent to minimize detrimental effects of hard water and to prevent mineral deposits from forming on equipment surfaces. These components act as sequestrants of calcium and magnesium. Commonly used water conditioners include sodium tripolyphosphate, sodium tetraphosphate, sodium hexametaphosphate, and tetrasodium pyrophosphate. Choice of the compound(s) to be used depends largely on the temperature at which the detergent is expected to function. If use of phosphates is not permitted in a given area, sodium gluconate can serve as a water conditioning agent.

Surfactants improve the wetting and penetrating properties of a detergent. They emulsify fat with water because the surfactants are molecules with lipophilic and hydrophilic parts. Four types of surfactants, anionic, cationic, non-ionic, and amphoteric—with the designation based on how they dissociate in an aqueous solution—are available for use in detergents. Quaternary ammonium compounds are cationic surfactants and germicidal. However, if they are combined with anionic surfactants, this germicidal activity is largely lost.

Although not used as commonly as alkaline detergents, acids can serve to clean food processing equipment, especially when mineral deposits are present. Organic acids, for example, gluconic, levulinic, glycolic, citric, lactic, and tartaric acids, are noncorrosive, effective, and easy to handle. Inorganic (mineral) acids, for example, hydrochloric, phosphoric, and nitric acids, can be used to remove extensive mineral deposits. However, they are corrosive and hazardous to handle and so should be used only with great care.

When equipment is to be cleaned, loose material should be removed first and then the equipment should be rinsed with warm, that is, 43°C (110°F), water to remove residual protein, fat, and other food constituents. Cool, that is, less than 32°C (90°F), or hot, that is, 71°C (160°F), water should be avoided to prevent solidifying fat (cool) or denaturing protein (hot). After rinsing, the hot detergent solution is used. If applied manually, the solution may be at 63°C (145°F), whereas it may be up to 82°C (180°F) if application is done mechanically. The detergent solution can be applied as a foam or gel and removed with hot water at high pressure. Alternatively, a clean-in-place (CIP) procedure can be used. To ensure success with the CIP procedure, equipment used for cleaning must be properly designed and concentration of detergent in solution must be carefully controlled.

C. Sanitizing Food Equipment

An effective cleaning program removes virtually all soil from food handling equipment, but will not eliminate many of the microorganisms that are present.

Consequently, cleaning must be followed by a suitable sanitization program which can use either physical or chemical methods.

Physical methods are largely restricted to heat or ultraviolet irradiation. Heat can be applied with steam (at atmospheric or higher pressure, depending on the equipment) or hot water [at 77–82°C (170–180°F)] and should be at least at 63°C (145°F) at the end of the sanitization process. When properly used, heat can be effective for sanitizing equipment. Commonly, disadvantages outweigh advantages so in practice it is used only occasionally. Ultraviolet irradiation has limited application for treating air and water.

Chemical methods are used widely and involve application of chlorine-bearing, iodine-bearing, or quaternary ammonium compounds to equipment surfaces (product contact) to inactivate most or all of the microorganisms that are present. The equipment surfaces must be clean before the sanitizer is applied. No sanitizer can effectively sanitize equipment surfaces laden with organic matter, especially if much of it is proteinaceous.

Chlorine is the most effective and economical sanitizer available. It is commonly used at 200–300 ppm and at pH values below 8.3. Both effectiveness as a germicide and corrosiveness to equipment increase as the temperature of the chlorine solution is increased. Chlorine is effective against spores and vegetative cells of bacteria, molds, and yeasts, provided it is in contact with the microorganism for at least 90–120 seconds. Various compounds can be sources of chlorine but, regardless of source, when in solution it acts as follows:

$$Cl_2 + H_2O \rightarrow HCl + HOCl \quad \text{(hypochlorous acid: germicidally active, unstable during storage)}$$

$$HOCl \rightarrow HCl + [O] \quad \text{(nascent oxygen)}$$

Iodine for sanitizing purposes is added to a surfactant, usually non-ionic, and this mixture is called an "iodophor." Iodophors can be used at pH values as low as 2.0 and thus can be effectively combined with acid detergents. Available iodine at 25 ppm is as effective against a wide spectrum of microorganisms as is 200-ppm available chlorine. Iodophors should not be used at or above 43°C (110°F) or free iodine is released and the sanitizer loses its effectiveness.

As mentioned earlier, quaternary ammonium compounds are cationic surfactants with germicidal activity. These compounds are more stable and costly than chlorine, are difficult to rinse from equipment surfaces, and are claimed to be more effective against gram-positive than gram-negative bacteria. Because of these limitations, use of quaternary ammonium compounds in the food industry is not as great as that of other sanitizers.

Use of hydrogen peroxide is restricted to "sterilizing" packaging material for ultraheated (UHT) products. Approval by the FDA to use hydrogen peroxide for this purpose made UHT processing a reality in the United States.

When cleaning and sanitizing equipment is completed, effectiveness of the procedures must be determined. This requires inspection—both visual and microbiological. Microbiological inspection is done to ensure that equipment surfaces are free from excessive numbers of microorganisms. Such inspection can be done by use of the swab technique, the reverse organism direct agar contact (RODAC) plate, the cellulose sponge technique, or passing an initially sterile liquid through equipment and then testing it microbiologically. Regardless of the method used, finding a few colonies on petri plates associated with the method is neither surprising nor a reason for concern. Finding hundreds of colonies suggests a failure in the sanitizing procedure (provided the test is done properly) and indicates the need to correct deficiencies that may exist.

V. Microbiological Criteria for Foods

A microbiological criterion tells the maximum level of some species or group of microorganisms that is permissible per unit weight of food. Specifically, a criterion comprises (1) the name of the contaminant of concern, (2) the analytical method to be used, (3) the plan for obtaining samples, and (4) how the pass–fail decision is to be made. Microbiological criteria are intended to control the risk of exposing the consumer to pathogenic organisms or their toxins, reveal whether gross contamination has occurred, and guarantee a reasonable shelf life of the food.

A. Types

At least three types of microbiological criteria are presently in use: standards, specifications, and guidelines.

Standards are established and enforced by a legal agency. They have the force of law, and violation is likely to result in imposition of a penalty. Microbiological standards should be used only when there is a definite need for them, and they should have some direct relevance to protecting the health of the consumer.

Specifications are established by a purchaser, to be met by a supplier, for example, of raw material for food. Some are relevant to health, for example, when the purchaser specifies that *Salmonella* shall not be detectable in some stated quantity of the material. Others may relate to fitness for processing, as when limits are placed on levels of thermophilic, sporeforming organisms in sugar or starch to be used in canning.

Guidelines are advisory or administrative criteria. They are norms that regulators or processors establish, to be applied in a specific context; they do not have the force of law. Whether used in regulatory or quality control activities, guidelines may apply to raw materials, foods during processing, or finished products.

B. Development

The great apparent success story in the history of microbiological standards for foods is that of Grade A pasteurized milk. The Grade A Pasteurized Milk Ordinance that is published periodically by the U.S. Public Health Service and widely (almost universally) adopted and enforced by states and sometimes by municipalities in the United States specifies that milk for pasteurization shall not contain more than 100,000 bacteria per milliliter before, nor more than 300,000 after, commingling.

After pasteurization, there must be no more than 20,000 bacteria and 10 coliform bacteria (100 in bulk transport tank shipments) per milliliter. Application of these standards has been accompanied by a dramatic drop in the previously high incidence of milk-borne disease, but it must be noted that a good deal more than just microbiological standards was at work. First, safety-related procedures are specified in the ordinance for every aspect of milk collection, transportation, processing, and vending; probably more significant, pasteurization is an extremely important deterrent to the transmission of disease agents via milk.

In contrast, standards for raw meats such as ground beef have been enacted by several cities and states and have a consistent record of failure. The State of Oregon withdrew its standards for fresh or frozen raw meat after 4 years of experience because the standards had not improved sanitation, reduced levels of bacteria in products, nor reduced the incidence of foodborne disease associated with these products. Oregon concluded that its public was being misled by the standards, since enforcement was not really leading to safer food and costs of enforcement were yielding no corresponding benefits.

C. Principles

When microbiological standards are being established for a food, some general considerations apply: (1) standards should be used only where needed; (2) standards should be attainable by following Good Manufacturing Practices; (3) the extent of testing to be done should be defined and not exceeded; and (4) the hazard associated with the food and the cost of applying the standard should both be taken into account. Food that is judged unfit for human consumption through not having met a standard may still be suitable for reprocessing, animal feed, or some other purpose.

Organisms for which tests are to be conducted should be relevant to the food in question, that is, an established indicator, pathogen, or spoilage organism for that food. For most organisms, low numbers in food are insignificant; there are some important exceptions.

Methods for microbiological analysis should be standardized as much as possible. Many government agencies (e.g., the U.S. Food and Drug Administration) and *ad hoc* national (e.g., the American Public Health Association) and international [e.g., the International Commission on Microbiological Specifications for Foods (ICMSF)] organizations propose, select, or adopt methods for microbiological examination of foods. It often is helpful if a method is tested collaboratively by several laboratories before adoption, although this is not always possible.

Limits should be based on microbiological data from various stages of processing and should, as has been stated, be attainable by use of Good Manufacturing Practices. The limit applied should, if it is said to be applicable to public health, be relevant to risk. Where a zero-tolerance limit is to be applied, as is often done with *Salmonella,* the quantity of food to be tested must be specified. Inevitably, the limits and the sampling plan often become intertwined.

Sampling plans should be administratively and economically feasible and should take into account the heterogeneity of distribution of microorganisms in foods. The ICMSF has proposed two-class and three-class sampling plans. In a two-class plan, the number of sample units which must be analyzed from a lot of food to satisfy the requirements of the plan is designated n, the maximum number of defective sample units is designated c, and the microbiological criterion of defectiveness is designated m. For example, a two-class plan might be used to specify that salmonellae not be detected in any of 10 sample units, by a prescribed testing method ($n = 10$, $c = 0$, $m = 0$). In a three-class plan, m is the microbiological criterion for marginally acceptable quality, whereas M is another microbiological criterion which separates marginally acceptable samples from those that are defective. For example, a three-class plan might specify that mesophilic anaerobic bacteria should not be recovered from any of 5 sample units examined in a number exceeding $10^6/g$, nor in a number exceeding $5 \times 10^4/g$ from 3 or more of the 5 sample units examined ($n = 5$, $c = 2$, $m = 5 \times 10^4$, $M = 10^6$). Implementation of sampling plans such as these allows more flexibility, probably with little loss in precision, in writing microbiological specifications when organisms are not uniformly distributed in the food—as they seldom are.

VI. Summary

Foods as raw materials have an indigenous microflora, some of which may cause spoilage and some of which may threaten human health. Other spoilage organisms and pathogens may be introduced as contaminants. Every food is an ecosystem in which some organisms will prosper more than others. Preservation methods are applied to prevent or delay spoilage, and sanitation is the means by which avoidable contamination is minimized. Nevertheless, the prudent consumer knows that foods are not sterile and assumes the presence of some agents that may be injurious if food is mishandled. Microbiological criteria are of value in assessing the safety or quality of some, but not all, foods.

Bibliography

Frazier, W. C., and Westhoff, D. C. (1988). "Food Microbiology," 4th Ed. McGraw-Hill, New York.

Imholte, T. J. (1984). "Engineering for Food Safety and Sanitation." Tech. Inst. Food Saf., Crystal, Minnesota, 1984.

International Commission on Microbiological Specifications for Foods (1980). "Microbial Ecology of Foods. Vol. 1: Factors Affecting Life and Death of Microorganisms." Academic Press, New York.

International Commission on Microbiological Specifications for Foods (1980). "Microbial Ecology of Foods. Vol. 2: Food Commodities." Academic Press, New York.

International Commission on Microbiological Specifications for Foods (1978). "Microorganisms in Foods. 1: Their Significance and Methods of Enumeration," 2nd Ed. Univ. of Toronto Press, Toronto.

International Commission on Microbiological Specifications for Foods (1986). "Microorganisms in Foods. 2: Sampling for Microbiological Analysis: Principles and Specific Applications," 2nd Ed. Univ. of Toronto Press, Toronto.

Jay, J. M. (1986). "Modern Food Microbiology," 3d Ed. Van Nostrand-Reinhold, New York.

Subcommittee on Microbiological Criteria, Committee on Food Protection, Food and Nutrition Board, National Research Council (1985). "An Evaluation of the Role of Microbiological Criteria for Foods and Food Ingredients." Nat. Acad. Press, Washington, D.C.

Troller, J. A. (1983). "Sanitation in Food Processing." Academic Press, New York.

PART II

INTOXICATIONS

CHAPTER 4

NATURALLY OCCURRING TOXICANTS IN FOODS

Steve L. Taylor

and Edward J. Schantz

I. Introduction

Since all chemicals are toxic at some dose, every chemical in foods, including all of the additive chemicals and all naturally occurring constituents, could be considered a foodborne toxicant. While this approach is philosophically correct, it is clearly impractical to view food constituents in that manner. In foods that are normal constituents of our diets, the component chemicals, both natural and synthetic, are usually present in doses that are insufficient to produce harmful effects when the foods are eaten in reasonable amounts and are prepared in a usual manner. Some exceptions exist to this statement, since atypical consumers with allergies to food constituents can experience adverse reactions to foods which are normally present in our diets. Also, this statement ignores any possible role of food components in cancer, heart disease, or hypertension, although the purported associations with these chronic diseases are controversial.

Thus, the degree of hazard associated with a chemical is more important than the chemical's toxicity. Toxicity is an intrinsic property of all chemicals. Hazard is the capacity of a substance to produce injury under the circumstances of exposure. Hazard takes into account the dose and frequency of exposure as well as the relative toxicity of the particular chemical. This chapter will focus on the naturally occurring chemicals in foods and their degrees of hazard.

II. Natural Sources of Toxicants in Foods

Two general classes of naturally occurring toxicants occur in foods: naturally occurring constituents and the contaminants that are produced in foods by various natural processes. The naturally occurring constituents of foods can be considered both normal and unavoidable. The naturally occurring contaminants are not always present and can be avoided, if the contamination is prevented.

A. Naturally Occurring Constituents of Food

Naturally occurring constituents are present in foods of animal, plant, or fungal origin. Most are not hazardous under normal circumstances of exposure. Foods of animal origin include meat, milk, cheese, eggs, fish, mollusks, and crustacea. The most hazardous chemicals occurring in this category are found in poisonous seafoods. Foods of plant origin include vegetables, fruits, grains, seeds, nuts, spices, and beverages. Most plant-derived chemicals are not particularly hazardous, but a few that are potentially hazardous will be discussed. The major food of fungal origin is mushrooms, many of which are hazardous.

B. Naturally Occurring Contaminants of Food

Foods can be contaminated naturally by bacteria, molds, algae, and insects. These biological contaminants can produce chemicals that remain in the food even after the biological source has been removed or destroyed. Contaminants from bacteria, molds, and algae are discussed in detail in other sections and chapters. Insects can also produce and secrete toxic chemicals into infested foods. Thus, prevention of insect infestation of foods may be more than merely an aesthetic consideration. Insect-produced chemicals will not be discussed further.

III. The Preoccupation with Natural Foods

In the past several decades, much attention has been focused on man-made toxicants, such as additives and pesticide residues, in foods. As a result, some consumers have accepted the notion that foods containing no added chemicals are safer than foods that contain added chemicals. It is impossible to demonstrate that natural is synonymous with safer, yet consumers are demanding such products.

A. Definitions of "Natural"

No legal definition exists for the word *natural* in United States food laws, so there are no legal limitations on the use of the term. The part of the definition in Webster's dictionary that is most relevant to food states: "planted or growing by itself; not cultivated or introduced artificially, e.g. grass; existing or produced by nature; consisting of objects so existing or produced; not artificial." Most consumers would likely define natural as being anything that is not artificial—another term that defies definition. To the food industry, natural can mean additive free, preservative free, or antioxidant free. It can also refer to foods derived from plant or animal materials, processed agricultural commodities, or raw, unprocessed agricultural commodities.

B. Concerns over Additives in Foods

Why are consumers concerned about chemicals added to their foods, and are their concerns justified? The concerns likely arose from notable government regulatory actions against certain food additives and incidental contaminants (pesticides), which contrasts with an absence of action against naturally occurring chemicals in foods. Also, the health foods industry promoted natural products as being beneficial to health and has been able to convince some consumers that natural products and supplements are valuable components of the diet. The reasons for consumer concerns seem clear, but are these concerns justified?

1. Regulatory emphasis on additives

The United States food laws assume natural foods to be safe, while most additives—including all newly developed ones—must be proven to be safe. The Food and Drug Administration (FDA) has rarely taken any action to limit the availability of naturally occurring foods because of the presence of toxic or carcinogenic chemicals of natural origin.

One exception was the FDA's decision in the 1970s to ban sassafras bark from sassafras tea, based on the demonstrated carcinogenicity of safrole, a naturally occurring component. Meanwhile, the FDA permits up to 20 ppb total aflatoxins, which are potent naturally occurring carcinogens, in peanuts.

In contrast to the general lack of regulatory activity on naturally occurring toxicants, the FDA has acted on numerous food additives because of concerns about their safety. The provisions of the Delaney clause have been used to ban cyclamate (a noncaloric sweetener) and FD&C Red #2 (a food dye) because of evidence for carcinogenic activity in animal feeding trials. Saccharin, another noncaloric sweetener, is allowed at present only because Congress enacted a moratorium. The FDA has required the specific declaration of FD&C Yellow #5 (tartrazine) and sulfites on food labels and has banned the use of sulfites on fresh fruits and vegetables because of concerns that these additives can trigger adverse reactions in some sensitive individuals. At the same time, the Environmental Protection Agency (EPA) has banned a number of pesticides, such as DDT and ethylene dibromide (EDB), because of their potential carcinogenicity. With all of these regulatory restrictions occurring, it is little wonder that consumers have developed a suspicious attitude toward chemicals added to foods.

2. Perspective on diet and health

The widespread use of additives and pesticides coupled with the regulatory actions just described has created concerns over chronic diseases such as cancer. However, health developments in the United States from 1970 to 1980 reveal that an epidemic of chronic disease is unlikely. During that decade, life expectancy increased by 2.7 years, the death rate from heart disease dropped 20%, the death rate from stroke dropped 33%, and fewer people under the age of 49 died of cancer. Meanwhile, the use of most chemicals in foods continued, and any benefits from the banning of chemicals such as cyclamate would be predicted to surface after a much longer delay.

C.   Hazards Associated with Naturally Occurring Substances

While consumer concerns about the safety of chemicals added to foods are understandable, consumers' lack of concern about naturally occurring chemicals in foods may not be justified.

1.   Naturally occurring acute toxins in foods

Certain foods naturally contain some rather well known toxic substances, such as mercury and arsenic in seafoods and cyanogenic glycosides, sugar derivatives that release cyanide on contact with stomach acid, in lima beans. Table I lists the estimated annual per capita intake of certain acute toxins among United States consumers.

While these chemicals are certainly toxic, several factors allow us to consume these foods with little chance of adverse reactions. First, the normal level of exposure to these toxins is usually below the threshold for toxicity. Second, the form of the chemicals may lessen their toxicity. For example, the mercury residues in fish may be bound to selenium, a form which is far less toxic than other forms of

Table I
Examples of Naturally Occurring Acute Toxins in Foods

Chemical	Source	Estimated yearly per capita consumption (U.S.) (mg)
Arsenic	Shellfish, seafood	50–332
Cyanide	Lima beans, cassava	40
Mercury	Tuna, swordfish	1.8–3.6
Myristicin	Nutmeg	44
Solanine	Potatoes	10,000

mercury. Third, these toxins, with the possible exception of mercury, do not accumulate in the body. Therefore, small doses from one meal are metabolized and excreted before another dose is consumed.

2. Toxicity of food nutrients

Since all chemicals are toxic, even the basic nutrients in foods are slightly toxic though not hazardous. Laboratory animals can be killed by feeding them glucose, sucrose, or salt, but only at rather high doses. However, some of the micronutrients such as vitamin A and some of the trace minerals (e.g., selenium) are hazardous if consumed in amounts only a few times greater than our requirements for these nutrients. With vitamin A, acute toxicity has been noted for adults ingesting 2–5 million International Units (IU); the recommended dietary allowance for vitamin A is 4000 IU for adult females and 5000 IU for adult males.

3. Chronic toxicity of naturally occurring substances

Numerous examples exist of naturally occurring carcinogens. Some of the mycotoxins, such as aflatoxin B_1 and sterigmatocystin, which can be natural contaminants of many foods, are carcinogenic. Some of the naturally occurring toxicants in plants including the pyrrolizidine alkaloids and safrole are carcinogenic. Many of the essential oils contain carcinogenic substances such as safrole. Even very common spices such as pepper have demonstrable carcinogenic activity. Aflatoxin B_1, which is allowed in foods at levels below 20 ppb, is a much more potent carcinogen than some of the additive substances that have been banned.

4. Hazards associated with alternatives to processed foods

As discussed previously, some consumers have become quite suspicious of chemicals added to their foods. Some of these consumers will seek alternatives, such as foraging for food in the wild or purchasing foods and remedies from health food stores.

a. Foraging in the forest

Foraging for foods in the forest can be hazardous for anyone not expert in the identification of edible species. The harvesting of plants and mushrooms in the wild is fraught with risks because toxic species are rather common and identification can be difficult. Mushroom poisoning occurs exclusively among individuals consuming mushrooms harvested in the wild. In the period of 1977 to 1981, the Centers for Disease Control reported 18 outbreaks of mushroom poisoning in the United States involving 48 cases. The ingestion of plants harvested in the wild also occasionally results in adverse reactions, often among campers or backpackers. Individuals harvesting their own herbs for the preparation of herbal teas are also victims on occasion. An elderly couple in the state of Washington in 1977 harvested what they thought were comfrey leaves for the preparation of herbal tea. They mistakenly harvested foxglove, a very toxic plant, and both individuals died as a result.

b.   Health food stores and their products

Health or natural food stores often have a limited array of products, which deters most consumers from purchasing all of their foods from these outlets. Most of the items sold are or are purported to be natural, and some are sold as health remedies. Because the natural chemicals present in these products are not legally required to be evaluated for safety, hazardous products may be more likely to be encountered in health food stores than in typical supermarkets.

Identity of ingredients   It is very difficult to verify the identity of the dried leaves in some herbal preparations.

Hazards associated with ingredients   A few health foods and remedies contain acutely toxic substances. For example, apricot kernels contain amygdalin, also known as vitamin B_{17} or laetrile. Amygdalin is purported to have anticarcinogenic properties, but in fact is a glycoside that releases HCN on contact with stomach acid. Cyanide is reasonably toxic and at least one death is attributed to ingestion of apricot kernels. Other fruit pits also contain cyanogenic glycosides and are hazardous to ingest in large quantities.

Many foods, including some health foods, contain substances that may pose a significant carcinogenic hazard, although there is no direct evidence that they do. Comfrey tea, for example, is widely recommended by health food stores for its general healing properties. It contains several pyrrolizidine alkaloids known to induce liver damage and tumors in laboratory animals. These alkaloids are potent carcinogens, and many consumers of comfrey tea ingest the product frequently.

Large doses of ginseng, a popular health food, have been reported to cause secondary female characteristics in men, including the loss of body hair and breast enlargement. Effects of high intakes of ginseng may also mimic corticosteroid intoxication, including high blood pressure, nervousness, and insomnia. The estrogenic effects are definitely due to chemicals present in ginseng. Other toxic effects may be due to other plants fraudulently sold as ginseng.

Some health food products can elicit allergic reactions in sensitive consumers. Chamomile tea can induce allergic reactions in individuals sensitive to ragweed (common in the United States), and individuals with pollen allergies may experience reactions after ingesting bee pollen.

Method of preparation   The method of preparation of health foods can be important in avoiding certain associated hazards. A few herbal teas require very careful filtration to remove potentially toxic components. Remedies containing valerian root are frequently marketed as tranquilizers, but active ingredients are easily inactivated by heat, acid, or alkali, so the commercial product is often worthless.

Dose of hazardous ingredients   The dose of the toxic constituents is always an important determinant of the hazard associated with a product. Because health foods are often harvested in the wild after growing under uncontrolled conditions, concentrations of toxic substances may be unpredictable. Tansy, a common ingredient of various remedies sold in health food stores, contains thujone, a convulsant and hallucinogen. The level of thujone varies widely in tansy, so consumers can never be certain how much of this toxic substance they are ingesting with the remedy.

Economic fraud   Fraudulent practices which are not hazardous themselves are common in health and natural food stores. The most common is the marketing of herbal remedies that have no actual therapeutic value. Applicable active ingredients are either absent or negligible in wild lettuce sold as a soporific, black cohosh for menstrual problems, red raspberry leaves (in herbal teas) as stimulants and smooth-muscle relaxants; and horsetail for the treatment of kidney and bladder ailments as well as tuberculosis. Federal law prohibits unfounded health claims on labels, so these claims are usually made in literature that accompanies the products, which is also available at the health stores.

Conventional medical therapy   Another risk associated with health food remedies is the avoidance of conventional medical therapy. Often consumers will use these products in an attempt to cure illnesses that would be much better treated by established medical means. As a consequence, the illness may worsen before suitable medical treatment is sought. Unnecessary complications and even death may occur.

IV.   Intoxications from Naturally Occurring Toxicants

Many naturally occurring, potentially hazardous chemicals exist in foods. Ingestion of these toxicants does not always cause illness, but intoxications can result under certain circumstances of exposure as indicated in Table II. Chronic illnesses, such as cancer, are difficult to correlate with foods or specific foodborne toxicants, since many confounding variables can affect the onset and course of the disease. Thus, the remaining examples discussed here will involve acute intoxications.

A.   Statistics on Chemical Etiology of Foodborne Disease

Chemical etiology accounted for 20–30% of all foodborne disease outbreaks reported in the United States from 1977 to 1981 (Table III). Staphylococcal food poisoning and botulism could be classified as chemical intoxications, but the Centers for Disease Control (CDC) record these in the category of bacterial infections. Foodborne disease, in general, is underreported; however, outbreaks of chemical

Table II

Intoxications from Consumption of Naturally Occurring
Foodborne Toxicants

Abnormal though natural contaminants that adversely affect *normal*
consumers eating *normal* amounts of the food
    Algal toxins in seafood
    Staphylococcal enterotoxins in various foods
    Botulinal toxins in various foods
    Mycotoxins in various foods
Unusual "foods" that adversely affect *normal* consumers eating
normal amounts of this "food"
    Poisonous mushrooms
    Poisonous plants such as foxglove and *Senecio*
    Poisonous fish such as pufferfish
Normal constituents of food that can cause illness if ingested by
normal consumers in *abnormal* amounts
    Cyanogenic glycosides in lima beans, cassava, and fruit pits
    Phytoestrogens in ginseng
Normal components of foods which, consumed in *normal* amounts,
are harmful to *abnormal* individuals
    Food allergies
    Lactose intolerance
    Celiac disease
Normal foods processed or prepared in an *unusual* manner and
consumed in *normal* amounts by *normal* consumers
    Lectins in underprocessed kidney beans
    Trypsin inhibitors in underprocessed legumes
    Heavy metals in acidic beverages stored improperly
Normal foods eaten by *normal* consumers in *normal* amounts over
an extended period of time (alleged)
    Cholesterol in atherosclerosis
    Saturated fats in atherosclerosis
    Dietary fat in cancer
    Caloric intake in cancer
    Sodium in hypertension

Table III

Reported Incidence of Foodborne Disease Outbreaks
of Chemical Etiology, 1977 to 1981

Year	Total number of outbreaks	Outbreaks of chemical etiology	
		Number	Percentage
1977	157	37	23.6
1978	154	37	24.0
1979	172	36	20.9
1980	221	66	29.9
1981	250	51	20.4

Table IV
Etiologic Agents in Reported Incidents of Chemical
Food Poisoning, 1977 to 1981

Agent	Outbreaks/Cases
Fish and shellfish toxins	
Ciguatera poisoning toxins	70/367
Scombroid fish poisoning toxins	68/461
Paralytic shellfish toxins	9/126
Tetrodotoxin	0/0
Heavy metals	13/394
Mushroom toxins	18/48
Monosodium glutamate	2/11
Miscellaneous chemicals	45/427

etiology probably would constitute 20–30% of the total number of outbreaks, even with complete reporting.

The agents involved in the foodborne disease outbreaks of chemical etiology in the period from 1977 to 1981 are listed in Table IV. Naturally occurring toxicants account for the majority of the outbreaks. Fish and shellfish toxins are the most prevalent causes of chemical intoxications. Ciguatera, paralytic shellfish, and tetrodotoxin poisoning will be discussed in this chapter. Scombroid fish poisoning is actually a microbial intoxication and is discussed in Chapter 9 on miscellaneous microbial intoxications. Mushroom poisoning is also a rather frequent form of foodborne chemical intoxication. Among the agents listed under miscellaneous chemicals in Table IV are several naturally occurring substances including marijuana and alkaloids from various plants. Some others listed are not naturally occurring. Most of the heavy metal intoxications are due to packaging errors. Monosodium glutamate is a food additive. Many of the miscellaneous chemicals are detergents, sanitizers, and other processing aids that are hazardous if used improperly.

B. Naturally Occurring Contaminants

As indicated in Table II, many examples exist of naturally occurring contaminants in foods. Separate chapters in this book are devoted to microbial toxicants. In this chapter, the algal toxins that occasionally contaminate seafoods will serve as examples. Considered together, these naturally occurring contaminants are a rather common cause of foodborne disease.

1. Algal toxins in seafoods

Seafoods are important food sources throughout the world, but poisons found at times in certain fish and shellfish cause death within minutes of eating. Other toxic substances found in certain fish cause illnesses that are disabling for weeks. These toxins are acquired by the fish and shellfish through the food chain after being produced by certain species of dinoflagellate algae. Seafood poisonings were once considered a public health problem only in coastal areas, but modern methods of freezing and shipping seafoods over long distances have made these a cosmopolitan concern.

a. Ciguatera poisoning

Occurrence and nature   Ciguatera poisoning is common throughout the Caribbean and much of the Pacific, particularly in areas between 35°N and 35°S latitude. Species of fish implicated include barracudas, surgeon fish, jacks, groupers, sea bass, sharks, trigger fish, wrasses, parrot fish, and especially red snappers and eels. Ciguatera poisoning is clearly the greatest hazard to public health among seafood intoxications. Almost all of the fish involved are palatable reef and shore species. As adults, they do not feed directly on plankton; rather, they acquire the poison through the food chain by eating smaller fish that feed on the poisonous algae or plankton. Most of the toxin is present in the liver and other viscera, rather than in the edible flesh.

The first symptoms of poisoning may be tingling of the lips, tongue, and throat, followed by numbness in these areas. In other cases, nausea, vomiting, metallic taste, dryness of the mouth, abdominal pain, diarrhea, headache, and general muscular pain are apparent. Weakness may progress until the person is unable to walk. Those afflicted usually recover within a few weeks, but in several cases death has resulted from various complications, mainly cardiovascular collapse.

The toxins   The first sign that fish in an area have become poisonous is illness among persons who eat the fish. Ciguatera toxin is detected in mice injected intraperitoneally with an ethanol–ether extract of the fish. Death in 1–6 hours indicates a poisonous fish, but false-positive deaths sometimes occur. If a mouse is unaffected after 36 hours, a nonpoisonous fish is indicated. Substances that cause ciguatera-like signs in animals are lipid soluble and withstand cooking and drying in fish.

The mechanism of action of the toxins and the doses required to cause sickness or death in humans are not known. Because ciguatera poisoning occurs only sporadically, public health measures comprise surveillance for cases in the fish-consuming population, verifying diagnoses by animal testing, and warning the public when a hazard is demonstrated.

b. Shellfish poisoning

Occurrence and nature   Many species of shellfish become poisonous through the consumption of toxic dinoflagellates. Paralytic shellfish poisoning—or mussel poisoning—is caused by eating shellfish that have fed on *Gonyaulax catenella* or *G. tamarensis*. Saxitoxin, the poison produced by these organisms, may cause death within an hour or two of eating poisonous shellfish.

First symptoms include a tingling sensation and numbness in the lips, tongue, and fingertips, sometimes within a few minutes of eating poisonous shellfish. This is followed by numbness in the legs, arms, and neck with general muscular incoordination. Victims often feel light, as though floating on air. Respiratory distress and muscular paralysis become increasingly severe, with death from respiratory failure within 2–12 hours, depending on the dose. If the victim survives 24 hours, the prognosis is good, and normal functions are regained within a few days. No effective antidote is known.

These intoxications were first investigated along the coasts of Germany and Belgium in 1885 and along the Pacific coast of central California in 1929. The poison in California mussels (*Mytilus californianus*) was due to the mussels feeding on a bloom of *Gonyaulax catenella;* the poison in the mussels and the dinoflagellate showed the same lethality in mice. Toxic dinoflagellates were later observed in other areas where people were poisoned from eating shellfish, particularly along the Pacific coast of North America from California to Alaska, Japan, and southern Chile, as well as the North Atlantic coast of North America, the coasts of the North Sea, and many other areas of the world.

The amount of toxin required to cause sickness and death in humans varies considerably. A mouse unit (MU) of poison is defined as the minimum amount of poison that will kill a 20-g white mouse 15 minutes after intraperitoneal injection of an acidic extract of mussel tissue. In California, sickness resulted from about 1000 MU and death from >20,000 MU. In the Maritime Provinces of Canada, sickness occurred after consuming about 600 MU and death at 3000–5000 MU.

When environmental conditions are right, poisonous dinoflagellates may reach concentrations >30,000/ml and persist for 1–3 weeks in a particular area. At a concentration of about 20,000/ml, the water becomes brownish red—thus the term *red tide*. California mussels become too toxic to be eaten safely when >200 *Gonyaulax catenella* cells are present per milliliter. Cell concentrations may be so high that eating one or two mussels will cause death. Mussels and most clams gradually destroy or excrete the poison, so that 1–3 weeks after the bloom of the poisonous dinoflagellate has subsided, the shellfish are safe to eat again. In the Alaska butter clam (*Saxidomus gigantus*), the toxin may be retained for many months before decreasing to safe levels. The shellfish seem not to be harmed by the poisonous dinoflagellates, so appearance is no indication of safety.

Saxitoxin is a neurotoxin; it specifically blocks the sodium pores of nerve and muscle membranes, thus preventing the passage of sodium ions into the cell, which is necessary for nerve conduction. The best treatment for poisoned persons is artificial respiration.

Detection and control   Saxitoxin is a tetrahydropurine base (Fig. 1) with a pK_a at 8.2 and 11.5. Its empirical formula as a free base is $C_{10}H_{17}N_7O_4$ (MW 300), but it was purified as the dihydrochloride salt (MW 372). It has a specific toxicity of 5500 MU/mg. Eleven derivatives, of which the 11-hydroxysulfate is most important, are known. One MU is equivalent to 0.18 μg of saxitoxin dihydrochloride, so amounts of toxin in a food can be estimated in micrograms directly from the mouse assay. The FDA's limit for toxin in marketable shellfish is 80 μg or about 400 MU/100 g of edible meats. In legal cases, several shellfish samples must be taken and at least 10 mice must be challenged per sample. Chemical tests have been developed for saxitoxin in shellfish, but these methods require partial purification of the poison and the use of special equipment.

In terms of the numbers of cases and deaths from consumption of shellfish, this is a very small public health problem. The toxins are very difficult to control from the food safety standpoint because of the sporadic occurrence of the organisms that

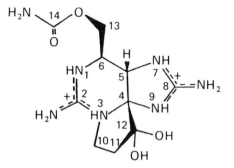

Figure 1 Structure of saxitoxin, a causative agent of paralytic shellfish poisoning.

produce them. Proper control by government agencies requires continuous surveillance of the seafoods that are at risk.

c. Pufferfish poisoning

Occurrence and nature Many deaths occur from eating pufferfish. The toxin occurs mainly in the ovaries, liver, intestine, skin, and roe of various species of puffers, sometimes called blowfish or globe fish. About 30 species of pufferfish are found worldwide, but the most poisonous occur along the coasts of Japan and China. Puffers in other areas are not poisonous. The choice edible species are the most poisonous; they are of the genus *Fugu* (family Tetraodontidae) and are considered a delicacy by the Japanese and Chinese. It was long believed that the toxin was produced by the fish, but there is now some evidence that a dinoflagellate may be the source.

Symptoms of pufferfish poisoning usually begin with a tingling sensation of the fingers, toes, lips, and tongue, much like that of shellfish poisoning, within a few minutes of eating poisonous fish. Nausea, vomiting, diarrhea, and epigastric pain may be evident in some cases. If the dose is sufficient, death results from respiratory paralysis as in shellfish poisoning. The mechanism of action of the toxin (tetrodotoxin) is identical to that of saxitoxin.

Detection and control Tetrodotoxin is an aminoperhydroquinazoline compound ($C_{11}H_{17}N_3O_8$, MW 319; Fig. 2). The toxin is unstable outside the pH range 3–7 but is not destroyed by cooking. Recognizing the poisonous species and proper removal of the roe and viscera before cooking are the best safeguards against poisoning. The Japanese government licenses people to perform these tasks. Still, many deaths occur in Japan and other countries of the Western Pacific because of ignorance and carelessness. It is also important for those who import and market fish in other countries to be able to recognize poisonous pufferfish. Puffers have been mistakenly mixed with angelfish from the Western Pacific and shipped to other countries where chefs were unaware of the hazard; many deaths resulted.

If necessary, the level of tetrodotoxin in fish can be determined by a mouse assay similar to that for shellfish poisons. It is assumed that the human lethal dose of tetrodotoxin is similar to that of saxitoxin.

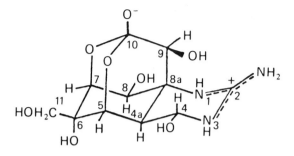

Figure 2   Structure of tetrodotoxin.

d.   Other seafood poisonings

All marine plankton feeders and animals that feed on plankton feeders may become poisonous when toxic dinoflagellates are blooming. Therefore, the study of marine seafood toxins mainly involves the study of poisonous dinoflagellates in certain areas and the feeding habits of edible shellfish and fish. Among more than 1000 species of dinoflagellates that may cause red tides, less than 10 have been shown to be poisonous and cause hazards in seafoods.

Several species of crab in waters around Japan and other parts of the world have been found poisonous, most likely from the consumption of small animals that have fed on poisonous dinoflagellates. The poison in one species of crab, *Zosimus aeneus,* that has caused sickness and death in areas around Japan has been identified as saxitoxin.

Another problem exists along the western coast of Florida, where the poisonous dinoflagellate *Ptychodiscus brevis* (formerly called *Gymnodinium breve*) blooms to heavy red tides and kills millions of fish. The results are pollution caused by decaying fish on the beaches and the loss of the fish as food. Shellfish in these red tides contain a poison that causes a condition similar to ciguatera poisoning, but they are not used commercially to any extent. The structure of one of the toxins from *P. brevis* is shown in Fig. 3.

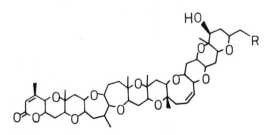

Figure 3   The general structure of the brevetoxins, causative agents of neurotoxic shellfish poisoning.

2. Naturally occurring constituents eaten in normal amounts

Some plants and a few animals contain hazardous levels of various toxicants. These plants and animals should not be eaten but are consumed intentionally or accidentally on occasion, resulting in foodborne chemical intoxications.

a. Animals

Most species of animal do not contain hazardous levels of toxicants. The only good examples are poisonous fish. Puffer fishes and the toxin they contain, which *may* be of algal origin, have already been discussed.

b. Plants

Many plant species contain hazardous levels of toxic constituents. Some of these plants, such as hemlock and nightshade, are classical agents used in early times to poison enemies. In modern times, intoxications from the ingestion of poisonous plants have resulted primarily from the misidentification of the plants by individuals harvesting their own foods in the wild. Less commonly, intoxications from poisonous plants occur with products purchased from retail outlets, as in the contamination of a retail herbal tea by *Senecio*.

Senecio longilobis (common name: thread-leaf groundsel) is a well-known poisonous plant. It was mistakenly included in a commercial herbal tea sold to the Mexican–American population in part of Arizona. This herbal tea, known as gordolobo yerba, was promoted as a cure for colic, viral infections, and nasal congestion in infants. The number of infants and others who ingested the hazardous herbal tea is not known, but six infants died.

Senecio longilobis (and many other plants) contains several of a group of chemicals known as pyrrolizidine alkaloids. Their general structure is shown in Fig. 4. Intoxications with the pyrrolozidine alkaloids can be acute or chronic, depending on the dose. Chronic low doses can produce liver cancer and cirrhosis. The acute symptoms include ascites (accumulation of fluid in the abdominal cavity), enlarged liver, abdominal pain, nausea, vomiting, headache, apathy, and diarrhea.

c. Fungi

Many species of poisonous mushrooms exist and may fool even expert mushroom hunters occasionally. Table V provides some examples of known poisonous mushrooms and their toxins. The toxins are grouped into seven categories, depending upon their structures and the symptoms produced.

The amatoxins of Group I are definitely the most hazardous of the mushroom toxins. *Amanita phalloides* contains 2–3 mg of amatoxins per gram of dry tissue. A single mushroom can kill an adult human. The amatoxins are cyclic octapeptides,

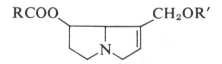

Figure 4   The general structure of the pyrrolizidine alkaloids.

Table V
Some Poisonous Mushrooms and Their Toxins

Species	Common names	Known toxins
Amanita phalloides	Death cap	Amatoxin (Group I)
		Phallotoxin (Group I)
		Lectins
Amanita muscarina	Fly agaric	Muscarine (Group III)
		Bufotenine (Group VI)
		Amatoxin (Group I)
		Phallotoxin (Group I)
		Ibotenic acid (Group V)
		Muscimol (Group V)
Clitocybe dealbata	—	Muscarine (Group III)
Coprinus atramen-tarinus	—	Coprine (Group IV)
Gyromitra esculenta	—	Gyromitrin (Group II)
Psilocybe mexicana	Mexican mushrooms, magic mushrooms, shrooms	Psilocybin (Group VI)
		Psilocin (Group VI)

while the related phallotoxins are cyclic heptapeptides. The phallotoxins are much less toxic than the amatoxins, perhaps due to poor absorption from the GI tract.

Symptoms of amatoxin poisoning begin within 6–24 hours of ingestion of the mushrooms. The first stage involves primarily the GI tract with abdominal pain, nausea, vomiting, diarrhea, and hyperglycemia. A short period of remission usually follows. The third and often fatal stage of the intoxication involves severe liver and kidney dysfunction. The symptoms experienced in this third stage include abdominal pain, jaundice, renal failure, hypoglycemia, convulsions, coma, and death. Death results from hypoglycemic shock, usually between the fourth and seventh days after the onset of symptoms. Recovery may require 2 weeks with intensive medical intervention.

The Group II toxins are hydrazines, such as gyromitrin. A bloated feeling, nausea, vomiting, watery or bloody diarrhea, abdominal pains, muscle cramps, faintness, and loss of motor coordination typically occur 6–12 hours after consumption of *Gyromitra esculenta* mushrooms. In rare cases, the illness can progress to convulsions, coma, and death.

The Group III toxins, characterized by muscarine, affect the autonomic nervous system. Within a few minutes to a few hours of consumption of mushrooms containing these toxins, the patient will experience perspiration, salivation, and lacrimation (PSL) syndrome, blurred vision, abdominal cramps, watery diarrhea, constriction of the pupils, hypotension, and a slowed pulse. Death does not usually occur when these are the only toxins in the poisonous mushrooms (e.g., *Clitocybe dealbata*). Fly agaric also contains Group I toxins, so a fatal combination of symptoms may occur.

Coprine is the classic example of a Group IV toxin. It causes symptoms only in conjunction with alcohol. Symptoms typically begin about 30 minutes after consuming alcohol and may occur for as long as 5 days after mushroom ingestion. The symptoms include flushing of the face and neck, distension of the veins in the neck, swelling and tingling of the hands, metallic taste, tachycardia, and hypotension, progressing to nausea and vomiting. These are the result of actions on the autonomic nervous system also.

The Group V and VI toxins primarily act on the central nervous system, producing hallucinations. The Group V toxins, isoxazoles including ibotenic acid and muscimol, cause dizziness, incoordination, staggering, muscular jerking and spasms, hyperkinetic activity, a coma-like sleep, and hallucinations within 30 minutes to 2 hours of ingestion. The Group VI toxins, including psilocybin and psilocin, are indoles. Symptoms begin about 30–60 minutes after ingestion and include pleasant or apprehensive mood, unmotivated laughter and hilarity, compulsive movements, muscle weakness, drowsiness, hallucinations, and finally sleep. Recovery is spontaneous. Mexican mushrooms have been used as recreational drugs for their hallucinogenic effects. However, the level of hallucinogens in these mushrooms is widely variable, so prolonged and severe side effects can be experienced. Death has occurred in small children who accidentally ate *Psilocybe* mushrooms. More commonly, patients experience persistent sequelae and are admitted to mental institutions.

Group VII toxins are not represented in Table V. However, it is known that many mushroom species will cause nausea, vomiting, diarrhea, and abdominal pain within a few minutes to a few hours of ingestion. The toxins responsible have not yet been identified.

3. Naturally occurring constituents eaten in abnormally large amounts

Since the dose of a toxic chemical is the major determinant of hazard, some foodborne intoxications occur only if unusually large amounts of the toxin-containing food are consumed. The cyanogenic glycosides in cassava and lima beans are examples.

Many plants contain cyanogenic glycosides, such as linamarin in lima beans (Fig. 5). Cyanide can be released from these compounds by enzymes present in plant tissues during storage and processing of the food or by stomach acid after the food has been ingested. The amount of cyanide present in plants varies with the species, variety, and part of the plant (Table VI). The commercial lima beans (white American) contain far less cyanide than some of the wild varieties.

Cyanide binds to heme proteins in the mitochondria and to hemoglobin in the blood, inhibiting cellular respiration. Cyanide prevents oxygen binding to hemoglobin, causing "cyanosis"—the skin and mucous membranes display a bluish coloration. The symptoms of cyanide intoxication include a rapid onset of peripheral numbness and dizziness, mental confusion, stupor, cyanosis, twitching,

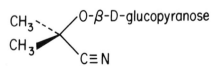

Figure 5 Structure of linamarin.

Table VI
Maximum Cyanide Yields of Various Plants[a]

Plant	HCN yield (mg/100 g wet weight)
Bitter almonds	250
Bitter cassava	
Dried root cortex	245
Whole root	53
Fresh root bark	89
Fresh stem bark	133
Leaves	104
Sorghum	
Whole plant, immature	250
Lima bean varieties	
Java, colored	312
Puerto Rico, black	300
Burma, white	210
Arizona, colored	17
America, white	10

[a]Adapted from R. D. Montgomery (1980). Cyanogens. *In* "Toxic Constituents of Plant Foodstuffs" (I. E. Liener, ed.), p. 143. Academic Press, New York.

convulsions, coma, and death. The lethal oral dose for humans is 0.5–3.5 mg/kg. Cyanide is rapidly absorbed from the GI tract.

Reasonable quantities of lima beans or cassava contain doses of cyanide insufficient to produce symptoms. Lima bean varieties used in the United States have low HCN yields—about 10 mg/100 g on a wet-weight basis. Assuming a lethal dose of cyanide is 0.5 mg/kg, a 70 kg adult would be unlikely to ingest 35 mg of cyanide or 350 g of lima beans. Cyanide is excreted from the body and so does not accumulate. Cassava has been associated with some cases of cyanide intoxication in parts of Africa and South America where people have little else to eat on occasion. Deaths have not been reported. Adverse reactions including deaths have occurred from the ingestion of fruit pits, because the level of cyanide found in these sources is much higher than that found in lima beans or cassava.

4. Naturally occurring constituents eaten by abnormal consumers

Some naturally occurring constituents of foods are hazardous only for consumers with enhanced sensitivities, such as those individuals with food allergies or metabolic food disorders discussed in Chapter 2 on foodborne disease processes.

5. Naturally occurring constituents from foods processed or prepared in an unusual manner

Humans have learned through the years how to detoxify many of the hazardous substances found in foods. For example, in the raw state soybeans contain trypsin inhibitors, lectins, amylase inhibitors, saponins, various antivitamins, and other potentially hazardous factors. The most important of these, the trypsin inhibitors and lectins, are inactivated by heating the soybeans. Fermentation can also destroy certain of these toxic factors, so fermented soybean products, such as soy sauce and tofu, are not hazardous. All other legumes contain similar toxicants. Many other foods contain toxicants that are removed or inactivated during processing. Food technologists should be aware of the naturally occurring toxicants in their raw materials and make certain that those toxicants do not appear in hazardous amounts in new food products.

An example is the presence of lectins in undercooked or raw kidney beans. Lectins bind to sugar residues on the surfaces of cell membranes, causing hemolysis of red blood cells and intestinal damage. Lectins from kidney beans cause nausea, abdominal pain, vomiting, and bloody diarrhea. The lectins are inactivated by thorough cooking. Problems have occurred among recent immigrants to England, who did not understand the importance of thorough cooking of kidney beans, a staple of the British diet. Consumers who soaked the raw beans and ate them with little or no cooking had a prompt onset of gastrointestinal symptoms.

Bibliography

Ayres, J. C., and Kirschman, J. C. (1981). "Impact of Toxicology on Food Processing." AVI, Westport, Connecticut.

Committee on Food Protection, National Academy of Sciences (1973). "Toxicants Occurring Naturally in Foods," 2nd Ed. Nat. Acad. Sci., Washington, D.C.

Harries, A. D., and Evans, V. (1981). Sequelae of a "magic mushroom banquet." *Postgrad. Med. J.* **57**, 571.

Liener, I. E., ed. (1980). "Toxic Constituents of Plant Foodstuffs," 2nd Ed. Academic Press, New York.

Mitchel, D. H. (1980). Amanita mushroom poisoning. *Ann. Rev. Med.* **31**, 51.

Montgomery, R. D. (1980). Cyanogens. *In* "Toxic Constituents of Plant Foodstuffs" (I. E. Liener, ed.), p. 143. Academic Press, New York.

Ory, R. L., ed. (1981). "Antinutrients and Natural Toxicants in Foods." Food Nutr. Press, Westport, Connecticut.

Peden, N. R., Pringle, S. D., and Crooks, J. (1982). The problem of psilocybin mushroom abuse. *Hum. Toxicol.* **1**, 417.

Peterson, J. E., and Culvenor, C. C. J. (1983). *In* "Handbook of Natural Toxins. Vol. 1: Plant and Fungal Toxins" (R. F. Keeler and A. T. Tu, eds.), p. 637. Dekker, New York.

Ragelis, E. P., ed. (1984). "Seafood Toxins." Am. Chem. Soc., Washington, D.C.

Tyler, V. E. (n.d.). "The Honest Herbal—A Sensible Guide to the Use of Herbs and Related Remedies." George F. Stickley Co., Philadelphia, Pennsylvania.

CHAPTER 5

STAPHYLOCOCCAL FOOD POISONING

Merlin S. Bergdoll

I. Introduction

Staphylococcal food poisoning, one of the most common types of foodborne disease, results from the ingestion of food containing a toxin produced by the staphylococci. The symptoms are characteristic in that they develop rather rapidly, are of relatively short duration, and have no lasting effects. A doctor is seldom consulted because of the relatively rapid recovery, so many cases are never reported.

A. Discovery of Cause

Apparently many cases of staphylococcal food poisoning were occurring long ago and were reported in the literature of the time. Little progress in identifying the causative factor had been made before 1914, when Dr. M. A. Barber reported his experiences with food poisoning from milk he obtained on a farm in the Philippines. He had made several visits to this farm, and on three occasions he became ill with gastroenteritis. He was able to eliminate all foods he had eaten on the farm except milk from the two cows. He noted that he did not become ill if he drank the fresh milk, but only after drinking the cream. He obtained milk directly from each of the two cows into clean bottles and took it to the laboratory, making sure that it was kept cold. He drank 30 ml of the cream from one bottle without any ill effects. After leaving the bottle of milk at room temperature (28–30°C) for 5 hours, he drank 40 ml of the milk and cream; he became ill in about 2 hours with nausea and diarrhea, the same symptoms he had experienced on the farm. He was able to isolate staphylococci from the milk which apparently came from the quarter of this cow's udder infected with mastitis. He inoculated some sterile milk with the staphylococci and incubated it for 8–9 hours at 36.5°C and drank some of it. He became ill with cramps, faintness, nausea, and diarrhea in about 2 hours. Two other volunteers became ill with the same symptoms after drinking the milk. Although Dr. Barber ascribed the illness to a toxin produced by the staphylococci, he did not demonstrate the presence of toxin in culture filtrates.

Dr. Gail M. Dack and his colleagues at the University of Chicago were able to demonstrate that the cause of staphylococcal food poisoning was indeed a toxin produced by the staphylococci. This was done by examining the remainder of two three-layer Christmas sponge cakes with thick cream fillings that had made 11 individuals ill with vomiting, mild cramping, and severe diarrhea. The research group demonstrated that the sponge cake substance was responsible for the illnesses when human volunteers became ill with nausea, vomiting, and diarrhea. Staphylococci were isolated from the cakes and grown in laboratory medium. The organisms were removed by centrifugation and the supernatant fluid was given to human volunteers. The presence of a toxin was demonstrated when the volunteers became ill with the same symptoms as those who had eaten the cake. The toxin, which was given the name enterotoxin, was the first foodborne disease toxin to be so designated. The results of this investigation were published in 1930.

B. Worldwide Occurrence

Staphylococcal food poisoning occurs worldwide but is seldom reported because of its relative mildness. Even so, there is great interest in carrying out investigations on this foodborne disease, as demonstrated by the many requests to the Food Research Institute for the reagents needed to identify staphylococcal strains as enterotoxin producers.

C. Incidence in the United States

The information available from the Centers for Disease Control on foodborne diseases for 1981 reveals that, of those illnesses due to bacterial causes, 17.6% (44 outbreaks) were due to staphylococcal food poisoning. In another 137 outbreaks, symptoms developed within the time limit of this type of food poisoning but with insufficient evidence to record them as staphylococcal.

D. Size of Outbreaks

The majority of staphylococcal food poisoning outbreaks involve a relatively small number of people, such as a family group or even only one individual, which accounts for many outbreaks never being reported. There have been very large outbreaks; the largest outbreak in the United States involved 1300 people attending a picnic in Indiana. An even larger outbreak occurred in Japan; it involved 1500 people who consumed contaminated rice balls contained in lunch boxes prepared at one location.

II. The Staphylococci

A. Nomenclature

The genus *Staphylococcus* has been subdivided into at least 23 species. The most important of these is *Staphylococcus aureus,* the species involved in essentially all of the staphylococcal foodborne disease outbreaks. The major characteristics of this species are coagulase and thermonuclease (TNase) production, which are primary in distinguishing it from the most important coagulase-negative species, *S. epidermidis* (Table I). In more recent years, two additional species have been inserted between these two species, namely *S. intermedius* and *S. hyicus;* most *S. intermedius* strains are positive for both coagulase and TNase while *S. hyicus* may be either positive or negative for these two substances (Table I). Both of these species have been reported to produce enterotoxin at very low levels but the frequency of their involvement in food poisoning is unknown, primarily because most often coagulase and TNase production are the only characteristics for which the offending organisms are tested.

Table I
Characteristics of *Staphylococcus* Species

Property	*S. aureus*	*S. intermedius*	*S. hyicus*	*S. epidermidis*
Pigment	+[a]	−	−	−
Coagulase	+	+	±	−
TNase	+	+	±	−
Hemolysis	+	+	−	±
Mannitol (an)[b]	+	−	−	−
Acetoin	+	−	−	+
Clumping	+	+	±	−
Hyaluronidase	+	−	+	−
Lysostaphin	HS[c]	HS	HS	SS[d]

[a]Over 90%.
[b]an, anaerobic conditions.
[c]HS, high sensitivity.
[d]SS, slight sensitivity.

B. Coagulase Production

Coagulase, a soluble enzyme that coagulates plasma, is produced by some strains of staphylococci. It clots purified fibrinogen in the presence of a factor in plasma (coagulase-reacting factor) that is indistinguishable from prothrombin and exists in higher concentrations in the plasma of some species (human, rabbit, horse) than others. Plasma is obtained by removal of the red blood cells from blood that has been treated with either citrate or oxalate to prevent the blood from coagulating; this is in contrast to serum, which is obtained by allowing the blood to coagulate before centrifugation.

Testing for coagulase production is done as follows. The staphylococcal strain to be examined is grown in brain heart infusion (BHI) broth at 37°C for 14–20 hours. One or two drops of the culture is mixed with 0.5 ml plasma in a 10 × 75 mm test tube and incubated at 37°C. Examination for coagulation is done periodically over a 24-hour period and the degree of coagulation is recorded as 1+, 2+, 3+, or 4+ (Fig. 1). A 3+ or 4+ reaction is considered positive, although on occasion a 2+ may be considered positive if the strain produces TNase.

C. Thermonuclease Production

Thermonuclease (TNase) is a heat-stable phosphodiesterase that can cleave either deoxyribonucleic acid (DNA) or ribonucleic acid (RNA) to produce 3′-phospho-mononucleosides. TNase is much more heat stable than ribonuclease and is useful in speciating staphylococci. There are two methods of equal sensitivity for the detection of TNase production. The first depends on the changing of toluidine blue to red by the splitting of DNA by TNase. Heated staphylococcal cultures are placed in wells in an agar layer containing toluidine blue and DNA. Development of red rings

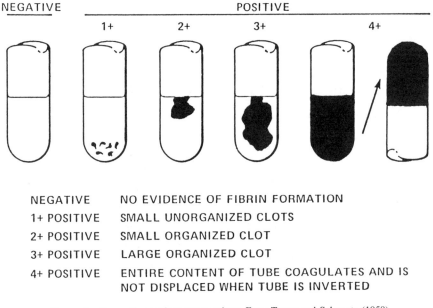

NEGATIVE   POSITIVE

        1+   2+   3+   4+

NEGATIVE   NO EVIDENCE OF FIBRIN FORMATION

1+ POSITIVE   SMALL UNORGANIZED CLOTS

2+ POSITIVE   SMALL ORGANIZED CLOT

3+ POSITIVE   LARGE ORGANIZED CLOT

4+ POSITIVE   ENTIRE CONTENT OF TUBE COAGULATES AND IS
                NOT DISPLACED WHEN TUBE IS INVERTED

Figure 1 Types of coagulase test reactions. From Turner and Schwartz (1958).

around the wells is a positive test for the production of TNase. The second method depends on the formation of a precipitate ring around wells in agar containing Trizma base and DNA when the plate is flooded with $4 N$ HCl. The precipitate ring should be separated from the well by a clear zone.

III. Causative Agents

A. Nomenclature

The agents responsible for staphylococcal food poisoning are a series of toxins given the name enterotoxins because of their effects on the intestinal tract. The enterotoxins are labeled enterotoxins A (SEA), B (SEB), C_1 (SEC$_1$), C_2 (SEC$_2$), C_3 (SEC$_3$), D (SED), and E (SEE). They are identified by their reactions with specific antibodies, with the exception of the SECs. All of the SECs react with the same major antibody but are distinguished by their reactions with specific minor antibodies.

B. Amount Necessary to Cause Illness

The amount of enterotoxin required to produce illness in a sensitive individual has been a matter of conjecture with estimates varying from 1 μg to 100 ng. The latest data, from an outbreak due to chocolate milk among school children, indicate that a dose of 100–200 ng may be sufficient to cause illness in sensitive individuals.

IV.   Chemical Nature of the Enterotoxins

A.   General Properties

The staphylococcal enterotoxins are single-chain proteins with molecular weights of 26,000–29,000. They are basic proteins with isoelectric points of 7.0–8.6. They are resistant to proteolytic enzymes such as pepsin and trypsin; this makes it possible for them to pass through the digestive tract to the site of action. The enterotoxins are relatively heat stable; heating at 100°C for 30 minutes is required to destroy the crude toxins.

Table II
Amino Acid Composition (g/100 g protein)
of the Staphylococcal Enterotoxins

Amino acid	SEA	SEB	SECs	SED	SEE
Alanine	1.9	1.3	1.7	2.0	2.4
Arginine	4.0	2.7	1.7	3.4	4.5
Aspartic acid	15.5	18.1	18.2	16.7	15.1
Cysteine	0.7	0.7	0.7	0.7	0.8
Glutamic acid	12.6	9.5	8.6	13.2	12.2
Glycine	1.0	1.0	3.1	2.7	4.1
Histidine	3.2	2.3	2.9	2.7	3.0
Isoleucine	4.1	3.5	3.8	6.0	4.3
Leucine	9.8	6.9	6.4	9.3	10.1
Lysine	11.3	14.9	14.0	12.9	10.8
Methionine	1.0	3.5	3.5	1.1	0.5
Phenylalanine	4.3	6.2	5.4	4.8	4.5
Proline	1.4	2.1	2.2	1.4	1.9
Serine	3.0	4.1	5.0	5.1	4.7
Threonine	6.0	4.5	5.7	4.5	6.4
Tyrosine	10.6	11.5	10.1	7.2	9.8
Tryptophan	1.5	1.0	1.0	0.6	1.7
Valine	4.9	5.7	6.0	4.1	4.4
Amide NH_2	1.8	1.7	1.5	1.7	1.7

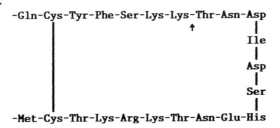

Figure 2 Cystine loop of enterotoxin B. Arrow indicates location of split by mild trypsin action.

B. Amino Acid Composition

The amino acid composition of the enterotoxins is similar in many respects; for example, they have a high lysine, aspartic acid, and tyrosine content (Table II). All of the enterotoxins have two half cystine residues that are joined into a cystine molecule to form a loop (cystine loop) which is located in the center of the molecule (Fig. 2). The amino acid sequences of SEA, SEB, and SEC$_1$ are known. SEB and SEC$_1$ have many areas of homology, but these enterotoxins have only one area of homology with SEA. This area of homology consists of five amino acid residues plus two additional common ones in the next four residues (Table III). This area of homology is proposed as the toxic site in the molecule.

C. Immunology

The enterotoxins are antigenic. Each induces production of specific antiserum when injected into rabbits. The antiserum produced against each enterotoxin, with the exception of the SECs, is specific for the enterotoxin used in the immunizations. Each of the SECs will react with the antiserum prepared against the other SECs; however, the structures of the SECs differ in that the reactions with the heterologous antisera show them to be slightly different antigenically, hence the terminology SEC$_1$, SEC$_2$, and SEC$_3$. There is a cross-reaction between SEA and SEE, that is, each of these enterotoxins reacts with the heterologous antiserum. It has been shown that the major antibody produced by both enterotoxins is specific for each of the enterotoxins, but each produces a minor antibody that is common. In some antisera produced against SEB, antibodies are present that react with both SEB and the SECs. Monoclonal antibodies have been produced that react with SEB and the three SECs. Other monoclonal antibodies have been prepared that react with both SEA

Table III

Common Amino Acid Sequence of the Enterotoxins

Type of enterotoxin	Amino acid sequence
SEA	—Thr—Ala—*Cys*—*Met*—*Tyr*—*Gly*—*Gly*—Val—*Thr*—Leu—*His*—Asp—Asn—*Asn*—Arg—Leu—Thr—
SEB	—Lys—Thr—*Cys*—*Met*—*Tyr*—*Gly*—*Gly*—Val—*Thr*—Leu—*His*—Gly—Asn—*Asn*—Glu—Leu—Asp—
SEC$_1$	—Lys—Thr—*Cys*—*Met*—*Tyr*—*Gly*—*Gly*—Ile —*Thr*—Lys—*His*—Glu—Gly—*Asn*—His—Phe—Asp—

and SEE. It has not been possible to produce antibodies that react with SEA and with SEB or the SECs.

V.   Mode of Action

A.   Effect on the Intestinal Tract

The site of action of the enterotoxins in the intestinal tract is not known, although the emetic reaction apparently is initiated there. This has been demonstrated by rendering monkeys refractory to the toxin given intragastrically by cutting the vagus and sympathetic nerves to the brain, where the vomiting center is located. It is known that the enterotoxins can produce pseudomembranous enterocolitis and apparently this does occur in staphylococcal food poisoning. Experiments with animals have shown that the growth of enterotoxigenic staphylococcal strains in the intestinal tract can produce enteritis; also, the injection of purified enterotoxin into the intestinal tracts of animals produces enteritis. Animal experiments have not indicated a site of attachment of the enterotoxins, but rather the enterotoxins pass through the intestinal tract rapidly and are removed from circulation by the kidney within a short period of time.

The diarrheal action is different from that of the so-called diarrheal toxins, such as *Salmonella* and *Clostridium perfringens,* in that the staphylococcal enterotoxins do not cause fluid accumulation when injected into experimental ileal loops in rabbits. Research has not revealed the action that stimulates the diarrhea.

B.   Effects on the Circulatory System

The staphylococcal enterotoxins are very potent toxins when injected intravenously into monkeys; however, the amount of toxin required to cause the emetic and diarrheal actions when the toxin is ingested is normally not sufficient to cause these more serious reactions. Among these reactions are high temperature, very low blood pressure, hypotension, decrease in urine output, pulmonary edema, pooling of blood in vascular beds, shock, and death.

C.   Other Effects

The staphylococcal enterotoxins have been responsible for the production of allergic effects in laboratory workers. Working with dried preparations of the enterotoxins has resulted in the development of sore throats and runny noses that may last for several hours. Occasional individuals have developed eye reactions similar to pinkeye, with the formation of matter that causes the eyes to swell shut. Another reaction that has affected some workers is the formation of blisters along the insides of the fingers, with a peeling of the palms of the hands about 1 week later.

VI.   Synthesis of the Enterotoxins

A.   Genetics

SEA, SEB, SEC$_1$, and SED have been cloned; this involves transferring the portion of the chromosome that carries the gene for production of the enterotoxin onto a plasmid which is subsequently transferred to *Escherichia coli*. If the gene for production of the enterotoxin is on the section of the chromosome transferred to the plasmid, production of the enterotoxin by the *E. coli* can be demonstrated.

B.   Defined Media

Laboratory experiments to determine the minimum growth requirements have shown that the amino acids arginine and cystine are essential for growth of the staphylococci and production of enterotoxin. Experiments with defined media to produce maximum amounts of enterotoxin show that several of the amino acids can serve as energy sources although they are not necessarily needed for the growth of the staphylococci and production of enterotoxin. Arginine was definitely necessary for the production of SEB, but was not utilized in very large quantities.

VII.   Factors That Affect the Production of Enterotoxin in Foods

A.   Temperature

The temperatures at which staphylococci grow and produce enterotoxin in laboratory medium were discussed previously. The same limitations apply to the production of enterotoxin in foods.

B.   pH

The pH range for the production of enterotoxin is very much the same as that in which staphylococci will grow, namely, pH 5.2–9.0. The staphylococci do not grow as well at the lower end of the pH range, hence, not as much enterotoxin is produced under those conditions. The optimum range appears to be pH 6.5–7.5. Although the staphylococci will grow at the higher pH range, laboratory experiments indicate that enterotoxin is not likely to be produced much above pH 8.0.

Staphylococci are more resistant to salt present in foods than other organisms, but the presence of salt does raise the pH at which the staphylococci will grow and produce enterotoxin, and the increase in pH is related to the amount of salt present.

C. Water Activity

Water activity (a_w) is defined as the vapor pressure of the water in a food divided by the vapor pressure of pure water. Staphylococci will grow at a_w values as low as 0.83, the optimum being >0.99. The production of enterotoxin varies; SEA is produced at somewhat lower a_w values than SEB. Laboratory experiments with foods have indicated that SEA can be produced in some foods at a_w values less than 0.90, whereas a_w values greater than 0.90 are necessary for the production of SEB; the optimum a_w value for both is >0.99.

D. Atmospheric Conditions

Staphylococci can grow under anaerobic as well as aerobic conditions, but growth is much slower anaerobically and, even after several days, cell numbers do not reach those attained under aerobic conditions. Although investigators have reported that enterotoxin can be produced in some foods under anaerobic conditions, other investigators have not been able to reproduce these results. There is no evidence to show that enterotoxin can be produced in vacuum-packed foods.

E. Presence of Other Organisms

Staphylococci do not grow well in the presence of other organisms unless the staphylococcal inoculum is larger than that of the other organisms present. Under raw food conditions, one would not expect staphylococci to grow appreciably because of the presence of other contaminants. In this connection, one would not expect raw milk to be involved in staphylococcal food poisoning unless the milk was from a cow with mastitis. Food poisoning from raw milk is rare, but has occurred when the milk was taken from a mastitic cow.

VIII. Demonstrating That an Outbreak Was Due to *Staphylococcus*

A. Symptoms

The usual symptoms of staphylococcal food poisoning—nausea, retching, vomiting, abdominal cramping, and diarrhea—develop within 1–6 hours; headache, muscular cramping, and marked prostration may be observed in more severe cases. Fever and blood pressure changes, if they do occur, are minor except in very severe cases; in severe cases the temperature may rise several degrees and the blood pressure may drop to quite a low level, 60/40 in one case. There have been deaths recorded, particularly in children and older individuals, but these are rare. Recovery is relatively rapid, from a few hours to one day or so, with no sequelae. There is no effective treatment, primarily because the illness develops so rapidly and is of such a short duration. In cases where excessive vomition and diarrhea occur, administration of fluids may be necessary to restore the salt balance.

B. Foods That Provide a Good Medium for Staphylococcal Growth

Staphylococcal food poisoning sometimes has resulted from the consumption of cheese. The last relatively large and widely distributed outbreak occurred in 1965. The cheese, manufactured with pasteurized milk in a modern plant over a several-month period, was contaminated with a common *S. aureus* strain that produced SEA and SED. The contamination occurred from a leaky valve in the line between the pasteurizer and the cheese vats. Analysis revealed that the only cheese containing enterotoxin was manufactured during a 2-month period in which there was a starter culture failure.

Milk has rarely been involved in this type of food poisoning, primarily because of the care which is used in handling the fluid milk supply. One outbreak did occur in 1985 from chocolate milk served to schoolchildren. The milk inadvertently had been held for several hours at a warm temperature before pasteurization because of a problem in the processing plant. No staphylococci were present in the pasteurized milk but SEA was detectable, indicating that the staphylococci had grown in the milk before pasteurization. The enterotoxins are relatively heat stable and will survive pasteurization.

Butter is generally considered to be exempt from staphylococcal food poisoning because of the small amounts consumed at any one time; however, two outbreaks from butter did occur in the United States. The last outbreak occurred in 1977 and resulted in over 100 cases of illness; all those who became ill had eaten at pancake houses. Staphylococci as well as SEA were detectable in the whipped butter manufactured in one plant. It is not certain how the contamination occurred, but the distribution of the enterotoxin in the butter indicated that the staphylococci had grown in the cream after it was pasteurized and before it was churned.

Ice cream is another product that seldom is involved in staphylococcal food poisoning in the United States, although it has been involved in other countries. An outbreak in the United States in 1984 was attributed to ice cream, but no enterotoxin or staphylococci were detectable in the ice cream. It is possible that the amount of enterotoxin was too small to be detectable even though concentration procedures were applied. One ingredient used in the ice cream that may have been the source of the enterotoxin was whey cream; whey cream that contained enterotoxin had been used in milkshake mixes that were involved in a staphylococcal food poisoning outbreak.

Raw meat is rarely involved in food poisoning because it does not provide a suitable medium for the growth of staphylococci. Cooking does increase the suitability of meat as a medium for the growth of staphylococci, but meat is usually consumed within a short period of time after being cooked. One exception is baked ham, primarily because of the manner in which this food item is often handled after baking. Baked ham sandwiches are a common picnic item and are frequently served at community dinners. Ham is easily contaminated by the food handler during the slicing operation. Nothing would be amiss if the ham were kept refrigerated in small lots until it was served, but this is not always done, particularly if it is taken to the picnic grounds in advance of the meal. Some of the largest outbreaks in the United States have been due to this food item, such as the one involving the 1300 picnickers in Indiana. Admittedly, it is quite difficult to provide adequate refrigeration at the picnic grounds for food for such a large group.

There have been three outbreaks of staphylococcal food poisoning from fermented sausage, all of the Genoa type, manufactured by three different companies. This type of sausage does not receive a heat treatment during the manufacture, hence, any staphylococci present in the meat used to make the sausage are not destroyed. The conditions of the fermentation were such that staphylococci grew to sufficient numbers to produce enterotoxin before the starter culture generated enough acid to prevent staphylococcal growth.

Another meat item involved in a number of food poisoning outbreaks, all of which occurred within the same year, was canned corned beef. The largest number of outbreaks occurred in England from corned beef canned in Brazil, although there were outbreaks in other places from corned beef canned in Argentina, Malta, northern Europe, and Australia. Essentially all of the outbreaks were from corned beef in large cans; contamination occurred by leakage through faulty seams during the cooling process.

A number of outbreaks have occurred from potato salad and various types of meat salads. One of the largest outbreaks involved over 600 high school girls in Indiana after they had eaten ham salad sandwiches. The ham used to make the salad was ground and left at room temperature at least overnight. Some of the students only tasted the sandwiches because of an off flavor, indicating that spoilage of the ham had begun. Sandwiches made from salads of egg, tuna, chicken, and other meats have been involved in staphylococcal food poisoning. Potato salad has frequently been implicated in this type of food poisoning. Usually the salad dressing that is used in the making of the salads is blamed for providing the conditions for the growth of the staphylococci and production of enterotoxin. It is not completely understood why the salad dressing should provide a good medium because usually it is sufficiently acid to prevent the growth of these organisms; in fact, staphylococci usually die off in such an acid environment. However, the ground-up major ingredient provides the medium for growth, because the acidity of the salad dressing is modified to such an extent as not to be inhibitory. Also, the major ingredient does provide a larger surface area for the growth of these organisms.

Custard and cream-filled bakery goods provide an excellent medium for growth of staphylococci and production of enterotoxin. Such items as cream puffs, eclairs, and cream pies were involved frequently in food poisoning before it was recognized that greater care was needed in handling this type of product. Symptoms characteristic of a large outbreak are illustrated by one due to cream puffs (Table IV). Another outbreak involving approximately 50 people occurred in Wisconsin from cream-filled coffee cake; it is used to illustrate the importance of refrigeration in preventing this type of food poisoning.

Any food that provides a good medium for the growth of staphylococci may be involved in food poisoning, and the type of food can vary from country to country For example, in Japan, rice balls are a major food item involved in this type of food

Table IV
Symptoms of Staphylococcal Food Poisoning from 122 Cases[a]

Symptom	Cases[b]	No reaction	Mild reaction	Severe reaction
Vomiting	122	15	12	95
Abdominal pain	122	6	40	76
Diarrhea	103	13	75	15
Headache	101	29	59	13
Muscular cramping	113	41	58	14
Sweating	100	33	67	0

[a]Includes 94 students who ate cream puffs at school, 8 lunchroom supervisors who took cream puffs home, and 20 cases from cream puffs sold at three cafes and from the bakery truck.
[b]Number of cases from which this information was available.

poisoning; they were the vehicle in an outbreak involving 1500 people. This item is prepared by hand and is quite moist, hence, if contaminated rice balls are kept at a warm temperature, the staphylococci will grow and produce enterotoxin. The lunch boxes in this outbreak were not refrigerated during a long train ride to the excursionists' destination.

Another item that is worth mentioning is Easter eggs. Three small outbreaks occurred in Wisconsin before an outbreak involving several hundred children occurred in California in 1983 following an Easter egg hunt. An experiment in the Food Research Institute demonstrated that water contaminated with staphylococci can be sucked into a boiled egg during cooling. If the eggs are allowed to stand at room temperature for a period of time, which is not unusual for Easter eggs, the staphylococci can grow to sufficient numbers to produce enterotoxin, in this case SEB. The individual who prepared the eggs had an infection on his hand by a staphylococcal strain that produced SEB.

Raw foods are less likely to be involved in food poisoning than cooked foods for four reasons: (1) raw meats are contaminated with mixed cultures that tend to prevent the growth of staphylococci, which are not good competitors; (2) raw meats do not provide as good a medium for growth of the staphylococci as do cooked meats; (3) raw meats are usually handled in large pieces, which provide less surface area for the growth of staphylococci; and (4) the temperature and the length of time of cooking tend to destroy any enterotoxin that may be present on the surface of the meat. The outstanding example of this is ham; all of the outbreaks due to this type of meat have been from ham that was baked and then sliced, which provided a much larger surface area for growth of the staphylococci. Although the baked ham would be virtually sterile, it is very easily recontaminated during slicing and subsequent handling.

Another factor that favors the growth of the staphylococci is that they are quite tolerant of salt, while competing organisms are not. Growth of staphylococci can occur in laboratory medium at salt concentrations up to 15%, although growth is slowed and less enterotoxin may be produced.

C. Presence of Staphylococci in Large Numbers

It is difficult to know how much growth needs to occur before sufficient enterotoxin is produced to cause illness. The figure of 10^5 has been used as a guideline, but in experiments with laboratory medium and foods, enterotoxin could not be detected before the count reached 10^6 or higher. However, in most food poisoning outbreaks, counts of 10^8 or even higher are not unusual. This does not mean that food poisoning does not occur with much lower counts, although we do not have adequate evidence to show this.

The Food and Drug Administration (FDA) method for determining the number of staphylococci present is as follows: (1A) 50 g of food is suspended in 450 ml of diluent; (1B) 10 ml of 1A is diluted to 100 ml with the diluent; (1C) 10 ml of 1B is diluted to 100 ml with the diluent; (2) 0.5 ml of each dilution (1A, 1B, and 1C) is spread on two Baird–Parker agar plates and incubated at 35°C for 40–48 hours; (3) a representative number of colonies is picked, regardless of colonial appearance, and each is suspended in 0.3 ml of brain–heart infusion (BHI) and incubated at 35°C for 18–24 hours; (4) 0.5 ml of plasma is added to each tube and incubated 1–6 hours; and (5) the *S. aureus* count = (1/dilution factor) × plate count × (coagulase positive/total picks).

D. Are the Staphylococci Enterotoxigenic?

1. Production of toxin

There are several methods used to grow staphylococci for the production of enterotoxin. The medium recommended is BHI + 1% yeast extract, with all incubations carried out at 37°C. The method used by the FDA laboratories is the semisolid agar method, in which the surface of semisolid agar medium in a Petri plate is inoculated with the staphylococcal strain to be tested. After incubation for 48 hours the agar is centrifuged to recover the liquid containing the enterotoxin. The amount of toxin produced with this method is comparatively small and requires the use of the microslide method to achieve adequate sensitivity.

The method used in the Food Research Institute is the membrane-over-agar method. In this method the surface of a membrane (from dialysis sac), placed over solid agar containing the medium, is inoculated with the staphylococcal strain to be tested. After incubation for 18–20 hours the surface of the membrane is washed with 2.5 ml of phosphate buffered saline (PBS; 0.02 M sodium phosphate containing 0.9 M NaCl at pH 7.4) divided into two portions. The wash is centrifuged to remove the cells and used in the optimum-sensitivity-plate (OSP) method to determine if toxin is present.

A third method, which is equal to the membrane-over-agar method in the amount of enterotoxin produced per milliliter, is the sac culture method. In this method the medium (50 ml) is placed in a dialysis sac which in turn is placed in a 250-ml Erlenmeyer flask and autoclaved. Twenty milliliters of sterile PBS is inoculated, placed in the flask, and incubated for 24 hours with shaking. The culture is removed from the flask, centrifuged, and analyzed by the OSP method.

A fourth method that is used primarily for the production of enterotoxin for purification is the shake-flask method. In this method the medium is placed in

Erlenmeyer flasks (25–50 ml in a 250-ml flask or a proportional amount in larger flasks), autoclaved, inoculated, and incubated on a gyrotory shaker at 280 rpm for 18–24 hours. After centrifuging, the culture supernatant is ready for the purification procedures.

2.   Enterotoxin detection methods

All laboratory methods for detection of the enterotoxins are based on the use of specific antibodies to each of the different enterotoxins. The methods most frequently used are those involving a reaction of the enterotoxins with their specific antibodies in some type of gel matrix. In these methods the toxin–antibody reaction results in the formation of a precipitate which can be easily observed in the agar and is quite specific.

a.   OSP method

In the OSP method, 3 ml of 1.2% agar in PBS containing thimerosal (1:10,000) is placed in a 50-mm plastic Petri dish and allowed to harden. Wells are cut into the agar layer according to the diagram in Fig. 3. The specific antiserum is placed in the center well and the standard enterotoxin is placed in the two smaller wells. Culture filtrates to be tested are placed in the four larger outer wells. Incubation is overnight at 37°C. If the enterotoxin being tested for is present in any of the culture filtrates, a line of precipitate will form and join with the line of precipitate formed between the standard toxin and its specific antibody (Fig. 3). The sensitivity of this method is about 100 ng/ml of culture filtrate, which is achieved by concentrating the culture filtrate fivefold.

b.   Microslide

The microslide method is not easy to perform, primarily because the reagents (toxin and antibody) are placed in funnel-shaped wells in an acrylic template placed over a very thin layer of agar—the thinner the layer, the more sensitive the method (Fig. 4). A layer of agar is placed between two bands of electrician's tape (two thicknesses) wound around a microscope slide and the template placed on the layer of agar with the edges resting on the edges of the tape layers, being sure that good contact of the template and the agar layer is made. The specific antiserum is placed in the center well, the standard enterotoxin in two wells diagonally opposite each other, and culture supernatant fluids being tested in the other two wells. After 3 days at 25°C or 24 hours at 37°C, the template is carefully removed without disturbing the agar layer and the presence of any precipitate lines is observed by holding the slide obliquely under a suitable light. Joining lines of precipitate with the standard toxin represents a positive reaction (Fig. 5). The sensitivity of this method is 50 to 100 ng/ml of culture supernatant; however, not all operators are able to achieve this degree of sensitivity. Any bubbles formed in the bottoms of the wells when the fluids are placed in them must be removed and care must be taken to avoid moving the template during the operations. The use of this method is limited primarily to the detection of enterotoxin in foods when the longer extraction and concentration procedures are employed.

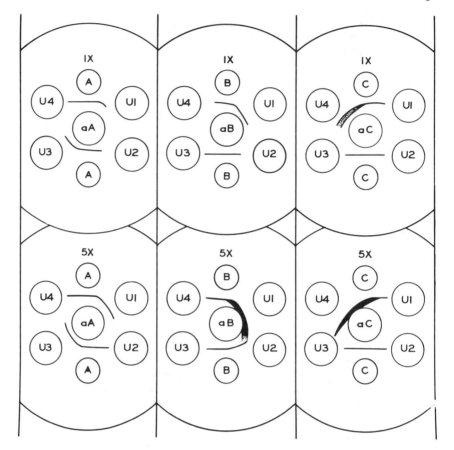

Figure 3 Enterotoxin analysis with optimum sensitivity plates (OSP). A, B, and C represent SEA, SEB, and SEC, respectively (4 μg/ml). aA, aB, and aC represent anti-SEA, anti-SEB, and anti-SEC, respectively. Unknown U1 contains approximately 0.5 μg A and 6 μg B per milliliter; unknown U2 contains no SEA, SEB, SEC; unknown U3 contains approximately 2 μg SEA per milliliter; unknown U4 contains approximately 16 μg C per milliliter. 1X, unconcentrated unknowns; 5X, 5 times concentrated unknowns. From Robbins, Gould, and Bergdoll (1974).

c. Monkey-feeding method

The biological methods for the detection of the enterotoxins are quite limited and are not very sensitive. The only specific biological method is the monkey-feeding test. In this method 50 ml of test sample is injected by catheter into the stomach of a young monkey (preferably Rhesus or cynomolgus); the animals are observed for 5 hours and, if vomiting occurs within that time, the sample is judged to contain enterotoxin. It is the only specific test for unidentified enterotoxins, since it is accepted that any staphylococcal product that produces an emetic reaction in monkeys is an enterotoxin. This method is seldom used now because of the cost of purchase and upkeep of monkeys.

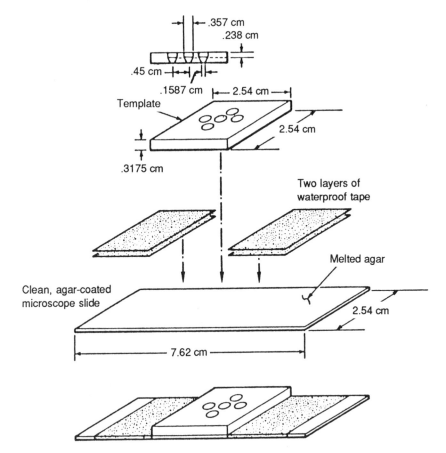

Figure 4   Microslide gel diffusion assembly with specifications for acrylic template.

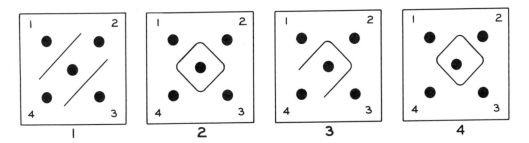

Figure 5   Enterotoxin analysis with microslide. The center wells contain antibody to SEA. Wells 1 and 3 contain SEA. Slide 1: Buffer solution in wells 2 and 4. Slide 2: The culture filtrates in wells 2 and 4 contain SEA. Slide 3: The culture filtrate in well 2 contains SEA; the culture filtrate in well 4 does not contain toxin. Slide 4: The culture filtrate in well 2 contains less SEA than the culture filtrate in well 4.

E.   Detection of Enterotoxin in Foods

As was related earlier, the amount of enterotoxin that may be present in foods can be as little as 50 ng/g of food. Normally the amount of enterotoxin present in foods that have been involved in food poisoning is easily detectable, since frequently it is 1–5 μg/g of food; however, in processed foods that are suspected of containing enterotoxin one needs to be sure that no enterotoxin is present before the food can be marketed. The more sensitive the method for detection the simpler the method needed for extraction of the enterotoxin from the food.

1.   Detection methods

a.   Microslide

The microslide method described previously has a sensitivity of 50–100 ng/ml and is the method used with the long extraction–concentration methods.

b.   Radioimmunoassay

The radioimmunoassay (RIA) method involves the use of ^{125}I-labeled enterotoxin in the detection of enterotoxin in unknown samples. The method is as follows: (1) the food extract (1 ml) being tested is added to a known amount of specific antibody in a reaction tube; (2) after the antibody reacts with any enterotoxin in the food extract a standard amount of the labeled toxin is added to the mixture; (3) after the labeled enterotoxin reacts with any unreacted antibody, staphylococcal cells containing protein A are added to precipitate the reaction product (protein A reacts non-specifically with the portion of the antibody that is not reactive with the enterotoxin); (4) the precipitate is collected by centrifugation; (5) the precipitate is counted in a scintillation counter; and (6) the amount of enterotoxin in the food extract is determined from a standard curve prepared from known amounts of enterotoxin. The larger the amount of labeled enterotoxin present, the smaller the amount of enterotoxin in the extract. The sensitivity of this method is 0.3 ng/ml or approximately 0.5 ng/g of food.

The RIA method is good but is used very little because of the necessity of handling radioactive materials along with the need for expensive equipment such as the scintillation counter. In addition, the purified enterotoxins are needed for preparation of the iodinated toxins.

c.   Enzyme-linked immunosorbent assay

The enzyme-linked immunosorbent assay (ELISA) method involves the use of an enzyme coupled either to the enterotoxin or to the specific antibody and depends on the development of a color by the reaction of the enzyme on a suitable substrate. The enzyme is most frequently coupled to the antibody so that the amount of enzyme–antibody conjugate bound is directly proportional to the amount of enterotoxin in the food extract; hence the amount of color developed is a direct measure of the amount of enterotoxin in the extract. If the enzyme is coupled to the enterotoxin, the amount of the enzyme–enterotoxin conjugate bound is inversely proportional to the amount of enterotoxin in the food extract; thus the amount of color developed is inversely proportional to the amount of enterotoxin present in the extract.

The method is as follows: (1) the surfaces of wells in a microtiter plate or of polystyrene balls are coated with the specific antibody; (2) the food extract is placed in the coated wells in case of the microtiter plate; if the ball method is used, the balls are placed in the food extract in a test tube; (3) after a suitable reaction time, the extract is removed from the wells and the enzyme-specific antibody conjugate is placed in the wells; in the ball method the balls are treated with the conjugate after they are removed from the extract and washed; (4) after a suitable reaction time, the conjugate is removed from the wells and the substrate is added; in the ball method the balls are treated with the substrate after the balls are removed from the conjugate and washed; (5) after a suitable reaction time, the colors developed in the wells of the microtiter plate are read in a microtiter plate reader; the color developed in the ball method is read in a colorimeter; and (6) the amount of enterotoxin in the extract is calculated from a standard curve developed using standard amounts of enterotoxin.

The microtiter plate method is the easier procedure to use because of the number of reactions that can be carried out in one plate; however, a plate reader is required to determine the amount of color developed. The ball procedure requires that each individual ball be handled separately and this becomes cumbersome if there are more than a few samples to be done; however, the advantage is that the color readings can be made with a simple colorimeter. The sensitivity of the ELISA method is essentially the same (0.3 ng/ml) as that of the RIA method. This method is the one that is being used currently for the detection of enterotoxins in foods.

d. Reversed passive latex agglutination

The reversed passive latex agglutination (RPLA) method involves the coating of latex particles with the specific antibody, followed by the addition of the food extract. If any enterotoxin is present in the food extract, the latex particles will agglutinate. This procedure is carried out in microtiter plates with the agglutination reactions observed visually. The sensitivity of the method is equivalent to that of the RIA and ELISA methods. However, to achieve this sensitivity with food extracts, the same extraction procedures used for the RIA and ELISA methods (1.0–1.5 ml/g of food) must be used. Unfortunately, it has not been demonstrated that such food extracts will be free of false-positive agglutinations. This method is not recommended until it has been demonstrated that false-positive reactions do not occur.

2. Extraction procedures

a. Extraction–concentration

The initial procedures developed for the detection of enterotoxin in foods were dependent on the use of the microslide as the enterotoxin detection procedure. In order to detect as little as 1 ng/g of food in food extracts with the microslide, it was necessary to concentrate the food extract about 500-fold. The recommended procedure for concentrating the food extract is as follows: (1) 100 g of food is ground to even consistency in 140 ml of water with the addition of 0.1 M HCl to bring the pH to 4.5–5.0; (2) the slurry is centrifuged and the supernatant fluid adjusted to pH 7.5 with 0.1 N NaOH; (3) the supernatant fluid is treated with $CHCl_3$ and filtered through cheesecloth to remove the $CHCl_3$; (4) the filtrate is adjusted to pH 4.5 and centrifuged to remove any precipitate; (5) the supernatant fluid is adjusted to pH 7.5

and stirred with CG-50 ion exchange resin at pH 5.4–5.9 at 4°C; (6) the resin is removed and extracted with 0.015 M sodium phosphate with 0.9% NaCl at pH 5.9; (7) the extract is dialyzed and concentrated in Carbowax (20 M polyethylene glycol); (8) the concentrated extract is centrifuged to remove any precipitate and lyophilized; (9) the lyophilized extract is dissolved in 0.2 ml of a 1% trypsin solution; and (10) after a 30-minute digestion period, the concentrated extract is analyzed by the microslide method.

b. Extraction procedure for RIA and ELISA

The extraction procedure for RIA and ELISA is as follows: (1) the food (any quantity; as little as 5–10 g can be extracted) is ground to a homogeneous slurry with 1 ml of water per gram of food (1.5 ml is used if the slurry is very viscous) and the pH adjusted to 4.5 with 6 N HCl; (2) the slurry is centrifuged and the supernatant fluid is adjusted to pH 7.5 with 5 N NaOH; (3) the extract is treated with $CHCl_3$ and centrifuged; and (4) the extract is ready for analysis by either RIA or ELISA.

F. Handling of Food during Preparation

1. Food handlers

The most frequent source of contamination of food is the food handler involved in preparing the food for serving. This subject will be discussed under source of contamination.

2. Temperature of storage

The cooking of food will destroy any staphylococci present in the food, since these organisms are destroyed by holding them for 30 minutes at a temperature of 60°C or above. Also, pasteurization of milk is adequate to destroy these organisms. The temperature limits for growth of staphylococci are 10–45°C, with the optimum at 37°C. The optimum temperature for the production of enterotoxin is 37–40°C, with production up to 45°C. Foods should be stored below 10°C or above 45°C when not being prepared or served. The other precaution needed is to store the foods in small lots in order to promote quick cooling. The best method for controlling this type of food poisoning is refrigeration.

3. Time foods held at warm temperatures

The time a food is held at a warm temperature before enterotoxin is produced is estimated to be 3–4 hours or longer. This is somewhat dependent on the inoculum size, for example, whether the inoculum came from a cough or sneeze from a healthy individual or whether it came from an individual with a sore throat or with an infection such as an infected cut on the hand. Contamination by a healthy individual is illustrated by an outbreak that occurred from sliced baked ham. The ham was sliced and packaged (8-oz [227-g] packages) on a Saturday morning and sold throughout the day without refrigeration. The ham remaining was placed in a deep pan and refrigerated overnight. The following morning the ham was removed from the refrigerator and warmed before continuing the sale at 11:00 A.M. Only those individuals who bought the ham the second day become ill with typical staphylococcal food poisoning. The source of the staphylococci was the throat of one of the persons who packaged the ham. This individual had no signs of illness or infection, hence, the inoculum must have been very small. This could be verified by the fact that the ham was kept for many hours during the day at room temperature without enough enterotoxin being produced to result in illness of those who bought the ham that day. Illness occurred only after the ham had been kept an additional several hours at a relatively warm temperature because placing the ham in a deep container did not allow quick cooling. In addition, more time elapsed after the ham was taken from the refrigerator and warmed before sale. This is in contrast to another outbreak in which a large number of people became ill after eating ham sandwiches at a picnic. The ham was contaminated from the lesions on the face of the individual who sliced the ham; he was observed to wipe his hands over his face during the slicing operation. The same staphylococcal organisms that were isolated from the ham were isolated from the lesions. The sliced ham was placed in the oven at 74°C until it was removed at 2 P.M. and taken to the picnic grounds, where it was served at about 6 P.M. It was a warm day (32°C) and the ham was not refrigerated. The people became ill 2–3 hours after eating the ham.

G.   Source of Contamination

1.   Possible sources

a.   Food handlers

A majority of the foods that have been implicated in staphylococcal food poisoning were cooked before the final preparation for serving was completed. In these cases the most likely source of contamination would be the food handler. Two examples of this were given earlier. A food handler with any type of infection on the hands, such as an infected cut, or with a sore throat or cold should not be allowed to prepare food, particularly for a picnic or dinner that is to involve a large number of people.

b.   Animals

Some believe that a major source of contamination is animals. It is true that most raw meats are contaminated with staphylococci, but it is unusual to serve these without adequate cooking, which would destroy any staphylococci present. Even if meats were served relatively raw, staphylococci are poor competitors and would not grow on the raw meat to produce enterotoxin. The one exception to this is possibly the fermented sausage that was involved in food poisoning; in this case the staphylococci responsible could have come from the animal because the meat was not heated. The other possibility is dairy products manufactured from milk that may have come from animals in the early stages of mastitis. In this case the staphylococci would need to grow and produce enterotoxin before processing because milk almost always is pasteurized before it is processed.

c.   Equipment

There have been outbreaks traceable to the equipment, such as meat slicers, used in handling the food. An outbreak due to baked ham resulted from contamination of the ham with the slicer; apparently there were time intervals between slicing operations because the ham was sliced only when a customer purchased it.

2. Determination of source of contamination

a. Phage typing

Many staphylococci are lysed by viruses known as phages; usually the phages that lyse a given staphylococcal strain are specific for that particular strain. The phages are divided into groups which are labeled Groups I, II, III, IV, and Miscellaneous. The phages lysing the staphylococcal strain isolated from the foods involved in any given outbreak are compared to the phages lysing the staphylococci isolated from the food handlers or other possible sources. If the pattern of the staphylococci from a particular food handler matches the pattern of the staphylococcal strain isolated from the food, it is concluded that this particular food handler was the source of the staphylococci causing the food poisoning.

b. Enterotoxin production

Another method for tracing the source of the staphylococci involved in a food poisoning outbreak is to compare the enterotoxin production by the staphylococci isolated from the food and those isolated from the possible sources of contamination. It is true that two strains lysed by different phages can produce the same enterotoxin and in such an instance the results would be inconclusive. However, there are two instances where the enterotoxin produced did indicate the source of the contamination. In an outbreak from cream-filled coffee cake, the staphylococci isolated from both the cake and the nose of the individual who put the cream filling in the cake produced SEE. The staphylococcal isolate from the nose of the individual who put the cream filling in the cake was the only isolate from those working in the bakery that produced SEE. In the case of the two food handlers who packaged the ham in another outbreak, the staphylococci carried by both individuals were lysed by the same phages, but only one of the staphylococcal strains produced SEA, the enterotoxin produced by the staphylococci isolated from the ham.

Bibliography

Bergdoll, M. S. (1970). Enterotoxins. *In* "Microbial Toxins. Vol. III: Bacterial Protein Toxins" (T. C. Monte, S. Kadis, and S. J. Ajl, eds.), pp. 265–326. Academic Press, New York.

Bergdoll, M. S. (1972). The enterotoxins. *In* "The Staphylococci" (J. A. Cohen, ed.), pp. 301–331. Wiley (Interscience), New York.

Bergdoll, M. S. (1979). Staphylococcal intoxications. *In* "Food-Borne Infections and Intoxications" (H. Reimann and F. L. Bryan, eds.), 2nd Ed., pp. 443–449. Academic Press, New York.

Bergdoll, M. S. (1983). Enterotoxins. *In* "Staphylococci and Staphylococcal Infections" (C. S. F. Easmon and C. Adlam, eds.), Vol. 2, pp. 559–598. Academic Press, London.

Bergdoll, M. S., and Bennett, R. W. (1984). Staphylococcal enterotoxins. *In* "Compendium of Methods for the Microbiological Examination of Foods" (M. L. Speck, ed.), pp. 428–457. Am. Public Health Assoc., Washington, D.C.

Minor, T. E., and Marth, E. H., eds. (1976). "Staphylococci and Their Significance in Foods." Elsevier, New York.

CHAPTER 6

BOTULISM

Hiroshi Sugiyama

I.   Introduction

Botulism is the syndrome of flaccid paralysis caused by a protein produced by *Clostridium botulinum*. The term *botulism* comes from *botulus,* the Latin for *sausage,* the food responsible for the first scientifically identified cases. Since a wide variety of foods is now known to cause the illness, botulism is a misleading name that continues to be used.

Botulism is divided into categories that differ in the way the toxin is acquired. The one of greatest interest has been the food poisoning, in which toxin is ingested with the food in which it is formed. The second category is the rare wound botulism, in which toxin is formed by *C. botulinum* infecting a tissue. The third category is infant botulism, in which toxin is also formed *in vivo* but by *C. botulinum* colonizing the lumen of the intestinal tract. The food poisoning is, therefore, a strict toxemia, while wound and infant botulism are toxemias from infections (toxicoinfections).

II.   Clinical

Since the toxin is responsible for all botulism signs, the three illnesses are clinically very similar. They result from progressive paralysis of the musculature innervated by cranial nerves.

Food poisoning botulism has an incubation period of 12–36 hours that tends to be shorter when more toxin is consumed. The illness may start with gastrointestinal problems such as nausea, vomiting, and diarrhea, but these effects may not be caused by toxin since they are not seen in infant and wound botulism. Constipation is a common symptom when typical botulism signs develop.

Fatigue and muscular weakness are the first indications of botulism. They are soon followed by ocular effects, such as droopy eyelids, sluggish response of pupils to light, and blurred and double vision. Effects in the mouth include dryness with difficulty in speech and swallowing. The musculatures controlling the limbs and respiration become progressively paralyzed, with death within 3–5 days from respiratory failure. The paralysis is bilateral but there is no fever unless a secondary infection occurs. Complete recovery from severe botulism may require many months.

Wound botulism is the counterpart of tetanus and usually involves an infection at a superficially located site. However, recent reports indicate that the intestinal wall itself can be infected by *C. botulinum*, particularly where surgery has been performed.

Infant botulism is characterized by an age dependence—it occurs only in babies 1 year or younger; victims in most cases are less than 6 months of age. This botulism also differs from the food poisoning in typically starting with a severe constipation that precedes the more obvious paralytic responses by one or more days. The two illnesses are otherwise basically similar, although infant botulism is more difficult to diagnose because of the inability of patients to communicate their symptoms. Breathing difficulty usually develops gradually over several days but has occurred within 5 hours or so after illness is first noted. When this is not seen, the unexpected death of such a rapidly developing case could be classified as a sudden infant death syndrome case since the toxin acts without leaving any telltale histological effects. Death from the gradually progressing infant botulism is rare. The low case-fatality rate arises because patients who reach the stage of requiring mechanical ventilation are already hospitalized so that this life-saving treatment is immediately available.

III. Organism

Members of the genus *Clostridium* are obligately anaerobic, gram-positive, rod-shaped, sporulating bacteria. Those that produce a neurotoxic protein, which elicits botulism, are all placed in the one species, *Clostridium botulinum*. The resulting species is composed of strains of diverse cultural properties. The toxin itself can be serologically different in that the toxicity of one toxin is neutralized only by the antitoxin for that particular antigenic type. Since the previously included C_2 toxin differs by being cytotoxic and should be placed in a different toxin category, there are at present seven neurotoxic types (A, B, C_1, D, E, F, and G).

Since a *C. botulinum* culture usually produces only one toxin type, it has been convenient to designate the strains as types that correspond to their toxin type. However, there are exceptions to the one culture–one toxin-type relationship. Many strains producing type C and D toxins produce these in mixtures; such strains are typed according to the toxin present in greatest (dominant) amount. Strains producing other pairs of toxin types are now being reported. The first of these was a soil isolate that produced a mixture of A and F toxins; it is called subtype Af since at least 90% of the total toxicity is type A toxin and the remainder is type F toxin. A subtype Ab or Ba has caused a food poisoning botulism outbreak; subtype Ba has caused one and subtype Bf, two infant botulism cases.

Another facet of botulinum toxigenesis is illustrated by the isolates from three illnesses which were clinically diagnosed as infant botulism. Two of the strains have the cultural properties of *Clostridium butyricum* except that they produce a toxin that is neutralized by type E botulinum antitoxin. This toxin has molecular properties identical or very similar to those of type E botulinum toxin. The other isolate is phenotypically *Clostridium barati,* but it produces a toxin that is neutralized by antitoxin raised against type F botulinum toxin. These unusual toxigenic strains probably arose when a normally nontoxigenic *C. butyricum* or *C. barati* acquired, respectively, the toxin gene of *C. botulinum* type E or F.

Clostridium botulinum strains differ in important phenotypic properties and could be separated into four species if production of a toxic protein were not used as the identifying property of the species. The difficulty of classification is avoided if the strains are first subdivided into groups whose index property is proteolysis—the digestion of meat particles or coagulated egg white irrespective of action on gelatin. The groups and their toxin types are as follows.

I. proteolytic; A, B, or F toxin, sometimes in pairs
II. nonproteolytic; B, E, or F toxin
III. nonproteolytic; C and/or D toxin
IV. weak or nonproteolytic and nonsaccharolytic; G toxin.

The groups bring out phylogenetic relationships. Cultures of the same group have common cultural properties even though their toxin types are different, and cultures of different groups are phenotypically different even when they produce the same toxin type. Thus a type B of Group I is similar to a type A culture but is quite distinct from a type B of Group II.

Their cultural properties, some of which are considered later, make Group I and II strains the important causes of human botulism. Group III strains are responsible for most botulism of birds and animals; the rare reports that they caused human botulism are not universally accepted. Type G has been indicated to be the pathogen responsible for several sudden and unexpected deaths in Switzerland, particularly of infants, but it has not been reported to have caused food poisoning botulism or the typical kind of infant botulism.

IV. Epidemiology of Food Poisoning

Although considerable publicity is generated when a commercially distributed food is involved, food poisoning botulism is a relatively rare illness in the United States (Table I). In the 1960 to 1977 period, an average of 10 outbreaks were reported per year and each outbreak averaged less than three cases. The 15–16 annual outbreaks for the 1978 to 1983 period represent a slightly higher average but the cases per outbreak have not changed significantly.

The outbreaks usually involve only a few cases since most are due to home-prepared products served only to family groups. In a summary covering the 1960 to 1977 period in the United States, home-prepared foods caused 119 outbreaks and commercially prepared foods caused 16. These numbers also indicate the successful preparation of safe products by commercial processors.

Commercially canned foods might be expected to cause large outbreaks since a large amount of food is prepared in one batch. They are, however, processed in

Table I
Food-Poisoning Botulism in the United States[a]

Period	Outbreaks	Cases	Deaths
1899–1977	766	1966	999
1960–1977	186	448	82
1978–1983	91	201	26

[a]From reports of the Centers for Disease Control, Atlanta, Georgia.

Table II
Recent Large Botulism Outbreaks
in the United States by Restaurant-Served Foods

Year	Cases	Type	Food
1977	59	A	Home-prepared peppers
1978	34	A	Potato salad[a]
1984	38	A	Sauteed onions[b]
1985	36	B	Garlic in oil[c]

[a]Most likely of two possible vehicles; made with
foil-wrapped baked potatoes held for several days
at room temperature.
[b]Prepared in a restaurant and served with meat-
patty sandwiches.
[c]Not refrigerated, although refrigeration specified
on label; Vancouver, Canada.

many small units and toxin is produced in only one or a few units. Also, early
publicity given to botulism caused by a commercially distributed food results in the
recall of unsold units and those already in homes not being used. Recent large
outbreaks in the United States and Canada have been caused by foods served at
restaurants (Table II).

The toxin types and food vehicles of botulism outbreaks in the United States are
given in Table III. Most outbreaks have been caused by type A toxin; fewer are
caused by B and E toxins. The type B is that of Group I strains. Of the food
vehicles, vegetables and fruits have been the most important, while meat products
have been responsible for relatively fewer outbreaks. Fish products have caused
most type E botulism outbreaks.

In contrast to the United States where vegetable and fruit products are most
important, meats in the form of ham are the most frequent cause of botulism in

Table III
Food Products Causing Botulism Outbreaks in the United States, 1899–1977[a]

Toxin type	Vegetables and fruits	Fish and fish products	Condiments[b]	Beef[c] and pork	Milk and milk products	Poultry	Other	Unknown	Total
A	137	11	17	8	3	2	8	9	195
B	38	4	5	2	2	2	3	3	59
E	1	25					3	1	30
F	—			1					1
A and B	2								2
Unknown[c]	2	1	1					6	10
Total	180	41	23	11	5	4	14	19	297

[a]Data from the Centers for Disease Control, Atlanta, Georgia.
[b]Includes tomato relish, chili peppers, chili sauce, and salad dressing.
[c]Includes type F from venison and type A from mutton; rabbit stew caused one type F outbreak after 1977.

several European countries. The difference has been attributed to the frequencies with which the two kinds of foods are preserved in homes. Home canning of the vegetable/fruit class is common in the United States, but home preparation of ham is infrequent. The reverse is the case in Europe. The toxin in European hams is usually type B toxin of Group II strains.

Botulism is being reported from countries where its occurrence was once unknown. Many cases have been reported in Iran; they are almost all type E illnesses caused by fish products. Botulism was thought to be rare in the Southern Hemisphere but canned foods have caused a number of outbreaks in Argentina. Botulism is an important problem in the People's Republic of China.

V. Infant Botulism

Group I strains have caused almost all cases of this illness. They are usually type A or B but subtype Bf has been responsible for two cases and subtype Ba for one case. Two cases were due to *C. butyricum* producing a toxin with molecular properties very similar but not identical to type E botulinum toxin, and one case was caused by *C. barati* producing what appeared to be type F botulinum toxin. There are more infant than food-poisoning botulism cases in the United States; during the 1977 to 1983 period, there were 403 infant botulism cases as compared with 311 food-poisoning botulism cases. The illness in other countries has been primarily in Argentina and Australia, but the incidence in these countries has been much lower than in the United States; lesser numbers have occurred in Canada, China, Czechoslovakia, Japan, and the United Kingdom.

Infant botulism occurs as individual cases. One possible exception is the illness of an infant whose crib had been previously used in a different house by an earlier case. The illness is more common where relatively high Group I *C. botulinum* levels are present in the environment. Type A cases predominate in areas such as California where type A strains are frequently present in soils. Type B cases predominate where type B organisms are expected to be common, such as in a belt area around Philadelphia, Pennsylvania.

Clinical diagnosis is confirmed by demonstrating *C. botulinum* and its toxin in the patient's feces. The high levels of toxin and cells in specimens from severe cases would not be possible unless the pathogen multiplied in the gut. There is no evidence that the intestinal wall itself is infected; growth occurs in the lumen, especially at the level of the large bowel.

Mice are susceptible to intestinal colonization by *C. botulinum* in an age-related fashion comparable to that in humans. Adult mice are naturally highly resistant but infants are susceptible during the 7- to 13-days-old age period. However, chronological age itself does not determine susceptibility or resistance since germ-free adult mice are even more susceptible than 9-day-old mice. The germ-free adults become resistant when they are exposed to normal mice so that they develop a complex gut flora.

These observations indicate that susceptibility or resistance to *C. botulinum* of the mouse gut is primarily determined by the nature of the intestinal microflora.

Additionally, conventional adult mice become susceptible when they are fed an antibiotic mixture that alters their gut flora. Since a similar effect is produced by metronidazole, obligate anaerobes are likely important to the natural resistance of adult mice. Infant mice change from the susceptible to the resistant state at the age when obligate anaerobes start to become part of the indigenous gut flora. Infant botulism can be considered an opportunistic event in which *C. botulinum* enters a large bowel lacking competitors of the pathogen. Since the competitors are normally absent during early infancy, this form of botulism would be most common in young babies.

If the large bowel is the principal multiplication site, the illness can be expected to be started by ingested spores; the infective dose, estimated to be as few as 100 spores, could be acquired with foods. However, honey produced in the United States is the only infant food in which *C. botulinum* spores have been consistently demonstrated. The organism appears to be quite rare in honey produced in other countries. Since infant botulism in this country is statistically related with feeding of honey, it is generally accepted that this food should not be given to infants less than 1 year old. *Clostridium botulinum* has been demonstrated in some corn syrup samples, but the importance of this food in causing infant botulism has not been firmly established.

Foods are undoubtedly important vehicles for transmitting the pathogen to infants, but there must be other means since as many as 50% of infant botulism cases occur among strictly breastfed infants. Epidemiologic evidence suggests that pathogens in soil habitats probably reach infants by the airborne route or by being carried on clothes. Spores could be swallowed when an infant licks the surface on which spores have settled. Spores, airborne in particles larger than aerosols, can be inhaled and thereby reach and colonize the large bowel of experimental mice.

If older individuals are normally resistant because their gut flora contains competitors of *C. botulinum,* a condition suppressing the competitors should result in a susceptible state. Several adult botulism cases described in the literature appear, upon review, to be the counterpart of infant botulism. One was a fatal case that developed several days after an adult consumed coconut milk which was later shown to contain *C. botulinum* type A but no toxin, The patient excreted pathogen and toxin over many days and the gut wall was not found to be infected at autopsy.

There have also been adult wound botulism cases in which the infection site is the gastrointestinal wall. These cases have generally followed abdominal surgery. Whether the toxin is formed in the lumen or wall of the gut, it is reasonable to assume that the infecting organism of the adult cases was acquired in a food.

VI.   Toxin Structure

A.   Structure–Toxicity

All toxin types except G have been purified. The primary molecular structures of the purified toxins are basically the same (Table IV). Recent findings indicate that C_2 toxin should be considered a different kind of toxin because of its cytotoxic activity.

Table IV
Molecular Properties of Botulinum Neurotoxins

Property	Specifics
Molecular weights	About 150,000
Intracellular	Intact protein chain
Extracellular	H and L subunits of about $2:1$ relative size, joined by disulfide linkage[a]; M_r same as intracellular
Toxicity	Originally low; toxins of proteolytics activated by endogenous protease; those of nonproteolytics activated experimentally with trypsin. 1×10^7–1×10^8 mouse LD_{50} per milligram of protein.
Complexes	Naturally as bimolecular complex (M_r about 300,000) with a nontoxic protein; some as trimolecular complex (M_r about 450,000) in which bimolecular complex associates with a second, different nontoxic protein (hemagglutinin).

[a]Either naturally or after trypsinization.

C_2 toxin also differs from the botulinum neurotoxins by being naturally composed of two separated molecules whose sizes are comparable to the covalently linked H and L subunits of the neurotoxins. This toxin is, therefore, a binary toxin.

Botulinum toxins purified from cell extracts are intact proteins with M_r of 150,000 and have low toxicities. When the culture is proteolytic, the toxin that becomes extracellular is exposed to endogenous proteases, among which is one that cleaves a peptide bond so that the intact protein is divided into two parts. One of these parts is the amino-terminal third of the original molecule and the other is the remaining two-thirds. The resulting molecule is, therefore, a two-subunit protein whose smaller (light or L subunit; M_r about 50,000) and larger (heavy or H subunit; M_r about 100,000) parts are about 1:2 in relative size. The subunits are held together covalently by an intersubunit disulfide bridge, which was originally intramolecular in the intact molecule, and by noncovalent forces. The M_r of the two-subunit molecule is indistinguishable from that of the intact protein. Although the molecular change by which the subunits are produced may not be responsible, the conversion into the two-subunit molecule is accompanied by activation of toxicity to the high level for which botulinum toxin is well known. The specific toxicities of the fully activated form of the several botulinum toxin types range from 10^7–10^8 mouse LD_{50} per milligram of protein.

Since type E strains are nonproteolytic, their intracellular or extracellular toxin is purified as an intact M_r 150,000 molecule comparable to the intracellular toxin of Group I strains. When the intracellular or extracellular toxin of type E is treated with trypsin to activate toxicity, it is converted into the two-subunit molecular form similar to that of toxins of Group I strains and the toxicity increase as much as several hundredfold. The trypsinization does not detectably change the size of the molecule. Recent findings indicate that toxicity activation results from cleavage of a lysyl peptide bond.

The subunits can be separated when the covalent connection is broken with a disulfide reducing agent (L subunit—S—S—H subunit into L subunit—SH + SH—H subunit) while the interchain, noncovalent attractions are minimized with a protein denaturant. The separated subunits are probably not toxic individually.

When an equimolar mixture of the subunits is held in certain condition, the subunits reconstitute into the two-subunit molecular form and toxicity reappears.

Toxic units in culture fluids act as molecules with an M_r of at least twice the 150,000 of pure toxin. The larger size is the result of the toxic molecule associating with a nontoxic protein of the culture about the size of the toxin molecule. These natural toxic entities are bimolecular association complexes since noncovalent attractive forces bring the component molecules together. Bimolecular complexes of Group I types A and B toxin can associate with a second, different nontoxic protein and become trimolecular complexes of M_r about 450,000. The bi- and trimolecular complexes are respectively called M (for medium) and L (for large) progenitor toxin since the isolated complexes can be used as the progenitor from which to obtain pure (derivative) toxin. Type A toxic crystals (M_r 900,000) are dimers of trimolecular complexes.

Specific toxicities determined by intraperitoneal (ip) injections into mice are inversely related to the degree of complexing. Since only one of the molecules of a complex is toxic, specific toxicity of pure (noncomplexed, M_r 150,000) toxin is about twice that of its bimolecular complex and, where applicable, three times greater than that of its trimolecular complex.

Intraperitoneally administered toxin rapidly enters the bloodstream so that most, if not all, of the dose contributes to the lethal effect. The situation is different for toxin given by mouth; only a small part of a dose is toxic since most is inactivated by conditions in the digestive tract or is not absorbed. Toxicity by this latter, peroral route is affected by the complexing of toxin. Toxin molecule in complexes is less easily inactivated; since the nontoxic molecule(s) helps protect the toxin molecule, more of the dose is absorbed from the gastrointestinal tract in a biologically active state. When the numbers of ip LD_{50} needed to give an LD_{50} effect by the peroral route are determined for the several complexed forms of toxin of the same culture, toxin in bimolecular complex is usually about 10 times more toxic than the corresponding pure toxin, and that in trimolecular complex is up to 10 times more toxic than the bimolecular complex. There are exceptions to these relative toxicities. In the case of toxin of one Group I type B strain, the trimolecular complex is 700 times more toxic than the bimolecular complex.

The composition of the food in which toxigenesis occurs affects the amount of toxin that can be produced as well as how the toxin is distributed between bi- and trimolecular complexes. The toxic dose for a human is not known for certain, but it has been estimated from the results of a study done on an adult who died of type B botulism. The toxin concentration in the food and the amount of food consumed indicated that 3500 mouse, ip minimal lethal doses (MLD) caused death. If an MLD equals two LD_{50}, the lethal dose was 7000 mouse LD_{50}. Since this toxicity is determined by ip injections while the human illness is due to toxin taken by the much less efficient peroral route, the observations indicate that humans are highly susceptible to botulinum toxin.

B. Pharmacology

Toxicity depends on the cooperative actions of the subunits. The H subunit has a property by which it binds to the receptors, which may be gangliosides, at endings of nerves which transmit messages from the central nervous system to muscles by releasing acetylcholine (ACh). This binding does not elicit a toxic effect, but the L subunit is now positioned so that it can exert its pharmacologic action. The binding of toxin to plasma membranes of these nerve endings has been visualized by autoradiographic methods.

The poisoning effect comes about because the stimulus reaching nerve endings does not release a normal quanta of ACh; it does not come from toxin acting on the muscle itself. Since smaller ACh quanta are released, muscles receive weaker stimuli so that their responses diminish. The poisoning seems to be the result of toxin interfering with the role played by intracellular Ca^{2+} in the ACh release process. The result is the flaccid paralysis that characterizes botulism.

VII. Microbiology in Foods

A. Prerequisites

Two prerequisite events for botulinum toxin to be formed in a food are *C. botulinum* getting into the product and the multiplication of the contaminant, during which toxigenesis occurs. The spore form is the important contaminant; it tolerates many conditions that kill vegetative cells and can remain dormant for long periods before germinating into vegetative cells and producing toxin when conditions become favorable.

Contamination may occur during the preparation of a food or during subsequent holding, but it is most likely to occur during the growth and harvesting of a product. It is, therefore, not surprising that botulism food poisoning vehicles often come from environments where *C. botulinum* is common. Their soil habitats give types A and B of Group I opportunities to contaminate vegetables and fruits so that these products are common causes of food poisoning. Type A is dominant in soils of the western United States and has been responsible for most botulism cases caused by foods grown in this geographic area. Type E strains are more likely to be present in freshwater and marine environments so that botulism from foods made of fish and aquatic mammals is predominantly type E.

Clostridium botulinum in a food is not dangerous unless it can develop into a toxin-producing vegetative culture. The growth depends on the food satisfying the nutritional requirements of the organism. The foods implicated as botulism vehicles, a few of which are listed in Table III, indicate that a wide range of food products is at least minimally adequate in this respect.

Growth of *C. botulinum* also depends on other factors. Since the organism is an obligate anaerobe, oxidation reduction (redox) potential is important. Oxygen inhibits *C. botulinum* by raising redox potential and by forming toxic radicals. *Clostridium botulinum* would not grow on the surface of a product exposed to air but could do so below the surface if there is a sufficient concentration of redox-reducing constituents such as thiol compounds. Meats and fish are examples.

The low redox potentials of canned foods favor toxigenesis. When a vegetable causes botulism, it is usually a canned preparation. The necessary anaerobic state can also develop in other situations. When a living tissue such as fresh mushrooms is packaged inside a plastic film limiting exchange of gases, respiration by the tissue uses up O_2 and redox potential falls to a level permitting growth of anaerobes. Toxin is formed when potatoes, surface-inoculated with *C. botulinum* spores, are wrapped in aluminum foil, baked, and held at room temperature for several days while still covered with the foil. The anaerobic conditions of sauteed onions causing a large type A outbreak probably developed because melted margarine formed a covering layer that prevented atmospheric O_2 from entering.

B.   Destruction of Spores

A food would not cause a botulism problem if all *C. botulinum* spores were destroyed before they could germinate into a vegetative culture. Since the most practical way of achieving this destruction is heating the food product sealed in a container, that is, canning, heat resistances of *C. botulinum* spores have been intensively studied.

The heat killing of bacteria occurs at a logarithmic rate that is expressed as a D value, the minutes of heating at a specified temperature (°F unless specified) that reduces the viable population by 90% or one logarithm. D is a measure of heat resistance; when heating temperature is the same, a lower D means less resistance than a higher D. Spores of *C. botulinum* Group I strains are among the more heat tolerant of bacterial spores. Their D_{212} is about 30 minutes; that is, 30 minutes at 212°F (100°C) inactivates 90% of the viable spores that are present. At 250°F (121°C), the reference temperature of the food industry, D is 0.21. Spores of Group II strains are less heat tolerant. Their D_{180} (180°F or 82°C) values are usually less than 2–3 minutes, although spores of some nonproteolytic type B strains have higher resistance.

Lethality increases with temperature so that D values are smaller at higher temperatures. This relationship is expressed as a Z value, the temperature difference that changes D by 10-fold. The Z of spores of Group I strains is 18 (10°C); that of spores of Group II strains is about 10–12 (6–7°C). Since it is the change of D with temperature, Z can be used to convert the D obtained at one temperature to the value at a different temperature. F_o is the total lethality at a temperature of 250°F (121°C) for spores whose Z is 18. Since the "botulinum cook" prescribed for low-acid foods (see Section VIII, C) is the reduction of viable Group I spores by a factor of 10^{12}, it is a treatment of F_o 2.5 (D_{250} of 0.21 multiplied by 12, the number of $\log_{10}$ of spores to be inactivated).

The intrinsic stability of spores is the most important factor, but heat resistance is also influenced by the medium in which spores are heated and by the culture medium used to demonstrate survivors. As an example, heated type E spores, apparently nonviable when cultured in a basal medium, germinate when the medium is supplemented with lysozyme. Reference heat resistance values are, therefore, obtained with known conditions such as heating spores in phosphate buffer (e.g., M/15, pH 7.0) and using a good culture medium to demonstrate heat-injured spores. The situation is different when a food is both the spore-heating medium as well as the recovery medium. The resistances determined in these cases would be lower than the reference value if the food is not an optimum recovery medium and/or increases the susceptibility of spores to heat inactivation.

Spores of Group I *C. botulinum* in a food could be destroyed by irradiation but this is not practical for most foods. They are among the most radiation resistant of bacterial spores, so that the necessary dosages result in organoleptically unacceptable products unless the irradiation uses a temperature far below freezing and O_2 is excluded. Present research focuses on using relatively low irradiation doses to obtain the economic benefits of extending the shelf life of perishable foods such as fresh fish. Since not all *C. botulinum* spores would be destroyed by these irradiation levels, some could remain viable in a food whose natural microflora has been greatly reduced by the irradiation. In this situation, *C. botulinum* faces less competition and the appearance of the usual spoilage signs that warn consumers is delayed. The practical usefulness of this process depends on the food undergoing an easily detected organoleptic change before botulinum toxin is formed.

C. Preventing Toxigenesis

Botulism-safe foods can be prepared without excessive heating by preventing multiplication of *C. botulinum*. This inhibition is primarily directed against spores, the important initial contaminants, whose transition from dormancy to a vegetative culture involves three successive stages called activation, germination, and outgrowth. Outgrowth (the emergence of a cell from a spore and its first division) seems most susceptible to inhibition, but toxigenesis can be prevented by interfering with any one of the three stages. The term *germination* is also used in a broad sense that includes breaking of dormancy through outgrowth. Germination is used in a broad sense in the following discussion.

Acidic pH is often used to prevent toxigenesis in foods. Germination of Group II spores is inhibited at pH 5.0, but the critical pH is 4.6, since this or lower pH is needed to inhibit germination of spores of Group I strains. Some products have enough organic acids that they have a natural pH of ≤4.6. When desirable, products of higher pH can be reduced to this level by acidification. Acidulants are usually short-chain organic acids whose pKa is in the pH 3.0 to 5.0 range since the undissociated acid is more inhibitory than the dissociated. The commonly used acids differ to some degree in their effectiveness; in a protein medium, the most to least inhibitory sequence of acids is acetic, lactic, citric, and hydrochloric.

Products of pH ≤4.6 are called high-acid foods to distinguish them from low-acid foods, which have higher pH. In canning, low-acid foods require a botulinum cook, while milder heating suffices for high-acid foods. The requirements differ because a viable spore in a low-acid food can germinate, multiply, and produce a food-poisoning amount of toxin, while the pH prevents toxigenesis in a high-acid food.

The experience of many years justifies separating foods into high- and low-acid categories. However, during the 1899 to 1975 period in the United States, 35 botulism outbreaks were attributed to high-acid foods, of which 34 were home-prepared products and 17 were some kind of tomato preparation. The toxin responsible for illness need not have been produced at the pH of high-acid foods. When a product with sizable pieces is acidulated, the target pH may not be reached inside the pieces for several days and toxin can be formed there before pH equilibration is complete, provided other conditions such as temperature are suitable. Secondly, toxigenesis could have occurred in the exceptions among what is accepted as a naturally high-acid food. Tomatoes are examples; fruits of some cultivars, especially when grown in particular locations, have a pH above 4.6.

The third and most important reason for toxigenesis in high-acid food is metabiosis, in which growth of a second organism creates conditions permitting toxigenesis. Yeasts, molds, or bacteria can have the metabiotic effect. For example, molds produce metabolites that can raise the pH of tomato juice. When the contaminating mold forms a mycelial mat, the pH of the juice immediately adjacent to the mat can be high enough for *C. botulinum* to produce toxin. If the toxic juice is mixed before taking a sample for pH determination, the average pH is measured and it appears as if toxin was produced at pH below 4.6.

The fourth possibility is toxin production by a pure *C. botulinum* culture at pH ≤4.6. This toxigenesis has been recently observed, but so far only in laboratory media whose high protein concentrations result in abundant precipitate and when strict anaerobic conditions are maintained. It may be that precipitates are microenvironments where the pH is higher than the average pH of the medium. If pure culture toxigenesis occurs in high-acid foods, a reassessment of the botulinum safety of high-acid foods may be needed.

All organisms require water for growth. Since water adsorbed to surfaces or bound to solutes cannot be used, available water is not moisture but equilibrium relative humidity/100, or water activity (a_w). The food preservative effect of brining comes primarily from the a_w-reducing action. If brining alone is used, ≥10% salt ($a_w \leq 0.95$) is needed to inhibit Group I strains while ≥5% ($a_w \leq 0.97$) suffices for Group II strains. High sugar concentrations also preserve food by their a_w effect; 30% sucrose is needed to inhibit Group I strains while about 15% sucrose is needed for Group II strains.

Clostridium botulinum grows reasonably well in the temperature range from 20°C to slightly above 45°C, but the low temperatures needed to inhibit Group I and II strains are different. Group I cultures do not grow at 10°C or lower, but Group II strains are psychrotrophic and can multiply and produce toxin at temperatures as low as 3.3°C. The different inhibitory temperatures mean that Group I strains will not be toxigenic in a refrigerated (4–6°C) food but Group II strains could form toxin in the same food.

Nevertheless, refrigeration importantly influences toxigenesis by Group II strains; it delays toxin production and raises the contamination level of the pathogen that can initiate toxigenesis.

Temperature abuse is frequently involved in toxin production. Outbreaks caused by commercial pot pies are examples, Botulinum toxigenesis is not possible while the pies are frozen, but at least two familial outbreaks have been caused when a pie was cooked and left at room temperature for about 24 hours before being consumed.

When one inhibitor is used to control toxigenesis, it must often be used at a level that reduces the acceptability of the product as a food. Such undesired organoleptic changes are less likely when toxin production can be prevented by a combination of several factors. The several inhibitions used together have their own anti-*C. botulinum* effect. These individual actions are cumulative so that the total antagonism of moderate levels of several inhibitors can prevent toxigenesis. These combinations can be made so that they have less unfavorable effect on the food than the extreme level of a single inhibitor. The total antibotulinum effect of a combination of factors is not changed if the effect of one factor is reduced and that of a different factor is proportionately increased. The inhibitions are considered hurdles or barriers that are placed in foods to make it difficult for *C. botulinum* to develop into a toxigenic culture.

Cured meats are a food category whose antibotulinum property derives from multiple inhibitions. They have an excellent safety record with respect to botulism, although they are low-acid foods which receive only a fraction of a botulinum cook. An important antibotulinum action comes from nitrite, which also imparts the cured flavor and keeps the color pink. Nitrite prevents growth of *C. botulinum* surviving the mild heat treatment by its iron chelating property, probably by inactivating some essential iron-containing enzyme of the organism. The antibotulinum effect of nitrite is supplemented by the inhibitory effects of moderate NaCl concentration, mild acidic conditions, other additives such as phosphates, and the mild heat treatment. The acidic pH also makes nitrite more effective by keeping it in the active nitrous acid form.

Carcinogenic nitrosamines may be formed when cured meats, especially bacon, are cooked. This finding has led to efforts to ban nitrite, use a substitute, or at least reduce the permissible nitrite level. A substitute having all the attributes of nitrite has not been found. However, bacon produced with 40–80 ppm of sodium nitrite is as organoleptically acceptable as that cured with the more normal 120 ppm of sodium nitrite. Fewer nitrosamines are produced in this bacon made with lower nitrite. The bacon is made botulism safe by having sucrose and *Pediococcus acidilactici* in the curing solution. When the bacon is temperature abused, the *P. acidilactici* grows and ferments sucrose so that the pH of the bacon rapidly falls to levels inhibiting *C. botulinum*.

Pasteurized cheese spread sealed in jars is a food that theoretically requires a botulinum cook that would ruin it as food. However, practical experience has shown that this product is safe with respect to botulism with only a pasteurization treatment. Its safety comes from the mild heating and a combination of several inhibitory effects, of which a pH of about 6.0, a_w of about 0.95, and phosphate are important.

The chance of *C. botulinum* breaking through an inhibitory system increases when the organism is present in higher numbers. Inoculated pack studies usually use spore concentrations that greatly exceed the maximum that might occur in practical situations. Toxigenesis is, therefore, more likely in experiments than in practice; the naturally low contamination levels of food is one reason for the low incidence of botulism. The heating of many foods before being served also contributes since toxin that may be present is likely to be inactivated.

VIII.   Laboratory Procedures

A.   Toxin

Toxin detection is the test most usually required of a laboratory dealing with a botulism outbreak. The one accepted procedure for this purpose is the biotest consisting of two steps: (1) a presumptive test which determines if a mouse lethal agent is present, and (2) confirming the lethal agent as botulinum toxin by neutralizing it with botulinum antitoxin.

Samples are usually foods, but feces and blood serum of patients would be tested in a clinical laboratory. If there is not enough liquid, the sample is homogenized in buffer–gelatin (e.g., 0.1 M phosphate–0.2% gelatin, pH 6.2) in which botulinum toxin is likely to maintain biological activity. The supernatant fluid obtained by centrifugation is used as the test extract. As small a volume of buffer as is practical is used so that a concentrated extract is available in case the sample has low toxicity. Samples should be kept cool during handling.

When toxin of a Group II strain is a possibility, the test extract is trypsinized so that the toxin to be tested will be near maximal toxicity. Trypsinization sometimes helps in looking for toxin of Group I strains, particularly if the sample is a poor medium for toxin production. On the other hand, the toxin-activation treatment cannot be used indiscriminately since it may give rise to nonbotulinum mouse lethal factors which interfere in the toxin test.

Routine toxin activation is done with a crude trypsin preparation such as the Difco 1:250 preparation. The enzyme solution is prepared by suspending 1.0 g in 10 ml of water at room temperature and later clarifying by centrifugation. For use, a mixture such as 1 volume enzyme:9 volumes extract is incubated at 37°C for up to 1.0 hour. Liquid obtained directly from sample can be similarly trypsinized, provided its neutral or adjusted pH is in the range of 6.0–6.6.

In its simplest form, the presumptive toxin test can be done with the undiluted extract. The sample is injected intraperitoneally, usually in a 0.5-ml volume, into white mice weighing 20–25 g. One mouse per sample may be used, but two animals are recommended. If trypsinization is done, a freshly trypsinized extract is tested undiluted in other mice. The injected mice are periodically observed during the next 3 days. Survival of all challenged mice indicates that the original sample does not contain botulinum toxin; death of any mouse indicates the presence of a toxic agent whose nature remains to be determined. Botulinum toxin would be suspected if death is preceded by signs such as wobbly gait, indrawn flanks, and labored breathing.

The lethal agent is shown to be botulinum toxin when it is made nontoxic by one or more of the typing botulinum antitoxins which react specifically with a particular toxin type. Since toxin types A, B, and E are responsible for almost all human botulism, the toxin test can be done with only antitoxins for these toxin types, although others such as type F and/or a mixture of all antitoxin types might be included in some circumstances.

The confirmation part of the toxin test determines the separate effect of the several antitoxin types or the pool of the antitoxin types on the lethal agent; extract treated with buffer instead of antitoxin is used as control. In the *in vitro* neutralization method, these mixtures of extract and individual antitoxin types are held up to 30 minutes at room temperature or 37°C and then injected intraperitoneally in 0.5-ml volumes into different pairs of mice. The mixtures can be equal volumes of extract and antitoxin and usually contain 1.0 international unit (IU) of antitoxin in 0.5 ml. The neutralization can also be done *in vivo*. In this method a prophylactic ip dose of 1.0 unit of one of several antitoxin types is given to separate pairs of mice; control mice are given buffer. All mice are then challenged 10–30 minutes later with a known volume (usually 0.5 ml) of test extract.

The lethal agent is shown to be botulinum toxin if it is neutralized by a particular antitoxin, used by itself or as one type in the antitoxin mixture. The antitoxin with the neutralization action indicates the botulinum toxin type. Two botulinum types are suggested when toxicity is neutralized only by the antitoxin mixture. The toxin types can be identified by using the possible pairs that can be made with the antitoxin types in the mixture.

Although satisfactory with many samples, the toxin test procedure using only undiluted extract is not suitable with other samples. The most frequently encountered difficulty is the death of all mice in the confirmation step. This kind of uninterpretable mouse death pattern is even possible when a botulinum toxin is the only toxic material in the extract and the corresponding antitoxin type is included in the test. The 1.0 IU of antitoxins routinely used in the test is such that 1 unit of A or B antitoxin neutralizes about 10,000 mouse LD_{50} of type-homologous toxin and 1 unit of E antitoxin about 1000 LD_{50}. More than these toxin amounts may be in the volume of a highly potent extract used in the test. In these situations 1 unit of antitoxin cannot neutralize all botulinum toxicity, so mice which must survive if the test is to be meaningful also succumb.

Similar uninterpretable toxin test results are given by nonbotulinum mouse lethal agents. When present with botulinum toxin, these "nonspecific" lethal agents interfere by killing mice which are protected from the effect of botulinum toxin by antitoxin. When present by itself, the nonbotulinum factor causes false-positive presumptive tests so that an unnecessary confirmatory test may be performed. These nonspecific lethal agents may be a food constitutent, such as NaCl of high concentration, but they are more usually products of food spoilage. Some nonspecific agents are heat stable so that their presence is demonstrated when a heated (100°C, 10 minutes) sample kills mice. The observation does not, however, prove that botulinum toxin is absent.

A simple and obvious way to avoid the problem of too much botulinum toxin is to dilute the extract so that the toxin is reduced to a level that one antitoxin unit can completely neutralize. Use of dilutions also avoids some of the interference caused by the presence of a nonspecific lethal agent. When botulinum toxin and a nonspecific agent are both present, the lethal levels of the two often differ. If botulinum toxicity is higher, it may be possible to dilute the nonbotulinum factor to below toxic level without similarly affecting botulinum toxin.

The toxin test is frequently done in situations in which the result is needed as soon as possible. When such urgency exists, time may be saved by use of dilutions early in the test sequence. Untrypsinized and trypsinized extracts are used in the presumptive test without dilution and also as $\frac{1}{2}$, $\frac{1}{10}$, and $\frac{1}{100}$ dilutions in phosphate buffer. These samples are all tested in different mouse pairs and those which are lethal are used in the confirmation step. The sample can be taken as being positive for botulinum toxin if one or more of the dilutions gives the proper mouse death pattern.

The toxin test can be modified according to the particular circumstance. The confirmation step might be done with only the highest dilution that is lethal in the preliminary test, provided this dilution has more than a barely lethal dose as shown by death of mice in less than 24 hours. If trypsinization does not increase toxicity, the confirmation test could be limited to the untrypsinized extract.

The nonspecific deaths that can make the biotest useless as well as the expense of maintaining mice are avoided in toxin test methods based on an *in vitro* toxin–antitoxin reaction. The toxin types causing human botulism have been assayed with enzyme-linked immunosorbent assay (ELISA) systems using antitoxins raised with immunizing agents made with purified toxins (M_r 150,000). The toxin detection limits are in the range of $50–100$ LD_{50}/ml. There is a minor cross-reaction problem in that a system intended for a given toxin type reacts to some extent with one or more of the other toxin types.

An amplified ELISA for type A toxin using a monoclonal antibody does not cross-react with other types and is positive when 10 type A LD_{50}/ml is present. Even the less sensitive ELISA using polyclonal antibodies may be useful if the sensitivity of the mouse test is not needed. However, toxicity levels reported for these *in vitro* tests can be misleading in some cases since toxin that has lost biological activity ("toxoid") still reacts in the test.

B. Organism

A food can be accepted as the vehicle of a food-poisoning botulism outbreak only when toxin is demonstrated; the presence of pathogen without toxin is not sufficient evidence by itself since the food poisoning is a toxemia. Detecting *C. botulinum* in a specimen does not require isolating a pure culture. If botulinum toxin is found in a medium that is incubated after being inoculated with the sample, the organism must have been in the inoculum.

The enrichment culturing is more likely to be successful when cultures are made with several small portions instead of one large sample. A recommended procedure uses about 2-g portions in about 15 ml of cooked-meat medium and/or trypticase–peptone–yeast extract–thioglycollate broth (TPGY). When type E is a possibility, filter-sterilized trypsin is added to some tubes of TPGY. The enzyme is used since type E may be accompanied by organisms which produce bacteriocins that are active against the pathogen. The inoculated media are incubated at 30°C; if type E is being considered as a possibility, both cooked meat and TPGY–trypsin are used; the former is incubated at about 35°C and the latter at about 27°C. After good growth occurs, which is usually about 5 days incubation, the culture fluid is tested for botulinum toxin. If growth does not occur, the enrichment cultures are incubated for at least an additional 5 days before being discarded.

Although the media are not selective for *C. botulinum*, enrichment culturing is surprisingly successful. When the pathogen cannot be demonstrated in a sample of special importance, a modification could be tried. A pair of tubes with cooked-meat medium is equilibrated at 80°C, a second pair to 60°C, and a third pair is at room temperature. After inoculating all tubes, those at 80°C are heated for 30 minutes and those at 60°C for 20–30 minutes. The heated tubes are rapidly cooled; one tube of each pair is incubated at about 35°C and the other tube at about 27°C. The preheatings select for spores of different heat resistances; those of Group I strains are likely to survive the 80°C treatment, while those of Group II survive the 60°C but not the 80°C treatment. Both preheatings destroy nonsporulating species and those organisms whose spores have low heat resistance. The two incubation temperatures are the optimum temperatures of strains of the two groups.

Clostridium botulinum cells can be microscopically demonstrated by immunofluorescent techniques using antibodies to somatic antigens. The method is not often used because many nontoxigenic organisms related to *C. botulinum* are frequent causes of false-positive reactions. The method does not determine *C. botulinum* type since the antibodies are group and not type specific.

Attempts should be made to obtain pure cultures. If pure isolates had not been studied, the toxigenic *C. butyricum* and *C. barati* as well as the *C. botulinum* subtypes producing two toxin types would not have been recognized.

Pure cultures are obtained by the usual approach of streaking a sample, usually a toxin-positive enrichment culture, on an agar medium and incubating the agar in an anaerobic environment. Agar media containing 5% egg yolk are recommended since *C. botulinum* produces a lipase which gives a surface "pearly iridescent" sheen over the colony and beyond. *Clostridium botulinum* strains are negative for lecithinase, an enzyme which forms a whitish precipitate in agar containing egg yolk. Colonies showing the lipase reaction are subcultured to see if the organism forms a botulinum toxin. If toxin is demonstrated, the isolate would be a gram-positive rod with an occasional spore. Those producing type A, B, or F toxin should be tested for proteolytic activity.

When enrichment cultures in nonselective media are streaked out on egg-yolk agar, *C. botulinum* may not develop because of the competition of other organism(s) which have reached high concentrations during enrichment and can grow well on the recovery agar. Chances for this kind of difficulty are reduced when the inoculum for the streak is a 1- or 2-ml portion of enrichment culture incubated with an equal volume of absolute ethanol for 1 hour. Chances of isolating Group I strains are increased by using an enrichment culture portion heated at 80°C for 10–15 minutes.

Egg-yolk agar containing 259 μg cycloserine, 4 μg trimethoprim, and 76 μg sulfamethazole per milliliter suppresses growth of many bacterial species in human feces without affecting growth of Group I *C. botulinum* strains. This medium has simplified the isolation of the pathogen from feces of infant botulism cases. The medium has also been useful in isolating Group I strains from some other kinds of specimens. It inhibits some Group II *C. botulinum* strains.

It is possible to identify suspect colonies as *C. botulinum* without the time-consuming subculturing to see if the organism produces botulinum toxin. If homologous type antitoxin is incorporated in an agar medium, toxin produced by cells forming a colony reacts with the antitoxin. Because of the low antitoxin concentration, the antigen–antitoxin precipitate that forms is usually not directly visible. It is made visible by a staining–destaining step. Since colonies would otherwise be washed off, the staining is done after plain agar is poured over the colonies to form a thin covering layer. This antitoxin agar medium would have greater practical use if it were possible to shorten or eliminate the staining step.

Bibliography

Hauschild, A. H. W. (1980). Microbial problems in food safety with particular reference to *Clostridium botulinum*. *In* "Safety of Foods" (H. D. Graham, ed.), 2nd Ed., pp. 68–107. AVI, Westport, Connecticut.
Kautter, D. A., and Lynt, R. K. (1984). *Clostridium botulinum*. *In* "Compendium of Methods for the

Microbiological Examination of Foods" (M. L. Speck, ed.), 2nd Ed., pp. 468–495. Am. Public Health Assoc., Washington, D.C.

Odlaug, T. E., and Pflug, I. J. (1978). *Clostridium botulinum* and acid foods. *J. Food Prot.* **41,** 566–573.

Roberts, T. A., and Ingram, M. (1973). Inhibition of growth of *C. botulinum* at different pH values by sodium chloride and sodium nitrite. *J. Food Technol.* **8,** 467–475.

Simpson, L. L. (1981). The origin, structure, and pharmacological activity of botulinum toxin. *Pharmacol. Rev.* **33,** 155–188.

Smith, L. D. S. (1977). "Botulism: The Organism; Its Toxins; the Disease." Thomas, Springfield, Illinois.

Sperber, W. H. (1982). Requirements of *Clostridium botulinum* for growth and toxin production. *Food Technol.* **36,** 89–94.

Sugiyama, H. (1986). Mouse models for infant botulism. *In* "Experimental Models in Antimicrobial Chemotherapy" (O. Zak and M. A. Sande, eds.), Vol. 2, pp. 73–91. Academic Press, New York.

CHAPTER 7

BACILLUS CEREUS FOOD POISONING

Eric A. Johnson

I. Introduction and Historical Background

The aerobic endosporeforming bacteria are classified in the genus *Bacillus*. Because of the ability of the aerobic bacilli to form resistant endospores and to synthesize a variety of extracellular enzymes and antibiotics, this group of bacteria is widespread and has successfully colonized a great variety of habitats. Of the 34 species in the genus, only 2, *B. anthracis* and *B. cereus,* are recognized as common pathogens. Some of the other *Bacillus* spp. may occasionally cause infections in humans. Although *B. cereus* was believed by certain microbiologists since early in the twentieth century to cause foodborne disease, it wasn't until 1950 that sufficient evidence was provided by Steinar Hauge in Norway to conclusively prove its pathogenesis. The recognition of this organism as an etiologic agent serves as an excellent example to demonstrate the evidence that is generally needed to recognize a bacterium as a new agent of foodborne disease.

The classic investigation of the illness was carried out by Hauge in Oslo, Norway from 1947 to 1949, and the results were published in 1955. He investigated four outbreaks of food poisoning that occurred in three hospitals and a convalescent home. Overall approximately 600 persons were affected. Interestingly, the food vehicle in all four instances appeared to be vanilla sauce. Since the four outbreaks were similar, only one of them, involving 400 people in an Oslo hospital, was investigated in detail. The Sunday dinner in the hospital consisted of a dish of meat and vegetables, and the dessert was chocolate pudding with vanilla sauce. Both items of the dessert had been prepared the previous day and stored in a large container at room temperature. The patients who were on special diets did not eat the main dish but had the same dessert as the others. Of 80 persons in a particular ward, all who ate the dessert contracted food poisoning. The disease was characterized by an incubation period of about 10 hours, and the patients suffered from diarrhea that was profuse and watery. Abdominal pain and nausea were also common, but vomiting was rare. Fever was distinctly uncommon. The symptoms subsided in 12 hours or less.

To provide evidence that *B. cereus* was responsible for the poisoning, Hauge took the following steps. Direct microscopic examination of the vanilla sauce revealed a heavy infection of a large gram-positive rod. To show that the bacillus was not an anaerobe such as *Clostridium perfringens,* Hauge prepared blood agar plates and incubated them aerobically and anaerobically, and after a suitable incubation time he exposed the anaerobic plates to air. On this medium, a nearly pure culture of a facultatively anaerobic sporeforming rod was obtained. The organism was strongly hemolytic and also tested positive for lecithinase on egg-yolk agar. According to taxonomic descriptions of *Bacillus,* which were at the time being developed by Gordon and her colleagues, the isolated sporeformer gave reactions typical of *B. cereus* (see Section III,A). Counts of 37 million organisms per milliliter of sauce were obtained. In the three other outbreaks, the dessert contained 25–110 million organisms per gram. Hauge found that the corn starch used in the preparation had approximately 10^4 spores of *B. cereus* per gram.

The findings of high numbers of *B. cereus* in the food did not convince several established bacteriologists that the aerobic sporeformer was responsible for the food poisoning. To reduce the skepticism surrounding his declaration, Hauge tried to find a test animal that was affected by feeding of the vanilla sauce. However, he was not successful in finding a susceptible laboratory model. Finally, he inoculated sterile vanilla sauce with the isolate from the food poisoning, let it grow for 24 hours at room temperature, then he consumed 200 ml of the sauce, which contained 92 million *B. cereus* per milliliter. After 13 hours the symptoms started, characterized by severe abdominal pain, diarrhea, and rectal tenesmus. Hauge stated that the symptoms lasted nearly continuously or 8 hours but subsided soon thereafter. In common with other *B. cereus* food poisonings, Hauge was unable to culture high numbers of the organism from his feces, but he noted that the numbers of enteric bacteria were quite low. With the few isolates he did obtain from his stool, he conducted similar volunteer experiments with personnel in his laboratory and found comparable results. Thus, the disease was apparently not psychosomatic in nature.

The connection of foodborne disease and a particular pathogen as shown by Hauge provides a good example of the kinds of evidence that are usually needed to recognize a "new" or "emerging" pathogen. Once a relationship between a food and a disease is established (epidemiological evidence) the investigator tries to satisfy the following criteria to prove the organism as the causal agent.

1. The organism is shown to be consistently associated with the disease. The organism is isolated from the food and the sickened host using artificial growth media.
2. The organisms isolated from the two sources are shown to be identical by phenotypic, immunological, and other tests.
3. Inoculation of the organism to an experimental animal or volunteer produces an identical or closely similar disease.
4. The organism can be recovered from the site of infection in the animal and the infectious cycle repeated.

These criteria, patterned after Henle–Koch's postulates, are useful in establishing the virulence of an emerging pathogen. The limitations of these experimental criteria are well recognized: certain organisms such as viruses cannot be cultured on artificial media, the etiologic agent does not cause sickness in experimental animals, or the illness is due to products of the organism such as toxins rather than to the organism itself. In practice, many recognized foodborne diseases are diagnosed by evaluating the symptoms and then isolating the etiologic agent or detecting the toxin from the sickened victim. Nonetheless, the elegant experiments and perseverance by Hauge exemplify the kinds of proof desired in designating a bacterium as a foodborne pathogen.

II. Nature of *Bacillus cereus* Foodborne Illness

A. Incidence

The first well-characterized outbreak of *B. cereus* diarrheal food poisoning in the United States occurred in 1969. In 1978, an outbreak involving 209 cases took place in North Carolina, and in the same year an outbreak involving 118 cases occurred in New York. Despite these large outbreaks, conclusively diagnosed food poisoning caused by *B. cereus* is relatively uncommon in the United States, but is common in England and is especially prevalent in Hungary. These geographical differences in incidence may be partly due to variations in foods consumed and also to greater surveillance and investigation in the European countries. In the 5-year period 1972 to 1978, the Centers for Disease Control (CDC) reported 13 *B. cereus* outbreaks or 1.2% of the diagnosed bacterial outbreaks in the United States. In 1982, 8 outbreaks were reported and diagnosed (3.6% of the total bacterial outbreaks reported by the CDC). The higher frequency in the latter year is probably mostly due to increased surveillance for *B. cereus*, which the FDA considers as an emerging pathogen.

The emetic syndrome (see Section II,B below) was first described in the United Kingdom in 1971. By 1982, more than 120 episodes had been reported. Similar outbreaks have occurred in Canada, India, Japan, Singapore, and the United States.

B. Description of the Illness

Two distinct types of illness have been attributed to the consumption of foods contaminated with *B. cereus*: (1) a diarrheal illness with an incubation time of approximately 4–16 hours and manifested as abdominal pain and diarrhea that usually subsides within 12–24 hours, and (2) an emetic illness with an incubation time of 1–5 hours with resulting nausea and vomiting. The incubation period and symptoms of the latter mimic those of *Staphylococcus aureus* food poisoning. The comparative symptoms and other properties of the illnesses are presented in Table I. In some *B. cereus* outbreaks there appears to be a clear overlap of the diarrheal and emetic syndromes.

Table I

Comparative Clinical and Epidemiological Data for Intoxications Caused by *Bacillus cereus,
Clostridium perfringens,* and *Staphylococcus aureus*[a]

Cause of illness	Onset of symptoms (hours)	Duration of illness (hours)	Diarrhea, abdominal cramps	Nausea, vomiting	Common food vehicles
C. perfringens	8–22	12–24	Prevalent	Rare	Cooked meat and poultry
B. cereus (diarrheal type)	8–16	12–24	Prevalent	Occasional	Meat products soups, sauces, vegetables
B. cereus (emetic type)	1–5	6–24	Fairly common	Prevalent	Cooked rice and pasta
S. aureus	2–6	6–24	Common	Prevalent	Cold cooked meat and poultry, dairy products

[a]From R. J. Gilbert and J. M. Kramer (1987). *In* "Progress in Food Safety" (D. O. Cliver, and B. A. Cochrane, eds.), pp. 85–93. Food Research Institute, University of Wisconsin, Madison.

C.   Foods Involved in the Outbreaks

The emetic syndrome is nearly always (118/120 diagnosed cases in one compilation) associated with the consumption of boiled or fried rice dishes, whereas foods involved in the diarrheal illness have been quite varied, ranging from vegetables and salads to meat dishes and casseroles. Since *B. cereus* is a sporeformer, the wide environmental distribution of spores probably gives it access to a variety of raw food materials. The frequent association of the emetic illness with rice dishes is not presently understood.

III.   Biological Properties of the Organism

A.   Species Description

The genus *Bacillus* comprises rod-shaped, gram-positive bacteria that aerobically form refractile endospores. The spores of the bacilli are more resistant than vegetative cells to heat, drying, food preservatives, and other environmental challenges. Strains of *Bacillus* produce catalase which, in addition to the aerobic production of spores, distinguishes *Bacillus* from *Clostridium*. The bacteria of the genus *Bacillus* are usually free living, that is, not host adapted, and their spores are widely distributed throughout nature.

The species in the genus *Bacillus* are classified into three groups depending on the shape of the spore and the swelling of the mother sporangium by the endospore. *Bacillus cereus* is easily designated to Group I; its spores are ellipsoidal, central to subterminal, and do not distend the sporangia. It is closely related to *B. megaterium* and to *B. anthracis*; *B. cereus* can be separated by anaerobic growth (positive), Voges–Proskauer reaction (positive), egg-yolk lecithinase reaction (positive), resistance to 0.001% lysozyme (resistant), and acid production from mannitol (negative). The cells of *B. cereus* are typically large, reaching 3–5 μm in length and 1.0–1.2 μm in width. The mol% G+C of the DNA has been reported to be approximately 32–38 for 11 strains and 35.7–36.2 for the type strain (ATCC 14579). DNA homologies with strains of *B. anthracis*, *B. mycoides*, and *B. thuringiensis* exceed 80%, suggesting a close relationship to these organisms.

B.   Reservoirs

Bacillus cereus is widely distributed in nature and in foods and is commonly found in soil, milk, cereals, starches, herbs, spices, and other dried foodstuffs. It is also found on the surfaces of meats and poultry, probably because of soil or dust contamination. Investigators in Sweden reported a *B. cereus* isolation rate of 47.8% from 3888 different samples of foods. In the United Kingdom, *B. cereus* was isolated from 98/108 (91%) rice samples. The organism is a problem in dairy products and is occasionally responsible for spoilage of raw and pasteurized milk.

Foods containing dried milks, such as infant formulas, may possess fairly high levels of spores or cells.

C.   Vegetative Growth Properties

Vegetative cells are gram-positive, motile by peritrichous flagella, and very large. The rods often occur in chains, and the colonies on agar media have a dull or frosted appearance.

The organism grows over the temperature range of approximately 10°C (50°F) to 48°C (118.4°F), with an optimum temperature of 28–35°C (82.4–95°F). The doubling time at the optimum temperature in a rich medium is 18–27 minutes. Several strains can grow slowly in sodium chloride concentrations of 7.5%. The minimum water activity for growth is 0.95. *Bacillus cereus* has an absolute requirement for amino acids as growth factors, but vitamins are not required. The organism grows over a pH range of approximately 4.9–9.3; of course these guidelines and other environmental limits for growth are dependent on water activity, temperature, and other interrelated parameters.

Strains of *B. cereus* produce a variety of extracellular enzymes, toxins, and antibiotics that have undoubtedly contributed to the success and wide distribution of the bacterium. It is known to secrete proteases, amylases, β-lactamases, peptide antibiotics, phospholipases, hemolysins, and toxins. The formation of extracellular enzymes enables it to use polymeric sources of carbon and nitrogen such as proteins and starch.

D.   Spores and Survival

Investigators in the United Kingdom have shown that spores from strains of serotype 1 (flagellar H antigen), which is a serotype commonly associated with food poisoning, have a D_{95} (95°C or 203°F) of approximately 24 minutes. Other serotypes were shown to have a wider range of heat resistances, with a D_{95} of 1.5–36 minutes. It has been suggested that the strains involved in food poisoning may in general have higher heat resistances and therefore be more apt to survive cooking.

Spore germination can occur over the temperature range of 8°C (46.4°F) to 30°C (86°F). Germination has an absolute requirement for glycine or a neutral L-amino acid and purine ribosides. L-alanine is the most effective amino acid stimulating germination.

IV.   Pathogenic Nature: Properties of Toxins

The rapid onset of symptoms and the short duration of the illnesses suggest that *B. cereus* food poisonings are mediated by toxins. At least two enterotoxins are be-

Table II

Properties of Diarrheal and Emetic Toxins of *Bacillus cereus*[a]

Property	Diarrheal toxin	Emetic toxin
Biological activity		
Monkey challenge	Diarrhea, 0.5–3 hours	Emesis, 1–5 hours
Rabbit ileal loop	Positive (ca. 150 μg)	Negative
Guinea pig skin	Positive (ca. 1 μg i.d.) vascular permeability	Negative
Mouse lethality	Positive (ca. 30 μg i.v.)	NA[b]
Inhibition of mammalian cells in culture (Vero)	Cytotoxic (0.1–0.5 μg)	NA
Structure and properties		
Biochemical structure	Multicomponent; probably consists of three proteins (43,000 MW; 39,000 MW; 38,000 MW)	Small protein (<10,000 MW)
Isoelectric point	~5.3	NA
pH stability	Unstable <4 and >11	Stable 2–11
Heat stability	Unstable; destroyed at 55°C (131°F) for 20 minutes	Resists heating at 126°C (259°F) for 90 minutes
Enzyme sensitivity	Inactivated by pronase and trypsin	Not inactivated by proteases
Synthesis in growth	Produced in log phase of growth cycle	Produced after active growth
Inhibitor sensitivity	EDTA resistant	NA

[a]Adapted from Gilbert and Kramer (1984).
[b]NA, data not reported.

lieved to be involved in causing the two distinct illnesses. The characterization of the toxins has been hindered by lack of convenient and reproducible assays of their activity. Investigators at the Food Research Institute (University of Wisconsin–Madison) demonstrated that the toxin responsible for the diarrheal syndrome is an enterotoxin. It causes fluid accumulation in rabbit ileal loops, alters vascular permeability in the skin of rabbits, and is lethal to mice when injected in very high quantities (approximately 30 μg iv). Another test for its activity shows toxicity for animal cells in culture (Table II). Antibodies have been prepared against the toxin and can also be used to detect enterotoxin protein.

Characterization of the emetic toxin has been slow due to the lack of a suitable animal model to test its activity. Cell-free filtrates cause vomiting in monkeys; obviously this assay is cumbersome and expensive. Other reported properties are presented in Table II.

V. Diagnosis of *Bacillus cereus* Foodborne Illness

Because the spores of *B. cereus* are widely spread in the environment, the incidental finding of this organism at low levels in foods should be expected. However, the isolation of high levels ($>10^5$ CFU/g of food) is suggestive of the organism's involvement in food poisoning. Selective and/or indicator media are commonly used for isolation of *B. cereus*; one medium is mannitol–egg yolk–polymyxin (MYP). Typically, *B. cereus* does not ferment mannitol, produces a positive lecithinase, and is resistant to polymyxin. During isolation and characterization, it is wise to compare the newly isolated strain with a standard culture to ensure that the phenotypic tests are giving the correct results. Following its isolation from food, various confirmatory tests are carried out including anaerobic glucose fermentation (*B. cereus* is facultatively anaerobic), nitrate reduction (positive), Voges–Proskauer test (positive), citrate utilization (positive), tyrosine decomposition (positive), gelatin or casein hydrolysis (positive), and resistance to lysozyme (resistant). Serological testing may be carried out in epidemiological studies. Those isolates that produce large gram-positive rods with central ellipsoidal spores that do not distend the sporangium, have a positive lecithinase, produce acid from glucose anaerobically, reduce nitrate, produce acetylmethylcarbinol (Voges–Proskauer), do not ferment mannitol, and grow in 0.001% lysozyme are very likely *B. cereus*.

To implicate *B. cereus* as the cause of food poisoning, high numbers of *B. cereus* ($>10^5$ CFU/g) should be isolated from the food and isolations should also be attempted from feces or vomitus of the victims. The isolates from the two sources should be identical in phenotypic properties.

VI. Prevention of *Bacillus cereus* Foodborne Illness

Because *B. cereus* is widespread in nature and survives extended storage in dried food products, it is not practical to eliminate low numbers of spores from foods. Control against food poisoning should be directed at preventing germination of spores and preventing multiplication of large populations of the bacterium. Foods should rapidly and efficiently be cooled to less than 7°C (44.6°F) or maintained above 55–60°C (131–140°F), and they should be thoroughly reheated before serving.

Bibliography

Gilbert, R. J. (1979). *Bacillus cereus* gastroenteritis. *In* "Food-Borne Infections and Intoxications" (H. Riemann and F. L. Bryan, eds.), 2nd Ed., pp. 495–518. Academic Press, New York.

Gilbert, R. J., and Kramer, J. M. (1984). *Bacillus cereus* enterotoxins: Present status. *Biochem. Soc. Trans.* **12,** 198.

Hauge, S. (1955). Food poisoning caused by aerobic spore-forming bacilli. *J. Appl. Bacteriol.* **18,** 591–595.

Johnson, K. M. (1984). *Bacillus cereus* foodborne illness—an update. *J. Food Prot.* **47,** 145–153.

Thompson, N. E., Ketterhagen, M. J., Bergdoll, M. S., and Schantz, E. J. (1984). Isolation and some properties of an enterotoxin produced by *Bacillus cereus. Infect. Immun.* **43,** 887–894.

CHAPTER 8

MYCOTOXINS

Elmer H. Marth

I. Introduction

Physical changes produced by mold growth in foods have been recognized for many years. Molds are generously endowed with extracellular proteolytic or lipolytic enzymes and so can cause softening of the product. Mold growth also causes off flavors or odors in food. Additionally, changes in appearance of food have been related to mold growth.

Nearly 30 years ago, we came to realize that molds can do more to food than produce these changes. We learned that molds can produce highly toxic substances during their growth on foods or feeds. These toxic metabolites are designated "mycotoxins," which is a collective term for the entire group of toxic substances produced by various molds. The diseases that mycotoxins cause are collectively called mycotoxicoses.

Two events that occurred in the early 1960s were responsible for bringing to our attention the fact that molds can produce toxic metabolites. The first occurred in Russia during the World War II. Although it occurred in the 1940s, information about the event was not commonly known until early in the 1960s. After the Germans invaded Russia, they headed toward Moscow in the fall of the year and drove the Russians off their fields before crops were harvested. One of these unharvested crops was the cereal millet. The Germans failed to capture Moscow because of the severe winter and then were driven back by the Russians. In doing this, the Russians recaptured the land and at this time many were hungry. Millet that had spent the winter under the snowdrifts was harvested and converted into baked products. These products were eaten and many people suddenly became ill. Thousands in a certain region of the Soviet Union died as a consequence of consuming the baked products made from the millet. An investigation revealed that the millet had supported growth of molds, principally in the genus *Fusarium,* and that these molds had produced toxic substances, probably trichothecenes, which caused the illness named alimentary toxic aleukia or septic angina.

The second event that caused concern about molds and the toxins they produce occurred in England in the early 1960s and was associated with illness in poultry, primarily in turkeys but also in ducklings and baby chicks. In turkeys, this disease was characterized by depression, a staggering gait, and sudden death. Examination of the carcasses revealed tissues to be congested and edematous. The liver invariably was enlarged, firm, and often pale yellow-red. Similar observations were made in ducklings, but in addition many had subcutaneous hemorrhages which appeared on the legs and back. Thousands of these animals died, which resulted in a serious economic loss for farmers.

Investigation of this problem revealed, first, that the sick and dead birds had consumed a diet containing peanut meal. Second, the peanut meal invariably was contaminated with *Aspergillus flavus.* Third, the peanut meal contained a toxic substance which had been produced by the mold. This material was given a trivial name by taking the "a" from *Aspergillus,* the "fla" from *flavus,* and adding "toxin" to get "aflatoxin." These two events clearly demonstrated that molds can produce substances highly toxic for humans or animals or both and prompted much concern and research activity in this area.

However, if we had given heed to history, it would not have taken us until the early 1960s to become concerned with molds that can produce toxic substances. We should have remembered the problem of ergotism, which for centuries has been associated with contaminated cereal grains. This disease, which will be described in greater detail later, is caused by toxic material produced by fungi in the genus *Claviceps.*

II. Ubiquity of Mycotoxin Biosynthesis by Molds

The first consideration is to answer the question, "Is the ability to produce mycotoxins limited to a few unusual species of molds, perhaps having to grow under unusual circumstances, or is this ability widespread among molds?" As it turns out, the ability to produce toxic substances is rather widespread among molds. Table I gives a partial list of molds able to produce such metabolites. Some of the molds and the toxins they produce will be considered later in this chapter. Brief comments will be made here about a few that will not be discussed later.

Paecilomyces variota which, depending on its stage of growth, also is called *Byssochlamys fulva* is of some concern. *Paecilomyces variota* (*B. fulva*) produces spores that, when compared with those of other molds, are rather heat resistant.

Table I
Some Molds Reported as Able
to Produce Mycotoxins

Alternaria, several species
Aspergillus, more than 20 species
Chaetomium globosum
Cladosporium, at least 2 species
Claviceps, at least 2 species
Fusarium, at least 6 species
Gibberella zea
Mucor hiemalis
Paecilomyces variota (*Byssochlamys fulva*)
Penicillium, more than 15 species
Pithomyces chartrum (*Sporodesmium bakeri*)
Rhizopus
Sclerotinia sclerotiorum
Stachybotrys atra
Trichoderma lignorum

These spores sometimes survive the relatively mild heat treatments given to fruit juices and then, through germination and growth, spoil products such as grape juice. The second concern is the ability of this mold to produce the mycotoxin byssochlamic acid, which is toxic to humans. Although the problem is minor, it should not be overlooked. *Pithomyces chartrum* produces a toxin of some importance in animal health. The genus *Rhizopus* includes the common bread mold, but some molds in this genus can produce toxins. *Sclerotinia sclerotiorum* finds its way onto celery and there produces a substance called psoralen. It has not been fully determined if the mold produces the psoralen or whether celery produces it in response to infection by the mold. In any event, psoralen is produced and the material can irritate the skin of persons who work with celery. *Stachybotrys atra* causes an animal health problem and *Trichoderma* is of minor importance. From these brief comments and from information in Table I, it is evident that numerous molds can produce toxic substances. Unfortunately, there also is considerable variability in the nature and activity of the toxic substances that are produced. Recently, it was claimed that about 80 different species of molds produced more than 100 different toxic substances, which indicates that some molds produce more than one toxin.

III.   Mycotoxins and Mycotoxicoses Produced by *Claviceps* Species

Ergotism is the first example of a mycotoxin-associated illness that will be discussed. This example is of particular importance because the disease has plagued humankind for many centuries. The organism primarily responsible for the problem is *Claviceps purpurea,* though *Claviceps paspali* also may be involved. Either of these fungi can infect the heads of rye and less often those of wheat, barley, and oats. There the fungus produces a structure called a sclerotium. This structure looks like a shriveled or incompletely formed rye kernel. It may be purplish-brown in appearance and it contains the toxic material.

Epidemics of ergotism have occurred among humans in Central Europe since the 1200s or earlier. Europe, including France, Germany, and Poland, as well as Great Britain and Ireland, tends to be cool and damp, conditions which favor growth of these fungi. The last major recognized outbreak of ergotism in Europe was as recent as 1951.

The *Claviceps* fungus also can grow on cereals in the United States although we have had no great problems with ergotism, at least none that we have recognized. This is true because cereals are cleaned before they are used as food and also because of regulatory control by the U.S. Department of Agriculture.

In humans, ergot, which is the common term for the toxic materials, has been used therapeutically to strengthen the tone of the uterine muscle during childbirth and also to control postpartum hemorrhaging. Currently purified preparations of the ergot alkaloid are preferred to the crude ergot. The therapeutic dose of ergot is in the range of 0.15–1 g/day. This range of values is important because it serves as the basis for specifying how much ergot is permissible in cereals. If much more ergot than the therapeutic dose is consumed, the disease "ergotism" results, in either the gangrenous or the convulsive form.

A. Gangrenous Ergotism

In the gangrenous form, initially there is a burning sensation in the the feet and hands. Because of the sensation, centuries ago this form of ergotism was called St. Anthony's Fire. There was once much mysticism associated with this disease. It was thought to be a punishment by God for having done something evil, religion became involved, and the term "St. Anthony's Fire" resulted. After the burning sensation has begun, there is a progressive restriction of the flow of blood to the hands and feet which leads to the onset of gangrene. In time, the extremities become sufficiently gangrenous so that limbs drop off or must be removed with considerable discomfort to the victim.

B. Convulsive Ergotism

The second type of ergotism is the convulsive form, which is associated with neurological involvement. The convulsive form begins with hallucinations. If consumption of ergot continues, the victim will suffer from convulsive seizures which may be fatal.

What are the active ingredients of ergot that are responsible for this problem? There are about nine different active compounds, which chemically are slightly different from one other. However, all are polypeptide derivatives of lysergic acid.

C. Control of Ergotism

Control of ergotism involves limiting the amount of ergot that can occur in cereals destined for human consumption. The tolerance in endemic countries is 0.10–0.15% sclerotia among kernels of grain. This is based on the premise that if a person were to consume, per day, 0.5 kg (approximately 1.1 lb) of bread made from such grain, from 0.5–0.75 g of ergot would be ingested. Since the maximum therapeutic dose is 1 g/day, the amount in acceptable grain would be too low to cause ergotism except possibly after prolonged exposure.

In the United States, control of this problem is a responsibility of the U.S. Department of Agriculture. The agency classifies grain as either "ergoty" or "not ergoty." Grain is considered ergoty if it contains more than 0.3% of *Claviceps* sclerotia by weight, and sclerotia must be removed before the grain can be used as food. This much ergot in the form of sclerotia is seldom found in grain in the United States. Also, current methods of cleaning grain, for example, the use of fanning mills and other devices, are fairly effective in removing sclerotia from grain.

Although problems with human ergotism are rare in the United States, sometimes ergotism occurs in livestock. If ergoty grain is cleaned through use of air separation techniques, both sclerotia and light kernels will be removed and may be used as animal feed. Since the ergot has become concentrated in such feed, animals may become ill. There also is the possibility that if ergoty feed is consumed by dairy cows some of these alkaloids could be transferred to the milk, as has been demonstrated for aflatoxin. This possibility should be investigated.

IV. Mycotoxins and Mycotoxicoses Produced by *Fusarium* Species

A. Trichothecene

The first toxin to be discussed is trichothecene, which causes alimentary toxic aleukia, the problem in Russia that was mentioned earlier. This problem seems to be associated primarily with cereals that have overwintered in fields, and this condition is not restricted to Russia during wartime. A variety of cereals is susceptible to infection by *Fusarium* spp., permitting production of the mycotoxin. It has been demonstrated that, besides millet, the toxin causing alimentary toxic aleukia, and believed to be of the trichothecene type, can be produced on wheat, oats, barley, rye, and buckwheat. Toxin production by the responsible *Fusarium* sp. (probably *F. sporotrichioides*) is stimulated at temperatures in the range of -1 to $-10°C$ and also by cycling of temperatures from below to above freezing.

The toxin in grains is destroyed at or above 200°C. This is much higher than the temperature attained in products during baking. As long as moisture is present in the product during baking there will be evaporation and the temperature of boiling water will not be exceeded on the inside of the baked product. Consequently, since a maximum of 100°C is reached during ordinary baking, the process will not inactivate the toxin. The toxin in grains retains its toxicity for as long as 6 years. Also, treatment with acid or alkali does not affect this trichothecene mycotoxin. The disease, alimentary toxic aleukia, has four stages that are identified on the basis of symptoms and pathology.

1. First stage

A person suffering from alimentary toxic aleukia initially experiences a burning sensation in the mouth and in pharyngeal tissue. This burning sensation signals the onset of the first stage and appears within a few hours after toxic grain is consumed. The burning feeling then progresses down the esophagus, and on to the stomach. One to three days after toxic grain is consumed, acute gastroenteritis develops which is accompanied by diarrhea, nausea, and vomiting. The gastroenteritis seems to be self-limiting and ceases after about 9 days even if the toxic cereal is still being eaten.

2. Second stage

The person, now free of gastroenteritis, enters the second stage of the disease and may be without symptoms from about 2 weeks to 2 months. During this time bone marrow is being destroyed, and at the end of this period there are marked abnormalities in the cellular composition of blood, such as leukemia, agranulocytosis, anemia, and a decrease in number of platelets. Toward the end of the second stage, petechial hemorrhages appear subcutaneously. Their appearance marks transition to the third stage of the disease.

3. Third stage

The third stage lasts from 5–20 days and symptoms reflect total atrophy of bone marrow. Included are necrotic angina, sepsis, total agranulocytosis, and a moderate fever of 38–40°C. The petechial hemorrhages that were mentioned earlier now become larger and confluent. This is followed by necrosis of the skin and of muscles which lie immediately below the skin where the necrotic lesions have appeared. After all this has happened, bronchial pneumonia appears and abscesses and hemorrhages may develop in the lungs.

4. Fourth stage

The third stage is now complete and the fourth stage can be characterized by one word—death. The mortality rate varies according to concentration of toxin in the cereal, amount of cereal (and hence of toxin) that is consumed, length of time toxic cereal is consumed, and general health of the person when he/she starts to ingest the toxic cereal product. Although the mortality rate can be as high as 80%, it need not be that high if consumption of the toxin stops before all the bodily changes occur.

B. Zearalenone

The other of the *Fusarium* toxins to be considered is zearalenone, which is produced primarily by *F. graminearum,* but also by other fusaria. Zearalenone is a problem of feed grains and hence can have an impact on the health of livestock. The mold grows on ears of corn in the field that may become inoculated when they are invaded by the corn earworm or the corn borer. Production of the toxin on corn or other cereals is favored by temperatures near freezing for an extended time and also by temperature cycling from a low to a moderate temperature and back again. The mold also can grow on corn during storage if the corn is harvested with too much moisture and is not dried properly before storage.

Although zearalenone primarily causes an animal problem, it can be a problem for people because of economic losses resulting from diseased livestock. This mycotoxin is unique because it has estrogenic properties. It causes the so-called "estrogenic syndrome" in swine and affects other animals in a similar manner. Symptoms of the estrogenic syndrome in swine primarily involve the genital system. In females, the vulva becomes swollen and edematous; in severe cases there may be vaginal prolapse. The uterus also becomes enlarged and edematous. The ovaries are shrunken, and the sow is likely to abort if she is pregnant when she ingests zearalenone. If males consume this mycotoxin, relatively young boars are likely to undergo a feminizing effect, including atrophy of the testes and enlargement of the mammary glands.

The empirical formula for zearalenone is $C_{18}H_{22}O_5$, its molecular weight is 318, its melting point is 164–165°C, and its structure is given in Fig. 1. Mycotoxins

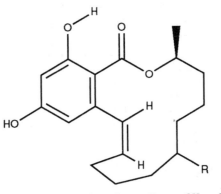

Figure 1   Structure of zearalenone. R = —OH, ═O.

generally are rather small organic molecules and are not proteins as are the staphylococcal enterotoxins and the botulinus toxin. Information about the melting point of mycotoxins is important because it indicates their stability to heat; commonly complete inactivation (loss of toxicity) results only when the melting point has been attained. However, this is not to suggest that a lesser heat treatment does nothing; it may reduce toxicity of the mycotoxin.

V.   Mycotoxins and Mycotoxicoses Produced by Penicillia

Next some of the mycotoxins produced by molds in the genus *Penicillium* will be considered.

A.   Rubratoxin

Rubratoxin is produced by *Penicillium rubrum*. About 20–30 years ago a disease of swine was observed that was caused by moldy corn consumed by the animals. A similar disease also was observed in cattle. The principal mold that was isolated from moldy corn associated with these problems was *P. rubrum*. After this mold had been isolated, corn was inoculated with it and was used to demonstrate that the mold did produce substances highly toxic to animals. In fact, consumption of 0.23 kg (0.5 lb) of corn made moldy by *P. rubrum* caused swine to die within a day. A few years later it also was noted that a hemorrhagic disease in poultry was caused by feed made moldy by *P. rubrum*.

Characteristically, *P. rubrum* produces a red or purple-red pigment. *Penicillium rubrum* is closely related to another mold, *P. purpurogenum*. This mold also can produce pigment and rubratoxin. Both species are widespread in nature; they can be found in soils and often on such plant products as peanuts, legumes, corn, and sunflower seeds.

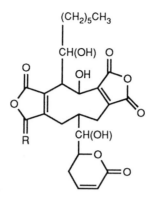

Figure 2 Structures of rubratoxins A (R = O) and B (R = H, OH).

Rubratoxin appears to be completely excreted into the medium and little or none is retained by the mold mycelium. This differs from some other mycotoxins such as aflatoxin (to be discussed later) that, to a considerable degree, are retained within the mycelium of the producing fungus.

There are two rubratoxins, designated A and B. The formula for rubratoxin A is $C_{26}H_{22}O_{11}$, its molecular weight is 510, and its melting point is in the range of 210–214°C. The LD_{50} value, determined by injecting mice intraperitoneally, is 6.6 mg/kg of body weight. Rubratoxin B is $C_{26}H_{30}O_{11}$, its molecular weight is 518, and the melting point is 168–170°C. In this instance, the LD_{50} value in mice is 3 mg/kg of body weight. The structure of both rubratoxins is given in Fig. 2. Cultures of *P. rubrum* commonly produce both rubratoxins, but rubratoxin B seems to predominate. Some cultures of *P. rubrum* produce only rubratoxin B.

B.   Patulin

Patulin is another mycotoxin produced by some penicillia, most commonly by *Penicillium expansum,* but sometimes by *P. claviforme* and *P. urticae.* There also are some aspergilli that can produce patulin. However, the major concern is with *P. expansum,* which often invades fruit. When fruit deteriorates (rots) through growth of *P. expansum* there is the likelihood that patulin is produced.

Patulin is toxic to some gram-positive and gram-negative bacteria. At one time patulin was thought to be useful as an antibiotic and was given such names as clavicin, claviformin, expansum, mycoin-c, and penicidin. Because of its toxicity, use of patulin as an antibiotic was abandoned.

The molecular formula for patulin is $C_7H_6O_4$ and its structure appears in Fig. 3. The mycotoxin is unstable in alkaline, but stable in acid conditions. It inhibits growth of tissue cultures and is toxic to certain bacteriophages. Patulin is toxic to some seeds when they germinate and also to some animals. The LD_{50} value for patulin administered intravenously to mice and rats is 15–35 mg/kg of body weight. Pasteurization does not destroy patulin, but fermentation of apple juice to produce hard cider eliminates the mycotoxin. What happens to the patulin during the fermentation remains unclear. Another means to eliminate it from apple juice is to add

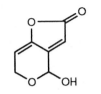

Figure 3   Structure of patulin.

vitamin C. As mentioned earlier, patulin is stable under acid conditions and, of course, fruit juices or other fruit products are acidic. Hence, it is evident that the activity of patulin, if present, will not be eliminated from such products even after extended storage.

C.   Yellow Rice Toxins

Next to be considered is a group of mycotoxins produced by penicillia and designated as "yellow rice" toxins. Rice is a major component of the Oriental diet, and sometimes the rice becomes moldy. Molds that grow on the rice frequently produce a toxin and a pigment that causes the rice to become yellow, hence "yellow rice" toxins. Species of molds that have been identified as involved in the yellow rice problem include *Penicillium toxicarium, P. islandicum, P. citrinum, P. rugulosum, P. tardum,* and *P. citreoviride.* Each of these produces one or several toxins, but they are all a part of the yellow rice problem. Two of the yellow rice toxins, citrinin and citreoviridin, will be considered in greater detail.

1.   Citrinin

This mycotoxin is produced by *Penicillium citrinum* and by several other penicillia. *Penicillium citrinum* is widely distributed in all the rice-producing areas of the world. Thus it has been isolated from rice produced in Burma, China, Egypt, Italy, Japan, and the United States. The mold commonly grows on stored rice, particularly on polished rice. Growth is accompanied by formation of the pigment which causes the surface of rice kernels to appear yellow. Exposure of the kernels to ultraviolet light results in fluorescence by the yellow areas. The formula of citrinin is $C_{13}H_{14}O_5$, it has a molecular weight of 259, its melting point is 172°C, and its

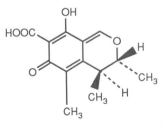

Figure 4   Structure of citrinin.

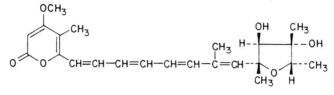

Figure 5 Structure of citreoviridin.

structure appears in Fig. 4. The LD_{50} value when the toxin is administered orally to mice is 50 mg/kg of body weight or more. The LD_{50} values are 19–58 mg/kg and 35–67 mg/kg when the toxin is administered intraperitoneally or subcutaneously, respectively. Citrinin affects the kidneys and causes tubular damage similar to that observed in the kidney diseases glomerulonephrosis or toxic nephrosis. Citrinin is antibacterial for gram-positive but not for gram-negative bacteria.

2. Citreoviridin

Another major yellow rice toxin is citreoviridin, which is produced by *Penicillium citreoviride*. The molecular formula of this toxin is $C_{23}H_{30}O_6CH_3OH$, its structure appears in Fig. 5, its melting point is 107–110°C, and the LD_{50} value is 20 mg/kg of body weight when administered subcutaneously to mice. When citreoviridin is ingested by an experimental animal, the initial symptoms of the disease it causes include paralysis of the hind legs and flank, vomiting, and convulsions. Later there are gradually developing respiratory disorders followed by cardiovascular disturbances, paralysis, decrease in body temperature, gasping, coma, and respiratory arrest.

D. Other Mycotoxins of the Penicillia

There are other mycotoxins produced by penicillia, and a few will be briefly mentioned. A mycotoxin of some importance is penicillic acid, which is produced by *Penicillium puberulum* and some other penicillia. *Penicillium puberulum* can grow with reduced oxygen tension and thus sometimes will grow on products when oxygen is limited in the atmosphere immediately surrounding the mold. Penicillic acid can occur in moldy corn and popcorn. The mold can invade kernels of corn and produce a condition called "blue-eye disease" of corn. The term results from the blue spot that develops when the mold grows just beneath the outer layer of the kernel.

Other mycotoxins produced by penicillia include luteoskyrin, cyclochlorotine, islanditoxin, erythroskyrine, rugulosin, mycophenolic acid, decumbin, β-nitropropanoic acid, cyclopiazonic acid, griseofulvin, xanthocillin, viridicatin, viridicatic acid, cyclopenin, and cyclopenol. The first five of these also are involved in the yellow rice problem.

VI. Mycotoxins and Mycotoxicoses Produced by Aspergilli

A. Ochratoxin

Ochratoxin was initially associated with moldy and toxic legumes and cereal products in South Africa. When the microflora of these products was studied, investigators regularly found *Aspergillus ochraceus*. Some strains of this mold produced
toxic material that killed ducklings. *Aspergillus ochraceus* is widespread in nature;
it can be found in soils, in decaying vegetation, and in stored cereals. In the United
States, ochratoxin has been found as a contaminant in poor-quality corn. There are
aspergilli other than *A. ochraceus* that can produce ochratoxin.

Some years ago ochratoxin caused a problem in Denmark. Apparently the toxin,
in feed consumed by pigs, carried over into the tissue and occurred in bacon from
these animals. The bacon was exported and was found to contain ochratoxin by the
importing country.

Aspergillus ochraceus has been isolated from numerous food crops including
peanuts, Brazil nuts, cereal grains (particularly if the moisture content is above
16%), red and black pepper, some Oriental fermented fish products, cottonseed, and
citrus fruit, and from flue-cured tobacco and cigarette tobaccos. There are several
ochratoxins produced; we will deal with the two that are designated A and B. Of
these, ochratoxin A is of greatest concern because it is most toxic.

The formula for ochratoxin A is $C_{20}H_{18}ClNO_6$, its melting point is 169°C, and
its structure appears in Fig. 6. The LD_{50} value of the toxin, when administered
orally to rats, is 20 mg/kg of body weight. This mycotoxin has been produced
experimentally on sterilized corn, shredded wheat, soybeans, rye, rice, buckwheat,
and peanuts. It also has been produced in semisynthetic and synthetic culture media.
Ochratoxin A affects both the liver and kidneys. In the liver, it causes an increase of
fatty vacuolation (e.g., more fat in the liver) and a swelling of mitochondria in liver
cells. In the kidneys, its principal effect is causing necrosis of the tubules, thus
obstructing them. Ochratoxin A is believed to be noncarcinogenic.

Ochratoxin B has a formula of $C_{20}H_{19}NO_6$, and its melting point is 221°C. It is
markedly less toxic than ochratoxin A and hence relatively less information about it
has been developed.

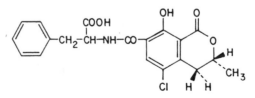

Figure 6   Structure of ochratoxin A.

Table II
Empirical Formulae, Molecular Weights, and Melting Points
of the Principal Aflatoxins

Aflatoxin	Formula	Molecular weight	Melting point (°C)
B_1	$C_{17}H_{12}O_6$	312	268–269
B_2	$C_{17}H_{14}O_6$	314	286–289
G_1	$C_{17}H_{12}O_7$	328	244–246
G_2	$C_{17}H_{14}O_7$	330	237–240

B. Aflatoxin

Aflatoxin is produced by many strains of *Aspergillus flavus* and *A. parasiticus*. Generally, when these molds grow on a suitable substrate, they produce a minimum of four different compounds, which are designated as aflatoxins B_1, B_2, G_1, and G_2. In cultures, generally aflatoxins B_1 and G_1 will predominate. There are some cultures of the molds that will produce more B_1 than G_1, and the reverse also is true. The B-aflatoxins are so designated because they emit blue fluorescence when viewed on a thin-layer chromatoplate exposed to long-wave ultraviolet light. The B_1 and B_2 designations refer to the different positions (R_f values) on a chromatoplate at which the two toxins appear. The G-aflatoxins emit a green fluorescence when viewed under long-wave ultraviolet light.

The empirical formulae, molecular weights, and melting points of the major aflatoxins appear in Table II, and their structures are in Fig. 7. Note that the melting

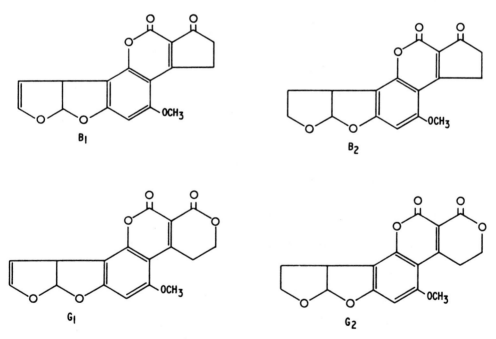

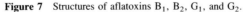

Figure 7 Structures of aflatoxins B_1, B_2, G_1, and G_2.

points are quite high. Another major form of aflatoxin is designated M_1 (milk toxin) and is the hydroxylated form of B_1. Aflatoxin M_1 was first isolated from milk and hence was given that particular designation. If a mammal such as a dairy cow consumes aflatoxin B_1 in its diet, about 1–3% of the amount of B_1 that is consumed will appear in milk as aflatoxin M_1. The toxicity of M_1 is about the same as that of B_1, but its carcinogenic potential is markedly less.

1. Conditions governing aflatoxin production

As is true of molds in general, the aspergilli are aerobic, although the amount of toxin they produce can be enhanced by slightly reducing the quantity of oxygen from that which is in air. If the atmosphere is fortified with additional carbon dioxide, it will have a negative effect on both growth and toxin production by the mold. Nitrogen can also be used to inhibit growth of the mold, but in this instance virtually all of the oxygen in the atmosphere has to be replaced with nitrogen.

The aspergilli produce toxin best at a temperature in the range of about 23–26°C. Both growth and sporulation of the toxic aspergilli are best at about 30°C. They can grow at temperatures in the range of about 2–45°C but do not produce toxin well at the extremes of temperatures that permit growth. In fact, it is generally thought that these molds will not produce toxin at temperatures below 8–11°C. Although aflatoxin production is favored by a medium high in carbohydrate content, substrates with considerable fat and protein (e.g., peanuts) also will support aflatoxin production.

2. Stability/degradation of aflatoxin

When the aflatoxins exist in a more or less pure form and are exposed to ultraviolet light, as might happen if thin-layer chromatography is used to measure presence and amount of the toxins, some of the toxins likely will be degraded. This knowledge also has been applied to food. Initially, irradiation of peanut meal with ultraviolet light was tried, and no apparent effect was noted, possibly because the ultraviolet light could not penetrate sufficiently into this kind of material. Use of ultraviolet light to eliminate aflatoxin M_1 from milk also has been tried and is successful, particularly if the milk is in a relatively thin film while it is exposed to the ultraviolet light. The effectiveness of ultraviolet light for inactivation of aflatoxin in milk can be enhanced by addition of a small amount of hydrogen peroxide. In the dairy industry there is historic precedent for treating milk with ultraviolet light (to add vitamin D) and for adding hydrogen peroxide (to avoid pasteurization when milk is to be converted into certain kinds of cheese). It is also possible to inactivate aflatoxin M_1 in milk by addition of hydrogen peroxide together with lactoperoxidase. This enzyme occurs naturally in milk, but the amount that is present is not enough to bring about the chemical reaction needed to inactivate the toxin. A combination of hydrogen peroxide and riboflavin, when added to milk, also will eliminate a major portion of the aflatoxin M_1 activity.

Another approach to eliminate aflatoxin from a liquid, reported more than 20 years ago, involves use of *Flavobacterium aurantiacum*. What happens to the aflatoxin is uncertain. From a practical viewpoint, use of *Flavobacterium* spp. in a food product may be unacceptable because this psychrotrophic bacterium is likely to synthesize proteolytic and lipolytic enzymes that can bring about unwanted changes in the substrate.

Heat can be used to inactivate aflatoxins, but their melting point must be reached to completely eliminate toxicity. Use of that much heat is unacceptable in processing of food. Lesser amounts of heat, however, will reduce their toxicity. For example, oil meals with 20% moisture have been held at 100°C for 2 hours, and this resulted in a reduction of activity of the toxin by 80%. Also, the common practice of roasting peanuts reduces the activity of aflatoxin B_1 by about 70% and that of aflatoxin B_2 by about 45%. In spite of this, use of heat generally is not a satisfactory way of minimizing or eliminating the toxicity of aflatoxin.

Oxidizing agents are effective in reducing toxicity of these mycotoxins. One of them, hydrogen peroxide, was mentioned earlier when reduction of toxic activity of aflatoxin M_1 was considered. Sodium hypochlorite also can inactivate the aflatoxins and should be available if one is working with them in the laboratory. If a solution of aflatoxins is spilled, the toxin can immediately be inactivated and rendered harmless through application of sodium hypochlorite.

Another approach for elimination of toxic activity is exposure to alkaline substances. Such a method has been developed by researchers at the Northern Regional Research Center of the U.S. Department of Agriculture in Peoria, Illinois, and consists of treating aflatoxin-containing corn with ammonia. Corn is placed in a steel building, ammonia together with moisture is added to the corn, and the ammonia is circulated through the system for an appropriate time. The ammonia reacts with the aflatoxin and neutralizes its toxicity. The corn is then dried to prevent further mold growth. Treated corn is brown in color and probably less palatable than it was originally, but it is apparently as nutritious as untreated corn. Animals will accept the treated corn. The same approach has been used to treat cottonseed, which sometimes can be contaminated with aflatoxin. Use of the ammonia process, as of early 1990, was not yet approved by the Food and Drug Administration.

Another treatment for corn employs sulfite or bisulfite and will eliminate much of the aflatoxin that might be present. In the corn-processing industry, corn is soaked in a bisulfite solution before products such as syrups or starch are produced. Although it is not done primarily for eliminating aflatoxin, this "fringe benefit" is likely to result if the corn contains some of the toxin.

The final comments about degradation of aflatoxin deal with the molds that produce the toxin. If a culture of *Aspergillus parasiticus* or *A. flavus* in a suitable medium is incubated at the right temperature, for example, 28°C, 2–3 days elapse before detectable toxin appears in the culture. Continued incubation for up to about 8 or 9 days is accompanied by a gradual increase in amount of toxin in the culture fluid. After about 8–9 days, the amount of toxin starts to decrease and continues to do so as incubation continues. The aspergilli degrade aflatoxin B_1 to form aflatoxin B_{2a} probably through activity of peroxidase enzymes. Aflatoxin B_{2a} is only minimally toxic.

3. Concerns about aflatoxin

Why are we concerned about aflatoxin in the food supply? There are two reasons for the concern: toxicity and carcinogenicity. Aflatoxin is acutely toxic to most animal species if enough is consumed. "Enough" is not very much; the LD_{50} value of aflatoxin B_1 for most young animals (ducklings, dogs, rabbits, guinea pigs, rainbow trout) is about 0.5 mg/kg of body weight. If this much is consumed, death of the animal commonly will occur in about 72 hours. If such animals are examined, it will be evident that they suffered from liver damage and hemorrhaging in the intestinal tract and peritoneal cavity. Most animals develop some resistance to the toxin as they grow older. For example, the LD_{50} value for a 1-day-old rat is 0.5–1.0 mg/kg of body weight. In contrast, the value for a 21-day-old rat is 7 mg/kg of body weight. For comparative purposes, the LD_{50} value of lead arsenate is 500 mg/kg of body weight. Thus aflatoxin B_1 is a rather toxic compound. Aflatoxin M_1 is essentially as toxic as B_1.

The second reason for concern is the carcinogenic property of aflatoxin. If an animal, or probably a human, consumes sublethal quantities of aflatoxin B_1 for several days to several weeks, moderate to severe liver damage is likely to result. This damage can take one of several forms. The most common is biliary hyperplasia, a condition in which there is excessive growth of cells in the bile duct region of the liver. This is the type of cancer that is initiated by aflatoxin, and the toxin is thought to be one of the most active of the carcinogens. However, this activity relates to a single form of cancer and not to all forms of cancer. The other major change in the liver associated with consumption of aflatoxin B_1 is accumulation of fat, which can be adequate to change the appearance of the liver from purple-red to yellow-red. In rats, consumption of as little as 10 µg of aflatoxin B_1 daily for perhaps several weeks can lead to biliary hyperplasia.

4. Determination of aflatoxin

Some brief general comments will be made about determination of aflatoxin. What applies to aflatoxin may apply, more or less, to some of the other mycotoxins. A suitable source of detailed information on methods, for example, the current edition of "Official Methods of Analysis" (Association of Official Analytical Chemists), should be consulted before doing tests for aflatoxin or the other common mycotoxins. Methods to determine the less common mycotoxins may have to be gleaned from individual research papers.

If an unknown sample is to be analyzed, first the aflatoxin must be extracted with an appropriate organic solvent system, which usually is a mixture of organic solvents rather than a single compound. An example is methanol plus chloroform. If the product to be analyzed is high in fat content, the fat may have to be removed before the toxin is extracted. Fat should be removed so it will not interfere later in the analysis of aflatoxin. If the sample contains little or no fat then this pretreatment can be avoided and one can go directly to extraction of the toxin. After extraction of the toxin the extract may have to be purified, depending on the nature of the material from which it is extracted. If it is plant material there are likely to be pigments present, which need to be eliminated because they too may interfere with later chromatographic procedures. Purification probably will involve liquid–liquid extraction or use of column chromatography depending on the mycotoxin involved and the kinds of impurities that need to be eliminated.

After purification, the next step is resolution of the toxin; this involves getting the toxin in a state so it can be measured. Initially, with aflatoxin, this was done with thin-layer chromotography. The preparation containing aflatoxin is placed on a layer of a suitable silica gel on a glass plate. The silica gel is treated with an appropriate solvent and the aflatoxin then migrates through the gel. The B_1 toxin stops at a certain point and B_2 at another. The same is true for the G-aflatoxins. The spots of aflatoxin will emit fluorescence and its intensity is related to the amount of toxin present. Initially fluorescence of unknown samples was visually compared with that of a series of standards and thus the amount of aflatoxin present was crudely estimated. Later intensity of fluorescence was measured with a fluorometer or a suitably modified densitometer. Currently, liquid chromatography is commonly used to make these measurements. High-performance liquid chromatography (HPLC) will resolve the toxin and also measure the amount of fluorescence. The HPLC device commonly will be attached to a recorder which will give a printout of the analytical results. The peaks on such a printout can then be compared with those of standards and thus the amount of toxin present can be determined. Methods based on antigen–antibody reactions can be used to obtain results more rapidly than is possible with HPLC, although such methods are not "official" and hence are most suitable for rapid screening of samples.

C. Other Mycotoxins of the Aspergilli

Several other mycotoxins produced by aspergilli will be mentioned. The first is aspergillic acid, which is unlikely to be of great concern. Another is kojic acid. The name of this toxin is derived from the word *koji,* which is the term for the inoculum used in some Oriental food fermentations. Kojic acid causes convulsions. Tremorgenic toxin is produced by some strains of *Aspergillus flavus.* This toxin does what the name implies—it causes tremors in experimental animals. The last to be mentioned is oxalic acid, which can be produced by several aspergilli. Oxalic acid is a toxic material also found in rhubarb, particularly in its leaves. There are still other toxic substances produced by the aspergilli, but they will not be considered.

VII. Biosynthesis of Mycotoxins

We shall now deal briefly with the biosynthesis of mycotoxins. When a mold grows, it does so in two phases. The first phase involves rapid mycelial growth and intensive dissimilation of glucose; it is designated as trophophase. The second phase occurs at the end of exponential growth by the mold. Onset of this phase, designated as idiophase, is accompanied by a reduced demand for oxygen and also by synthesis of products that are called secondary metabolites. When a mold colony is growing, these two phases can occur in that single colony. Growth is mature where spores are located in the colony, but the mold is actively growing where sporulation has not occurred. Hence, both primary metabolism (trophophase) and secondary metabolism

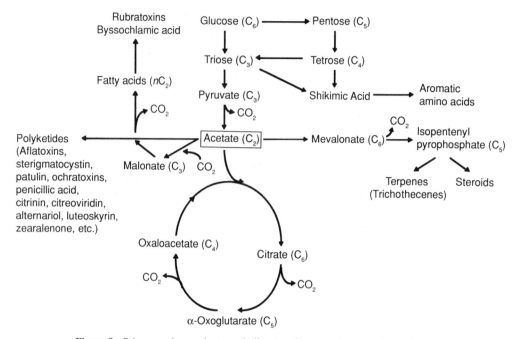

Figure 8 Primary and secondary metabolism together result in biosynthesis of mycotoxins via several pathways. Adapted from J. Reiss, ed. (1981). "Mykotoxine in Lebensmitteln." Fischer, Jena.

(idiophase) can be proceeding simultaneously. The onset of secondary metabolism is usually accompanied by development of spores or sclerotia.

There is a series of metabolic pathways involved in the biosynthesis of mycotoxins. These processes and some mycotoxins arising from each are illustrated in Fig. 8. General descriptions, but not details, of these pathways will follow. The first of these is the so-called polyketide pathway. This involves two-carbon fragments which have their origin in acetic acid and malic acid as a consequence of other metabolic events in the mold. These two-carbon fragments undergo head-to-tail condensation, followed by reduction, cyclization, oxidative coupling, and alkylation of the carbon atoms of methylene groups which may be present. The polyketide pathway is the way most of these secondary metabolites, for example, mycotoxins, are produced.

Another biosynthetic process is the terpenoid pathway. In this pathway, acetyl CoA from primary metabolism goes through several steps and is converted to mevalonate, from which terpenes and steroids are ultimately formed.

The third possible process involves the citric acid cycle. Commonly, acetic acid and oxaloacetic acid condense to form citric acid. In the synthesis of rubratoxin and byssochlamic acid, acetic acid is replaced by longer-chain acids.

Finally, some synthetic processes involve amino acids that can originate in various places in metabolic processes and serve as starting material for synthesis of certain mycotoxins. Often amino acids will combine with metabolites such as polyketides.

VIII.   Universality of the Mycotoxin Problem

It is necessary to recognize the worldwide nature of the mycotoxin problem. There is probably no place which is totally free of this difficulty, because molds can grow almost anywhere. Consequently mycotoxin-containing products have been found all over the world: Africa, Europe, India, the Philippines, Taiwan, Thailand, the United States, and elsewhere. The extent of the problem is greater in some parts of the world than in others because their climatic conditions are more favorable for mold growth and thus synthesis of mycotoxins. Furthermore, the degree of care which is exercised in producing, processing, and storing foods varies from country to country. Hence, wherever care is lacking, thus facilitating growth of mold, the problem will be greater than in places where greater care is taken to protect food from invasion by and subsequent growth of mold.

In the United States control of aflatoxin contamination in food products is the responsibility of the Food and Drug Administration (FDA) and the U.S. Department of Agriculture (USDA). The USDA oversees peanut products, which in the past have been a major concern. The FDA is concerned with other foods. In the United States, the action level for aflatoxin in food is 20 ppb except for aflatoxin M_1 in milk, where the action level is 0.5 ppb. From time to time consideration has been given to reducing the 20-ppb value, but as of early 1990 it had not been done. The original 20-ppb value resulted because it was the smallest amount that could be detected conveniently at the time the guideline was established. In the meantime, methods have become far more sensitive, so from that standpoint the limit could be reduced. Lower values have been established in some countries.

IX.   Factors That Control Mycotoxin Production

Finally, some comments will be made about the major factors that control mycotoxin production. The first to be considered is temperature. Some information about this factor appears throughout this chapter and will not be repeated. It should be emphasized, however, that some molds can produce toxins at lower temperatures than others. For some molds, temperature cycling can enhance toxin production. Furthermore, for each mold there is a low temperature beyond which it will not produce toxin; likewise, there is a high temperature beyond which the mold will not produce toxin and ultimately will not grow. These temperatures vary from mold to mold.

Moisture is the second factor which must be considered. It is well known that molds require less moisture for growth than do yeasts or bacteria. The moisture in a product must be available, and this availability can be expressed as water activity (a_w). The optimal a_w value for toxin production by toxigenic fungi is in the range of

0.93–0.98. The limiting a_w value, the value below which they do not produce toxin, is in the range of 0.71–0.94, depending on the mold in question.

Another factor is degree of aeration or amount of oxygen that is present. This has also been considered elsewhere in this chapter and so will not be discussed further here.

The pH value of the substrate also can affect production of mycotoxins. Generally toxin production is favored by pH values in the range of about 3.4–5.5. Some toxigenic molds can grow over a much wider range of pH starting at about pH 2 and continuing to about 10, depending, in part, on the acid present in the substrate. Many of the toxigenic molds can initiate growth at the low pH values and then will cause the pH value of the substrate to increase so it becomes more favorable for toxin production. However, a low pH, within reasonable limits, does not preclude toxin production.

We also need to be concerned with the substrate. A substrate high in carbohydrate content is most suitable for toxin production. However, molds also can produce toxins on substrates that are relatively high in their content of protein or fat, as is evident from production of aflatoxin in peanuts and cheese. In spite of this, the ideal substrate for maximum yield of mycotoxins generally is high in carbohydrate content and relatively lower in content of fat or protein.

The final consideration is that of microbial interaction. In the real world, toxigenic molds seldom exist on products as pure cultures. Instead, they probably occur together with other molds, with yeasts, and with bacteria. These other microorganisms can have an impact on the amount of toxin that is produced by the toxigenic mold and also on stability of the toxin in the substrate. There are some molds or bacteria that can stimulate toxin production, whereas others tend to inhibit toxin production. Some molds, at least one bacterium, and at least one yeast (baker's yeast) can reduce the amount of certain mycotoxins in the substrate. Unfortunately, the exact effect of a given microorganism on a toxigenic mold is not predictable with certainty.

The best way to control the mycotoxin problem is to prevent biosynthesis of these secondary metabolites in foods or feeds. An understanding of the factors just described and application of the information in ways suitable to a given food (or feed) processing, storing, and distributing system should help to minimize contamination of our foods with mycotoxins.

Bibliography

Applebaum, R. S., and Marth, E. H. (1981). Biogenesis of the C_{20} polyketide, aflatoxin. A review. *Mycopathologia* **76**, 103–114.

Applebaum, R. S., Brackett, R. E., Wiseman, D. W., and Marth, E. H. (1982). Aflatoxin: Toxicity to dairy cattle and occurrence in milk products—A review. *J. Food Prot.* **45**, 752–777.

Bauer, V. H. (1973). "Das Antonius-Feuer in Kunst und Medizin." Springer-Verlag, Berlin.

Bullerman, L. B. (1979). Significance of mycotoxins to food safety and human health. *J. Food Prot.* **42**, 65–86.

Doyle, M. P., Applebaum, R. S., Brackett, R. E., and Marth, E. H. (1982). Physical, chemical and biological degradation of mycotoxins in foods and agricultural commodities. *J. Food Prot.* **45**, 964–971.

Reiss, J., ed. (1981). "Mykotoxine in Lebensmitteln." Fischer, Jena.

Rusul, G., and Marth, E. H. (1988). Food additives and plant components control growth and aflatoxin production by toxigenic aspergilli: A review. *Mycopathologia* **101,** 13–23.

Yousef, A. E., and Marth, E. H. (1989). Aflatoxin M_1: Stability and degradation. *In* "Mycotoxins in Dairy Products" (H. P. van Egmond, ed.), pp. 127–161. Elsevier, London.

CHAPTER 9

OTHER MICROBIAL INTOXICATIONS

Steve L. Taylor

I. Introduction

Microbial intoxications are diseases caused by toxins elaborated by microorganisms, usually bacteria. In the case of foodborne microbial intoxications, the toxin is
usually produced during the growth of the bacteria in the food. The bacteria are
often destroyed by subsequent processing or preparation of the food, but the toxin
may remain depending on its stability. The intoxication occurs when sufficient
quantities of active toxin are ingested regardless of whether viable bacteria are
consumed at the same time.

Microbial intoxications share several common features. As just mentioned, a
microbially produced toxin is the causative agent. The onset time, the time between
ingestion of the incriminated food and the onset of symptoms, usually is relatively
short, ranging from minutes to several hours. The severity and duration of the
symptoms are variable depending on the nature of the toxin. Preventive measures
typically involve destruction or hindering the growth of the responsible bacteria.

Several microbial intoxications, staphylococcal food poisoning, and botulism
have been discussed in previous chapters. Several other microbial intoxications can
be foodborne, and one of these illnesses, histamine poisoning, occurs frequently.

II. Monoamine Intoxications

A. The Formation of Monoamines

Monoamines are formed by the decarboxylation of amino acids. A general amino acid
decarboxylation reaction is depicted in Fig. 1. These decarboxylation reactions are
catalyzed by amino acid decarboxylase enzymes found in certain bacteria. Small
quantities of the monoamines also exist in plants, probably the result of their
formation by plant amino acid decarboxylases. The majority of monoamine intoxications have been associated with tyramine, the decarboxylation product of tyrosine.
Other monoamines of some importance in monoamine intoxications include 2-
phenylethylamine (derived from phenylalanine), tryptamine (derived from tryptophan), and serotonin and dopamine (naturally occurring plant monoamines). The
structures of tyramine, 2-phenylethylamine, and tryptamine are shown in Fig. 2.

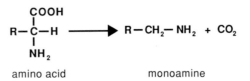

amino acid   monoamine

Figure 1   General reaction for the decarboxylation of amino acids.

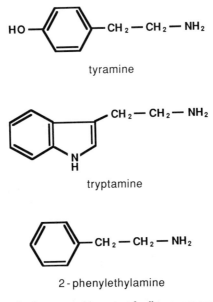

Figure 2 Structures of important foodborne monoamines.

B. Clinical Features

The symptoms of monoamine intoxications typically appear within minutes to a few hours after ingestion of the incriminated food. The duration of symptoms usually ranges from 10 minutes to about 6 hours.

The symptoms of monoamine intoxication include palpitations, severe headache, hypertension, flushing, profuse perspiration, stiff neck, nausea, vomiting, and prostration. It is unlikely that all of these symptoms will be observed in every case. The most typical symptoms for making a tentative diagnosis of monoamine intoxication are severe headache and hypertension, which are also among the most commonly encountered symptoms. These monoamines are often known as pressor amines because they will cause an increase in blood pressure. The hypertension likely leads to the development of the headache.

C. Occurrence

Monoamine intoxications occur infrequently. Most individuals can ingest rather large quantities of these monoamines with no ill effects. For example, up to 80 mg of tyramine can be taken orally with no elevation in blood pressure. Foodborne monoamines are not hazardous to most individuals, because the monoamines are detoxified in the gastrointestinal tract. However, individuals taking certain types of therapeutic drugs have a diminished capability for detoxifying the monoamines. These individuals are at risk for monoamine intoxications if they consume certain types of food while taking these medications. The association between the ingestion of certain foods and hypertensive crises immediately after meals for patients taking these medications was first made in the early 1960s. Several severe reactions and deaths occurred before the association with intake of certain foods was made. These drugs now contain a warning to avoid eating foods that serve as significant sources of monoamines. As a result of this increased awareness, incidents of monoamine intoxications have declined considerably.

D. Bacterial Sources of Monoamines

Tyrosine decarboxylase, the enzyme involved in the formation of tyramine, is found in several types of bacteria that commonly occur in foods. The Group D streptococci are the most important tyramine-producing bacteria. Other bacteria possessing tyrosine decarboxylase include most clostridia, especially *Clostridium perfringens* and *C. sporogenes,* a few lactobacilli, *Leuconostoc cremoris,* some strains of *Escherichia coli,* and some strains of the various *Proteus* species.

Phenylalanine decarboxylase, the enzyme that catalyzes the formation of 2-phenylethylamine, is not widely distributed in bacteria. This enzyme is known to exist only in some strains of *Streptococcus faecalis* and a few unusual *Pseudomonas* species.

The distribution of tryptophan decarboxylase, the enzyme that catalyzes the conversion of tryptophan to tryptamine, in bacteria has not been studied. However, small quantities of tryptamine are found in certain fermented products, such as cheeses.

E. Foods Associated with Monoamine Intoxication

The food most commonly involved in episodes of monoamine intoxication is cheese, particularly aged cheddar cheese. Numerous incidents of hypertensive crises associated with cheeses were recorded in the medical literature of the early 1960s. Tyramine is the primary monoamine responsible for these cheese-associated episodes, although cheeses may also contain small amounts of tryptamine and 2-phenylethylamine. Cheddar cheese can contain up to 1800 ppm tyramine, while other cheeses typically contain somewhat lesser amounts of tyramine (Table I). The Group D streptococci frequently proliferate during the fermentation of cheeses and are likely responsible for most of the tyramine formation. Because tyrosine decarboxylase is more widely distributed in bacteria than either phenylalanine or tryptophan decarboxylase, tyramine is the monoamine that is most frequently implicated in episodes of monoamine intoxication. Tyramine intoxication has also been observed to occur with pickled herring, yeast extract (commonly eaten as a condiment in England), and chicken livers.

Other monoamines have been implicated in a few episodes of monoamine intoxication, including 2-phenylethylamine in chocolate and dopamine, a naturally occurring monoamine, in broad beans. The "Physician's Desk Reference" lists a variety of other foods that should be avoided by individuals taking the drugs that interfere with the ability to detoxify the monoamines. Included in this list in addition to the foods mentioned above are sour cream, wine, beer, sherry, canned figs, raisins, bananas, avocados, soy sauce, and meats treated with tenderizer.

Table I
Monoamine Levels in Cheeses

Type of cheese	Monoamine level (ppm)		
	Tyramine	Tryptamine	Phenylethylamine
Camembert	70–660	ND–60[a]	ND
Cheddar	ND–1800	ND–2	ND–303
Cottage	6–13	—	ND
Danish blue	166	—	ND–10
Gouda	80–670	ND–200	ND–4
Processed	11–72	ND–1	ND–155
Roquefort	50–1100	ND–1100	—
Swiss	ND–276	ND	ND–78

[a]ND, not detected.

F.   Detoxification of Monoamines

Monoamines, such as tyramine, are detoxified by the enzyme monoamine oxidase (MAO), which converts the monoamines to less toxic aldehyde products. The detoxification of tyramine by MAO is depicted in Fig. 3. Monoamine oxidase is present in all tissues. The activity of MAO is very high in the gastrointestinal tract, which may be important for the detoxification of foodborne monoamines. Monoamine oxidase is a mitochondrial marker enzyme. Two distinct types of MAO, namely MAO-A and MAO-B, are known to exist. These different forms of MAO are distributed somewhat differently in tissues and have somewhat different substrate specificities. Together, the two forms of MAO display a very wide substrate specificity and will act on all of the major foodborne monoamines including tyramine, tryptamine, 2-phenylethylamine, dopamine, and serotonin.

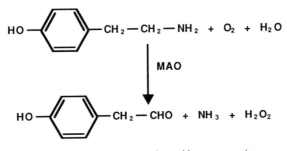

Figure 3   Action of monoamine oxidase on tyramine.

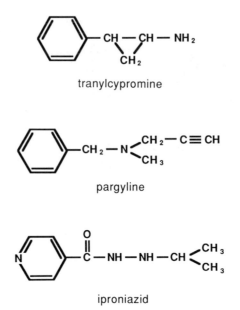

Figure 4   Structures of monoamine oxidase-inhibiting drugs.

G.   Monoamine Oxidase Inhibitors

Several drugs are monoamine oxidases inhibitors (MAOI), including tranylcypromine, pargyline, and iproniazid (Fig. 4). Tranylcypromine and pargyline were introduced as antidepressive drugs in the late 1950s. They are extremely potent MAOI, and it is that property which is responsible for their pharmacological efficacy. The widespread use of tranylcypromine and pargyline after their introduction was soon followed by the observations of hypertensive crises in patients who consumed cheeses while taking these drugs and led to the discovery of this classical food–drug interaction.

H.   Preventive Measures

Individuals taking MAO-inhibiting drugs should be informed of the hazards of eating foods that contain high levels of monoamines such as tyramine. Where possible, other drugs without these side-effects should be substituted for the MAO-inhibiting drugs. Of course, such substitutions may not always be possible, because the MAO-inhibiting drugs are extremely effective in the treatment of certain conditions.

III.   Histamine Intoxication

A.   Formation of Histamine

Histamine is formed from the amino acid histidine by the action of the enzyme histidine decarboxylase (Fig. 5).

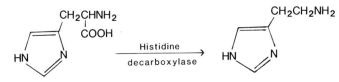

Figure 5 Histidine decarboxylase reaction. Reprinted with permission from S. L. Taylor (1986). Histamine food poisoning: toxicology and clinical aspects. *CRC Crit. Rev. Toxicol.* **17**, 91–128.

B. Clinical Features

The symptoms of histamine intoxication, or scombroid fish poisoning, usually begin within minutes to a few hours of ingestion of the incriminated food. The duration of the symptoms is usually less than 12 hours. The symptoms include intense headache, flushing, dizziness, nausea, vomiting, diarrhea, oral burning sensation (peppery taste), abdominal pain, palpitations, hypotension, edema, hives, and itching. Individuals suffering from histamine intoxication will usually have only a few of these symptoms.

The symptoms of histamine poisoning are not particularly definitive. Consequently, this illness is frequently misdiagnosed. The most characteristic symptoms, such as hives, do not occur in many cases of histamine intoxication. Histamine intoxication is frequently confused diagnostically with an allergic reaction. Many of the same symptoms are observed in an allergic reaction, since histamine is the primary *in vivo* mediator of allergic disease. Also, antihistamine therapy will be equally effective in allergies and histamine intoxication. However, histamine poisoning can be easily distinguished from a food allergy by (1) the lack of a previous history of allergic reactions to the implicated food(s), (2) an attack rate of nearly 100% in group outbreaks of histamine intoxication, and (3) the detection of high levels of histamine in the incriminated food.

C. Occurrence

Table II shows the number of outbreaks and cases of histamine intoxication reported in the United States for the years from 1976 to 1981. Outbreaks of histamine intoxication have also occurred with some frequency in England and Japan. In all likelihood, many small outbreaks of histamine intoxication are either misdiagnosed or unreported because of its mild and transitory nature. Large outbreaks occur rarely in the United States, but a large outbreak did occur in 1973 involving more than 230 cases in four states associated with ingestion of commercially canned tuna.

D. Bacterial Sources of Histamine

Histidine decarboxylase is not widely distributed among bacteria. Bacteria known to produce high levels of histamine include *Morganella morganii*, some strains of *Klebsiella pneumoniae*, *Enterobacter aerogenes*, *Clostridium perfringens*, some strains of *Hafnia alvei*, *Lactobacillus buchneri*, and *Lactobacillus delbreuckii*. The enteric bacteria, such as *M. morganii* and *K. pneumoniae*, are responsible for

Table II
Outbreaks of Histamine Intoxication in the United States
(1976–1981)

Year	Outbreaks	Cases	Implicated food (number of outbreaks)
1976	3	43	Tuna (1)
			Mahi mahi (1)
			Swiss cheese (1)
1977	13	71	Tuna (5)
			Mahi mahi (3)
			Bluefish (3)
			Yellowtail (1)
			Anchovies (1)
1978	7	30	Mahi mahi (7)
1979	12	132	Mahi mahi (5)
			Tuna (2)
			Other fish (5)
1980	29	153	Mahi mahi (21)
			Tuna (3)
			Other fish (5)
1981	7	67	Tuna (4)
			Mahi mahi (2)
			Other fish (1)

histamine formation in fish, while the lactobacilli are likely responsible for histamine formation in cheeses.

E. Foods Associated with Histamine Intoxication

Fish are the foods most commonly implicated in outbreaks of histamine intoxication. This foodborne disease is sometimes referred to as scombroid fish poisoning because of the frequent involvement of the families Scomberesocidae and Scombridae including tuna, mackerel, and bonito. However, nonscombroid fish are also widely implicated in outbreaks of histamine intoxication. The nonscombroid fish include mahi mahi, sardines, bluefish, yellowtail, and herring. Bacterial formation of hazardous levels of histamine can occur during the spoilage of any fish that has appreciable levels of free histidine in its tissues, as is the case with all of the fishes mentioned above.

Cheese, especially Swiss cheese, has been implicated in a few outbreaks of histamine intoxication.

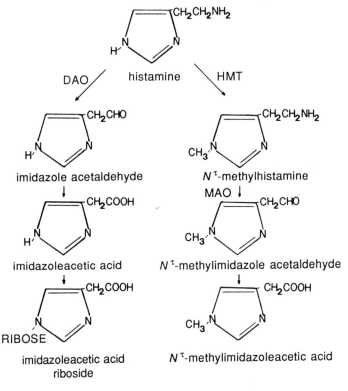

Figure 6 Histamine metabolism pathways.

F. Detoxification Mechanisms

Histamine is metabolized by two enzymatic pathways catalyzed by diamine oxidase (DAO) and histidine N-methyltransferase (HMT). These pathways are illustrated in Fig. 6; the major products, imidazoleacetic acid and N-methylimidazoleacetic acid, are much less toxic than histamine and are readily excreted in the urine. In humans, DAO is localized almost exclusively in the small intestine. Orally administered histamine is metabolized predominantly by the DAO pathway in humans. Diamine oxidase is a nonspecific enzyme that catalyzes the oxidation of a variety of diamines. In contrast, HMT has very strict substrate requirements and acts only on histamine. The HMT pathway predominates in all human tissues except the intestinal tract.

Humans can tolerate a dose of 150 mg of histamine orally with only mild or no adverse reactions. However, humans eating spoiled tuna containing in excess of 50 mg of histamine per 100 g will always develop more serious symptoms of the type described earlier. In all likelihood, these symptoms are developing at doses below 150 mg of histamine. Diamine oxidase and HMT will detoxify histamine ingested with food, but factors must exist in spoiled tuna which interfere with the detoxification process.

G. Inhibitors of Histamine-Metabolizing Enzymes

Spoiled fish and other foods may possess inhibitors of DAO and HMT that interfere with the detoxification of histamine and potentiate the toxicity of histamine. Several other putrefactive amines commonly found in spoiled food, including cadaverine, putrescine, and tyramine, will inhibit DAO and HMT and increase the intestinal absorption and urinary excretion of unmetabolized histamine. Some pharmacologic agents including isoniazid are also inhibitors of DAO and HMT; isoniazid therapy has been implicated as a factor in several outbreaks of histamine intoxication.

H. Preventive Measures

The key to prevention of histamine intoxication is to prevent histamine formation in foods. Holding fish at temperatures below 5°C after catching them will prevent histamine formation. Control of histamine formation in cheese is tied to reduction of the numbers of histamine-producing bacteria in the raw milk.

IV. Bongkrek Food Poisoning

Bongkrek food poisoning was once common in Indonesia but has not occurred in the United States. The symptoms of this foodborne disease include hypoglycemia, severe spasms, convulsions, and death.

This illness is associated with the consumption of bongkrek, which are flat white cakes made from pressed coconut and fermented with the fungus *Rhizopus oryzae*. The cakes are wrapped in banana leaves during the fermentation. The toxin known as bongkrek acid (Fig. 7) is produced by *Pseudomonas cocovenenans,* which overgrows the fungus under some conditions. Bongkrek acid is a heat stable, unsaturated fatty acid. The bacterial overgrowth can be prevented by use of oxalis leaves rather than banana leaves. The oxalis leaves contribute to a rapid drop in pH to about 5.5, which prevents the growth of *P. cocovenenans*. The substitution of oxalis leaves has largely eliminated bongkrek food poisoning.

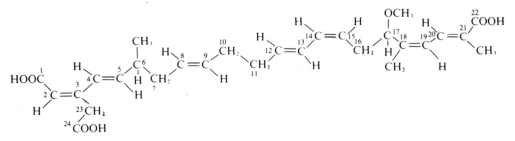

Figure 7   Structure of bongkrek acid.

V.   Fermented Corn Flour Poisoning

Between 1961 and 1979, 327 known cases of intoxication with 101 deaths were reported in the People's Republic of China associated with the ingestion of fermented corn flour. The disease had a short onset period and was characterized by abdominal discomfort, mild diarrhea, and vomiting. In severe cases, the disease progressed to jaundice, coma, delirium, oliguria, hematuria, rigidity of the extremities, urinary retention, toxic shock, and death.

The toxin responsible for this illness is produced by *Flavobacterium farinofermentans*. The toxin was recently identified as bongkrek acid (Fig. 7). This foodborne illness can be prevented by properly controlling the fermentation of the corn flour by ensuring that the pH of the fermentation is sufficiently high. The fermented corn meal produced in the affected regions of China was made under conditions of neutral pH. Under alkaline conditions, the growth of *F. farinofermentans* would be discouraged, and the toxin is unstable.

VI.   Intoxications Caused by Nitrate-Reducing Bacteria

The reduction of nitrate produces nitrite, which can be acutely toxic to humans. The symptoms of nitrite intoxication are methemoglobinemia, nausea, vomiting, headache, weakness, shortness of breath, cyanosis, collapse, and occasionally death. Most cases of nitrite intoxication involve inadvertent addition of meat-curing salts containing nitrite to other foods; these outbreaks do not involve bacterial conversion of nitrate to nitrite.

Nitrate occurs in plants naturally but levels can be increased as the result of application of nitrogen-based fertilizers. Some plants will accumulate more nitrate/nitrite in their edible tissues than others; but considerable variability is observed depending on species, variety, plant part, stage of maturity, and environmental conditions such as drought, harvest temperatures, nutrient deficiencies, insect damage, use of herbicides and/or insecticides, and fertilizer application. Some plants possess the enzyme nitrate reductase, which will convert nitrate to nitrite, but in most plants, the majority of the nitrate/nitrite remains in the nitrate form, which is less toxic.

Bacteria can also possess nitrate reductase and convert the nitrate in plant tissues to nitrite. Improper storage of spinach and carrot juice at elevated temperatures, which encourages bacterial growth, has contributed to cases of nitrite intoxication involving bacterial formation of nitrite. Many common bacteria possess nitrate reductase including pseudomonads, Enterobacteriaceae, staphylococci, and *Clostridium perfringens*. Proper storage of nitrate-containing plants at refrigerated temperatures will prevent bacterial nitrite formation.

Bibliography

Fassett, D. W. (1973). Nitrates and nitrites. *In* "Toxicants Occurring Naturally in Foods" (Natl. Acad. Sci., Comm. Food Prot., ed.), pp. 7–25. Natl. Acad. Sci., Washington, D.C.

Hu, W. J., Zhang, G. S., Chu, F. S., Meng, H. D., and Meng, Z. H. (1984). Purification and partial characterization of flavotoxin A. *Appl. Environ. Microbiol.* **48,** 690–693.

Keating, J. P., Lell, M. E., Straus, A. W., Zarkowsky, H., and Smith, G. E. (1973). Infantile methemoglobinemia caused by carrot juice. *N. Engl. J. Med.* **288,** 825–826.

Marley, E., and Blackwell, B. (1970). Interactions of monoamine oxidase inhibitors, amines, and foodstuffs. *Adv. Pharmacol. Chemother.* **8,** 185–249.

Taylor, S. L. (1986). Histamine food poisoning: toxicology and clinical aspects. *CRC Crit. Rev. Toxicol.* **17,** 91–128.

van Veen, A. G. (1967). The Bongkrek toxins. *In* "Biochemistry of Some Foodborne Microbial Toxins" (R. I. Mateles and G. N. Wogan, eds.), pp. 43–50. MIT Press, Cambridge, Massachusetts.

CHAPTER 10

CHEMICAL INTOXICATIONS

Steve L. Taylor

I. Introduction

In this chapter, the potential hazards associated with man-made chemicals in foods will be discussed. Naturally occurring toxicants have already been addressed.

A. Incidence of Foodborne Disease Outbreaks of Chemical Etiology

Chemical intoxications account for about 20–30% of all acute foodborne disease outbreaks according to statistics compiled by the Centers for Disease Control (CDC). However, many of the causes of these chemical intoxications are naturally occurring chemicals. In the previous chapters, the importance of the seafood toxins such as ciguatera toxins, paralytic shellfish toxins, and histamine was emphasized. Mushroom toxins are another common cause of acute chemical intoxications associated with foods. Man-made chemicals actually account for a very small percentage of the foodborne disease outbreaks reported to the CDC. Most of these incidents have involved inadvertant or accidental contamination of foods with heavy metals or detergents.

Of course, not all foodborne disease outbreaks of chemical etiology will be reported to the CDC. Reporting is not mandated. Some of the illnesses are either mild and short-lived or difficult to ascribe to particular man-made chemicals in foods. Thus, incomplete reporting of acute intoxications associated with foodborne chemicals of man-made origin is a certainty. Also, the CDC do not attempt to define cause-and-effect relationships between man-made chemicals in foods and chronic diseases such as cancer.

B. Types of Chemicals Involved in Chemical Intoxications Associated with Foods

The major categories of man-made chemicals that can occur in foods are agricultural chemicals (insecticides, herbicides, fungicides, fertilizers, feed additives, and veterinary drugs), food additives, chemicals migrating from packaging materials, and inadvertant or accidental contaminants including industrial and environmental pollutants. Chemicals produced by reactions occurring during the processing, preparation, storage, and handling of foods could also be considered man-made, because these processes occur through the intervention of humans. Table I lists some examples of chemicals in each of these categories that will serve as examples in this chapter.

II. Agricultural Chemical Residues

A. Insecticides

Insecticides are added to foods and feeds to control the extent of insect contamination. In areas of the world where insecticides are not widely used, a substantial

Table I

Examples of Man-Made Chemicals Found in Foods

Agricultural chemicals

  Insecticides

    Organochlorines (DDT, heptachlor)

    Organophosphates (malathion, parathion)

    Carbamates (aldicarb, carbaryl)

    Botanicals (pyrethrum, nicotine)

    Inorganics (arsenicals)

  Herbicides

    Chlorophenoxy compounds (2, 4-D)

    Dinitrophenols

    Bipyridyls (paraquat, diquat)

    Substituted ureas (monuron)

    Carbamates (propham)

    Triazines (simazine)

  Fungicides

    Captan

    Folpet

    Dithiocarbamates

    Pentachlorophenol

    Mercurials

  Fertilizers

    Nitrogen fertilizers

    Sewage sludge

  Feed additives and veterinary drugs

Food additives

  GRAS ingredients

  Direct additives

  Color additives

Chemicals migrating from packaging materials

  Monomers, plasticizers, and stabilizers

  Compounds from printing inks

  Inorganic chemicals—lead and tin

Chemicals produced during processing, preparation, storage, and handling of foods

  Nitrosamines

  Mutagens from heat processing of meats

  Polycyclic aromatic hydrocarbons

  Lipid oxidation products

Inadvertant or accidental contaminants

  Industrial/environmental pollutants

    PCBs and PBBs

    Mercury

  Chemicals from utensils

  Accidents and errors

portion of the food is lost to insects. The major types of insecticides added to food crops in the United States are organochlorine compounds (e.g., DDT and chlordane), organophosphate compounds (e.g., parathion and malathion), carbamate compounds (e.g., carbaryl and aldicarb), botanical compounds (e.g., nicotine and pyrethrum), and inorganic compounds (e.g., arsenicals). The Environmental Protection Agency (EPA) regulates the manner in which insecticides can be used. Insecticides are approved for use on only certain crops. The EPA also establishes tolerances for the amounts of insecticide residues allowed on raw food crops. The Food and Drug Administration (FDA) has tolerances for the amounts of insecticide residues that can exist on processed foods.

Several characteristics of insecticides merit consideration when one is trying to compare their safety. Some insecticides will accumulate in the environment. DDT and the other organochlorine compounds are good examples of insecticides that accumulate in the environment. Concerns were voiced about this environmental accumulation because DDT is a weak animal carcinogen and because it may have adverse effects on certain types of wildlife. For example, DDT residues may have interfered with the reproductive efficiency of certain birds. Therefore, DDT use was banned in the United States. The alternative has been to use insecticides which do not accumulate in the environment. However, these insecticides tend to be more acutely toxic to humans and other animals. Certain of the organophosphate insecticides such as parathion pose a substantial hazard to farm workers because of their degree of toxicity in humans and because they can be absorbed through the skin. However, the organophosphates and carbamates are widely used because they do decompose rather rapidly in the environment. Insects can develop resistance to various insecticides. Thus, the arsenal of insecticides must be rather large to prevent the recurrent exposures of the insects that would result in the development of resistance.

While the exceedingly low residue levels of insecticides found in most foods are not particularly hazardous, large doses of insecticides can be toxic to humans and other animals. Many of the common insecticides are neurotoxins. The organophosphates and carbamates are cholinesterase inhibitors. Cholinesterase is a key enzyme involved in the transmission of nerve impulses at the synapse. The neurotoxic mechanism of the organochlorines is unknown. The arsenicals are a particularly hazardous class of insecticides which are fairly toxic to humans and which also tend to accumulate in the environment.

No food poisoning incidents have ever been attributed to the proper use of insecticides on foods. Several incidents have occurred as the result of improper use of insecticides, however. Several reasons exist for the low degree of hazard posed by insecticide residues on foods: (1) the level of exposure is very low if the insecticides are used properly; (2) some insecticides are not very toxic to humans; (3) some insecticides decompose rapidly in the environment; and (4) many different insecticides are used, which limits our exposure to any one particular insecticide. Problems can arise from the inappropriate use of certain insecticides. A good example is the outbreak of aldicarb intoxication from watermelons that occurred on the West Coast several years ago. It is illegal to use aldicarb on watermelons because excessive levels of the insecticide are concentrated in the edible portion of the melon. Several farmers used aldicarb on watermelons illegally, resulting in several cases of aldicarb intoxication and the recall and destruction of thousands of watermelons.

B. Herbicides

Herbicides are applied to agricultural lands and crops to control the growth of weeds. Many different types of herbicides are used. Among the more important classes of herbicides are chlorophenoxy compounds (e.g., 2,4-D and 2,4,5-T), dinitrophenols (e.g., dinitroorthocresol), bipyridyl compounds (e..g, paraquat and diquat), substituted ureas (e.g., monuron), carbamates (e.g., propham), and tri-azines (e.g., simazine). Again, the EPA controls which herbicides can be used on various crops and establishes limits on the allowable residue levels.

In assessing the potential risks from the use of herbicides on foods, the toxicity of the herbicides, their environmental half-lives, and the presence of toxic impurities must be considered. Most herbicides are selectively toxic toward plants. Thus, they present very little hazard to humans. Exceptions are the bipyridyl compounds, such as paraquat and diquat. These bipyridyl compounds are nonselective herbicides; they are usually used to kill all vegetative growth in an area. For example, they were sprayed on marijuana fields in Mexico as a means of reducing illegal shipments of that recreational drug into the United States. However, the bipyridyl compounds are also rather toxic to humans, and their use should be closely monitored. Most herbicides do not accumulate in the environment. Highly toxic impurities have not been identified in most herbicides. An exception is the chlorophenoxy compound 2,4,5-trichlorophenoxy acetic acid or 2,4,5-T. During the Vietnam War, large quan-tities of this herbicide, known as Agent Orange, were sprayed as part of the defolia-tion program. Some batches of Agent Orange contained a highly toxic class of impurities, the dioxins, including tetrachlorodibenzodioxin (TCDD).

Generally, herbicide residues in foods do not represent any hazard to consumers. No food poisoning incidents have ever resulted from the proper use of herbicides on food crops. The lack of hazard from herbicide residues is associated with the low level of exposure, their low degree of toxicity and selective toxicity toward plants, and the use of many different herbicides which limits exposure to any particular herbicide.

C. Fungicides

Fungicides are used to prevent the growth of molds on food crops. Some of the more important fungicides are captan, folpet, dithiocarbamates, pentachlorophenol, and mercurials. The hazards associated with fungicides are miniscule because our ex-posure to these chemicals is very low, most of the fungicides do not accumulate in the environment, and most fungicides are not very toxic to humans. Pentachloro-phenol and the mercurials do persist in the environment. The mercurials are often used to treat seed grains to prevent mold growth during the storage of these grain seeds. The seed grains treated with the mercurials are usually colored pink or some other noticeable color. These treated grains are clearly intended for planting and not for direct consumption. On several occasions, consumers have eaten these seed grains and developed mercury poisoning. The mercurials are quite hazardous to humans and care must be taken to avoid the consumption of seeds treated with these fungicides.

D. Fertilizers

The most commonly used fertilizers are combinations of nitrogen and phosphorus compounds. Nitrogen fertilizers stimulate the growth of plants but must first be oxidized to nitrate and nitrite in the soil. Both nitrate and nitrite can be hazardous to humans if ingested in large amounts. The major problem is the contamination of ground water with nitrate. This ground water is often used as drinking water on farms and in farming communities. Infants can suffer from methemoglobinemia, a blood disorder associated with an inability of hemoglobin to carry oxygen, if they routinely consume water that has nitrate residues exceeding 10 ppm. Some plants can accumulate nitrate. An example is spinach. If spinach or other nitrate-accumulating plants are allowed to grow on soil overly fertilized with ammonia or other nitrogen fertilizers, the spinach can accumulate hazardous levels of nitrate. This situation can become even more serious if nitrate-reducing bacteria are allowed to proliferate on these foods. In that case, some of the nitrate is converted to the more hazardous nitrite. A discussion of the hazards associated with nitrite produced by bacteria can be found in Chapter 9 on other microbial intoxications. Only a few instances of food poisoning have occurred in this manner, and all of these incidents have involved infants eating spinach or other plants containing excessive nitrate and/or nitrite. Actually, these incidents are the result of the inappropriate use of excessive amounts of nitrogen-based fertilizers.

An increasingly important fertilizer is sewage sludge. Sewage sludge has the potential to carry any toxic chemicals that might be dumped into the sewage system. Most of the concerns have centered around residues of heavy metals, such as cadmium, from industrial activities. The residues of heavy metals are concentrated by some plants. Thus, sewage sludge should be monitored periodically for certain types of toxic chemicals.

The degree of hazard associated with the use of fertilizers on food-producing land is quite low. The few incidents that have occurred have involved excessive use of the fertilizers.

E. Feed Additives

Some chemicals are added to feed to serve as growth stimulants. Diethylstilbestrol (DES) was once allowed to be used as a growth promoter with beef cattle. However, when DES was shown to be carcinogenic, its use as a feed additive was banned. Diethylstilbestrol is definitely carcinogenic to humans; its use as a drug to prevent miscarriages in pregnant women has been directly linked to certain types of cancer in their offspring. However, no evidence exists to demonstrate that the extremely low levels of DES found in edible beef after its use as a growth promoter pose any carcinogenic hazard to humans.

F. Veterinary Drugs and Antibiotics

Antibiotics are widely used with food-producing animals. Penicillin is often used to treat mastitis in cows. Concerns over the effects of penicillin residues in milk on consumers with penicillin allergy led the FDA to enact a zero tolerance for penicillin in milk. That action has not prevented penicillin use, but has resulted in the dumping of milk from treated cows during the treatment period and for a short time thereafter. The hazards associated with other antibiotics are generally limited to concerns about their role in the development of antibiotic-resistant bacteria. That particular concern is beyond the scope of this chapter.

III. Food Additives

Numerous ingredients are knowingly added to foods to provide a wide variety of technical benefits. Several thousand food additives exist, but many of these chemicals are used in rather small amounts. Food additives can be classified on the basis of their regulatory standing: (1) generally recognized as safe (GRAS) substances, (2) flavors and extracts, (3) direct additives, and (4) color additives.

Generally recognized as safe substances are those food ingredients that were in common use before the latest version of the Food, Drug, and Cosmetic (FD&C) Act which was enacted in 1958. The 1958 Act required FDA approval of any newly developed food additives but recognized the long history of safe use of many additives. Over 600 chemicals are on the GRAS list including such materials as sucrose, salt, butylated hydroxytoluene (BHT), and spices. Most of the common food additives are on the GRAS list because they were in common use before 1958. From a legal standpoint, GRAS chemicals are not actually additives, but that distinction is seldom made by the consumer. Reviews of the safety of the GRAS substances have been conducted since 1958 and deficiencies in our information on their toxicity have been identified and corrected in some cases. Substances or certain uses of substances can be removed from the GRAS list if the FDA acquires evidence of some hazard to consumers.

A large number of food additives would fall into the category of flavors and extracts. The Flavor and Extract Manufacturers Association (FEMA) keeps a list of accepted flavors and extracts. FEMA evaluates the safety of the chemicals on the list. In essence, the FEMA list is a GRAS list for flavors and extracts. Over 1000 chemicals are on the FEMA list, although some of these chemicals and extracts are no longer used.

Direct food additives are those new food additives that have been approved by the FDA since 1958. Actually, very few approvals for new food additives have been granted in recent years. Extensive safety data are required, so the process of obtaining FDA approval for a new food additive can be rather costly. Aspartame, a nonnutritive sweetener, is perhaps the most notable direct food additive in use in the United States. Since approval of aspartame as a sweetener for certain types of uses a few years ago, the consumption of this new additive has become substantial.

Color additives are regulated in a separate part of the FD&C Act. New color additives must be approved by the FDA in much the same way that new food additives are approved. Some color additives in common use before 1958 have been banned because of more recent concerns about their chronic toxicity. A good example is FD&C Red #2.

The degree of hazard associated with the presence of additives in our foods is quite small. Several factors account for the low degree of hazard. First, our level of exposure to most food additives is rather low. This is especially true for many of the flavoring ingredients. Second, the oral toxicity of food additives tends to be extremely low, especially with regard to acute toxicity. Some concerns have arisen about the chronic toxicity of some food additives. The so-called Delaney clause to the FD&C Act prohibits the use of any additive that causes cancer in laboratory animals. High doses of some food additives have been shown to cause cancer in animals. One of the best examples is saccharin. Questions exist regarding how properly to extrapolate to humans, who typically ingest much lower levels of the ingredient, the results of feeding high levels of an ingredient to animals. Thus, the carcinogenicity of saccharin to humans at typical levels of intake is uncertain. A third reason for the low hazard associated with food additives is the established safety of many additives. Most food additives have been subjected to some safety evaluations in laboratory animals. Thus, the toxicity of food additives is often well known and exposure can be limited to levels far below any dose that would be hazardous. By contrast, the toxicity of naturally occurring chemicals in foods is often not known, and we cannot be certain that hazardous circumstances will not exist.

The safety of some food additives has been questioned. Most of the questions have revolved around evidence for weak carcinogenic activity in laboratory animals. Some additives such as FD&C Red #2 and cyclamate have been banned. Warning labels are required for saccharin. These are but a few examples. In addition to carcinogenicity, other concerns have arisen such as the role of sugar in dental caries and abnormal behavioral reactions, the role of salt in hypertension, and the role of aspartame in headaches and other behavioral and neurological reactions. While a detailed discussion of these issues is beyond the scope of this chapter, suffice it to say that many of these assertions have been questioned and remain to be validated.

A few food additives have caused acute illness under certain conditions of exposure. These intoxications are usually the result of either excessive consumption of the additive or ingestion by an individual who has an abnormal sensitivity to the additive. Misuse of food additives by consumers or food processors has also created hazardous situations on occasion. These types of situations will be discussed later in this chapter.

Dietetic food diarrhea is a good example of an intoxication resulting from the excessive consumption of a food additive. The hexitols and sorbitol are widely used sweeteners. They are especially common in candy and chewing gum because they are noncariogenic. These sugar alcohols are not as easily absorbed as sugar but, once absorbed, they are equally as caloric as sugar. Because of their slow absorption, these sweeteners can cause an osmotic-type diarrhea when excessive amounts are consumed. Several cases have been reported where consumers were ingesting more than 20 g of these sweeteners per day. The levels of hexitols and/or sorbitol used in foods will vary, but in one case the ingestion of 12 pieces of hard candy over a short period of time provided 36 g of sorbitol and resulted in diarrhea.

Sulfite-induced asthma is a good example of an extreme sensitivity to a food additive that afflicts only a small percentage of the population. Sulfites are widely used food additives with a number of desirable technical properties. The acceptable daily intake for sulfites is 72 mg/kg body weight/day. However, a small percentage of asthmatics, perhaps 1–2% of the 9 million asthmatics in the United States, are exquisitely sensitive to sulfites. Ingestion of some typically sulfited foods induces an asthmatic episode in these individuals; other consumers eat these same foods with no ill effects. A few deaths have been attributed to the ingestion of sulfites by such consumers. As a result, the FDA rescinded the GRAS status of sulfites for use on raw vegetables other than potatoes in 1986, because the use of sulfites on these products was often not labeled and sensitive individuals would not be aware of the hazard. Sulfite-sensitive individuals can avoid many of the hazards associated with sulfited foods by reading labels and avoiding foods that contain this additive.

IV. Chemicals Migrating from Packaging Materials

Chemicals migrating from packaging materials do not represent a significant hazard. A variety of chemicals can migrate from packaging materials into foods, including plastics monomers, plasticizers, stabilizers, printing inks, and others. However, the level of exposure to these chemicals is extremely low and most of these chemicals are not particularly toxic. United States law requires that packaging materials be tested to determine the degree of migration.

Concerns have arisen about residues of lead migrating into foods from soldered cans. Lead is a well-known toxicant that can affect the nervous system, the kidney, and the bone. Lead does exist in the solder used to seal can seams. Extensive migration of lead does not occur in most situations because access of acid to the solder is prevented. However, lead-soldered cans are being phased out as a result of this concern.

V. Chemicals Produced during Processing, Preparation, Storage, and Handling of Foods

Countless chemical reactions occur during processing, preparation, storage, and handling of foods. Literally millions of chemicals are formed as a result of these reactions. The toxicity of these chemicals has not been established in most cases. A thorough discussion of this subject is beyond the scope of this chapter. However, the formation of nitrosamines should serve as a good example of this type of situation.

Nitrosamines are formed by the reaction of nitrites with secondary amines. The amines are common, naturally occurring components of many foods. Nitrite is a food additive used in the curing of meats, but the majority of nitrite entering the gastrointestinal tract arises from other sources such as water, plants (especially if fertilized with nitrogen-based fertilizers), nitrogen oxides in polluted air and the open flames used in some types of food processing, and saliva. Nitrosamine formation is favored by heating and by acidic conditions. Among the cured meats, nitrosamine formation in bacon is most critical because of the high temperatures used in frying. Most nitrosamines are carcinogenic. Nitrosamines can alkylate DNA and act as initiators of the carcinogenic process. The risk associated with nitrosamines in foods can be lessened by lowering the nitrite levels used in the curing of meats and by the addition of vitamin C, vitamin E, or antioxidants to cured meats. These antioxidants diminish nitrosamine formation. The removal of nitrites entirely from cured meats would not eliminate this possible hazard because many other sources of nitrite exist. Also, the removal of nitrite from cured meats would increase the risk of botulism.

VI. Inadvertent or Accidental Contaminants

A. Industrial and/or Environmental Pollutants

Industrial and/or environmental pollutants often migrate into foods in small amounts Occasionally hazardous levels of such chemicals enter the food supply, causing foodborne illness. Obviously such gross cases of pollution should be prevented, but occasional incidents are likely to occur even with diligent preventive measures.

The contamination of foods with polychlorinated or polybrominated biphenyls (PCBs or PBBs) has occurred on several occasions. The most infamous incident involved the accidental inclusion of PBBs in dairy feed in Michigan. The PBBs are lipid soluble so they were concentrated in the milk. As a result of this incident, many cows and their milk had to be destroyed. Consumers of this milk continue to have PBB residues in their fatty tissues many years later. The ultimate consequences of this incident remain unclear, but it was obviously unfortunate and unnecessary. A separate incident involving a leaking transformer in a facility that produced poultry feed resulted in the contamination of the feed with PCBs. This incident resulted in the destruction of chickens, eggs, and egg-containing products. Pollution of Lake Michigan by PCBs has reached such a level that fish in that lake are routinely contaminated with PCBs. Commercial fishing on Lake Michigan has ceased as a result. Recreational fishing continues, even though the consequences of frequent consumption of these fish are uncertain.

Perhaps the most famous incident involving industrial pollution occurred in Minamata Bay, Japan. An industrial firm was dumping mercury-containing wastes into the bay. Bacteria in the sediment converted the inorganic mercury to highly toxic methylmercury. Fish in the bay became contaminated with the methylmercury. The ultimate result was over 1200 cases of mercury poisoning among consumers of these fish. Symptoms included tremors and other neurotoxic effects and kidney failure.

B. Chemicals from Utensils

Potentially toxic heavy metals will leach from containers and utensils into beverages if the beverages are acidic. Acute heavy metal intoxication is a relatively common cause of foodborne disease. It almost always results from the contact of acidic beverages with containers or utensils containing heavy metals such as copper, zinc, cadmium, or tin. Lead contamination can also occur but does not usually result in acute intoxications.

Copper poisoning, characterized primarily by nausea and vomiting, can occur from faulty check valves in soft-drink vending machines. The check valves prevent contact between the acidic, carbonated beverage and the copper tubing that delivers the water. Several outbreaks have resulted from faulty check valves, and each outbreak has the potential to involve hundreds of people. Zinc intoxication can result from the storage of acidic beverages in galvanized buckets. Refrigerator shelves containing cadmium residues have caused problems when the shelves were employed as barbecue grills. Tin intoxication has resulted from the placement of acidic juices in unlined cans. Juices are usually packaged in cans with a lining that prevents contact between the acidic beverage and the tin plate. Glazed pottery and painted glassware have been recalled from sale because of the presence of lead in the glazes and paints and the fear of lead poisoning.

C. Accidental Contaminants

Occasionally, accidents will result in foodborne intoxications. Some of these accidents are errors of ignorance such as the use of galvanized containers to store acidic beverages. These accidents could be avoided if the individuals involved were aware of the risks. Other accidents are not so clearly preventable.

Several foodborne intoxications have resulted from confusion about the identity of food ingredients. Sodium nitrite can easily be confused with other salts, including sodium chloride, which is much less toxic. In one incident, a small grocery store was repackaging additives such as sodium chloride, sodium nitrite, and monosodium glutamate (MSG) from bulk containers. Somehow, sodium nitrite was labeled as MSG. The mislabeled product was used in hazardous amounts by consumers, resulting in acute methemoglobinemia and at least one death.

Sometimes it is less clear if the mistake was entirely accidental. In 1983, an outbreak of niacin intoxication occurred among consumers of pumpernickel bagels in New York. Niacin intoxication is a rather mild, short-term illness involving rash, pruritis, and a sensation of warmth. The bagels had been excessively enriched with niacin, one of the B vitamins; they contained about 60 times the normal amount of niacin. This incident likely resulted from an accident, although intentional use of megadoses of vitamins is considered desirable by some consumers.

One very serious outbreak was clearly an error of ignorance on the part of the processor. A manufacturer of a soybean-based infant formula wished to decrease the sodium content of the formula despite a lack of evidence that such action would prevent the development of hypertension in the infants later in life. The manufacturer removed the NaCl from the formula. Most infants receiving soybean formula survive on that formula alone because of allergies to formulae based on cows' milk. The removal of NaCl resulted in a deficiency of chloride in the formula. The result was a condition known as metabolic alkalosis, characterized by lethargy, poor appetite, failure to gain weight, vomiting, and diarrhea. Several infants died as a result.

More often, such errors of ignorance are perpetrated by consumers. A good example was a small outbreak of vitamin A intoxication. Two twin infants were provided a diet consisting largely of pureed chicken livers, pureed carrots, milk, and vitamin supplements. The mother of these infants stated that she did not trust commercial baby foods. After several weeks on this diet, the infants began to vomit and developed a skin rash. The symptoms disappeared when a more normal diet was instituted. The estimated intake of vitamin A and carotene was 44,000 IU/day compared to the RDA of 1500–4500 IU/day for infants.

Bibliography

Archer, M. C. (1982). Hazards of nitrate, nitrite and N-nitroso compounds in human nutrition. *In* "Nutritional Toxicology" (J. N. Hathcock, ed.), Vol. 1, pp. 327–381.

Coats, J. R. (1987). Toxicology of pesticide residues in foods. *In* "Nutritional Toxicology" (J. N. Hathcock, ed.), Vol. 2, pp. 249–279. Academic Press, Orlando, Florida.

Irving, G. W., Jr. (1982). Determination of the GRAS status of food ingredients. *In* "Nutritional Toxicology" (J. N. Hathcock, ed.), Vol. 1, pp. 435–450. Academic Press, New York.

Linshaw, M. A., Harrison, H. L., Gruskin, A. B., Prebis, J., Harris, J., Stein, R., Jayaram, M. R., Preston, D., Diliberti, J., Baluarte, H. J., Elzouki, A., and Carroll, N. (1980). Hypochloremic alkalosis in infants associated with soy protein formula. *J. Pediatr.* **96,** 635–640.

Munro, I. C., and Charbonneau, S. M. (1981). Environmental contaminants. *In* "Food Safety" (H. R. Roberts, ed.), pp. 141–180. Wiley, New York.

Roberts, H. R. (1981). Food additives. *In* "Food Safety" (H. R. Roberts, ed.), pp. 239–293. Wiley, New York.

Taylor, S. L., and Bush, R. K. (1986). Sulfites as food ingredients. *Food Technol.* **40**(6), 47–52.

Taylor, S. L., and Byron, B. (1984). Probable case of sorbitol-induced diarrhea. *J. Food Prot.* **47,** 249.

PART III

INFECTIONS

CHAPTER 11

SALMONELLA

Michael P. Doyle

and Dean O. Cliver

I. Introduction

The natural habitat (therefore, original source) of *Salmonella* is the intestinal tract of humans and other animals. Both water and foods of animal origin have been identified as vehicles for transmission of the organism. Of the known species of *Salmonella*, our present understanding is that all are pathogenic to humans. The degree of virulence of *Salmonella* is strain dependent, and the susceptibility of the individual depends on the state of health. For individuals in poor health, it appears that relatively low doses of *Salmonella* can produce illness.

The salmonellae can be either host adapted or non-host adapted. Most species of *Salmonella* are non-host adapted, meaning that they are carried by a variety of animals; less than 1% of the known *Salmonella* serotypes are host adapted. Certain serotypes are principally associated with specific animals or humans. For example, the reservoir of *S. typhi* and *S. paratyphi* A and C (also known as *S. hirschfeldii*) is humans. *Salmonella pullorum* and *S. gallinarum* are the organisms responsible for bacillary white diarrhea and fowl typhoid, respectively, in poultry—they generally are not found in other animals or humans. Other examples include *S. typhisuis* and *S. choleraesuis*, principally associated with pigs. *Salmonella dublin* has been an increasing cause of foodborne disease; it is principally associated with cattle. *Salmonella abortusequi* is principally associated with horses, and *S. abortusovis* is principally associated with sheep. In addition to these examples, several other types of *Salmonella* are principally host specific.

II. Salmonellosis

A. Syndromes

The disease caused by *Salmonella* is generically called "salmonellosis." Three different syndromes in humans are caused by different types of *Salmonella*. The most severe is typhoid fever, caused by *S. typhi*. Fortunately, this is an infrequent disease in the United States—less than 2.5% of the human salmonellosis in the United States is typhoid fever. Humans are the only reservoir for *S. typhi*, so instances of typhoid fever imply human fecal contamination of water or food. *Salmonella typhi* gets into water and food via raw sewage or by direct contamination by a food handler who has typhoid fever and sheds the organism in feces.

The signs and symptoms of typhoid fever are quite severe. They include septicemia (i.e., the organism gets into the bloodstream and grows), high fever, headache, constipation, vomiting, and diarrhea. Frequently rose spots appear on the chest and trunk, and there is bleeding from the bowel as well as from the nose.

Infection begins when the organisms are ingested and reach the small intestine. There they penetrate the epithelial cells of the villi. This principally occurs in the lower small intestine. They invade the lamina propria within the villi and ultimately get into the host's lymphatic system. Once in the lymphatic system, they are phagocytosed by macrophages and multiply within the macrophages. Macrophages are a defense mechanism that normally ward off infection by killing invading organisms, but *S. typhi* can resist the bactericidal properties of macrophages and survive and grow within them. After the *S. typhi* multiply they spill out of these macrophages into the blood and travel to the liver, spleen, gall bladder, and other organs to set up a systemic infection.

During the time that the bacteria are within the macrophages, they are thought to be resistant to antibiotics, which explains the high relapse rate in cases of typhoid fever treated with antibiotics. Often the first dose of antibiotic is not entirely effective in eliminating the illness, so that multiple treatments are required.

As has been stated, the reservoir for *S. typhi* is the human carrier. Some are long-term carriers, as was true of the infamous Typhoid Mary. The organism can be excreted not only in the feces, but also in the urine, a characteristic fact that is used in diagnostic testing.

Both water and food have been vehicles for transmission of *S. typhi*. Raw milk has been involved in outbreaks of typhoid fever. Milk has been eliminated as a vehicle of *S. typhi* in developed countries by pasteurization, but in developing countries where raw milk is served, typhoid fever is still a problem. Shellfish and raw salads have also been identified as vehicles of typhoid fever. Foods that are handled by an infected individual and are not given some subsequent heat treatment are most often involved.

The second syndrome in the category of salmonellosis is enteric fever. Three types of *Salmonella* are principally responsible for enteric fever—*S. paratyphi* A, B, and C. *Salmonella paratyphi* B is now called *S. schottmuelleri*, and *S. paratyphi* C is now called *S. hirschfeldii*. Less than 0.5% of the cases of salmonellosis that occur in the United States are of the enteric fever type.

The symptoms of enteric fever are very similar to those of typhoid fever but less severe. There is generally septicemia, fever, headache, and abdominal pain. The illness usually lasts anywhere from 1–3 weeks, whereas typhoid fever may last from 1–8 weeks.

The sources of *S. paratyphi* A, *S. schottmuelleri*, and *S. hirschfeldii* organisms are the same as for typhoid fever—humans. The foods that are involved are also very similar—raw milk, raw salads, eggs, and shellfish.

The most common type of salmonellosis that occurs in the United States is a gastroenteritis syndrome (food poisoning) caused by all the other types of *Salmonella*. More than 2300 serotypes of *Salmonella* are presently known, but only about 150 have been associated with human disease. The remaining types are still considered to be pathogenic, even though they have not been shown to cause human disease.

The symptoms of *Salmonella* food-poisoning syndrome include diarrhea, abdominal pain, chills, fever, vomiting, dehydration, and headache. The severity of these symptoms varies depending on the host's immunocompetence and many other variables. The mortality rate for salmonellosis of this type is in the range of 0.1–0.2%. Those that are fatally afflicted are principally the elderly and the very young. The incubation period for this syndrome can be in the range of 5–72 hours, but is usually 12–36 hours. The duration of illness is usually from 1–4 days.

Once the organisms are ingested in sufficient numbers, they will penetrate the epithelial cells of the villi, usually at the distal or lower end of the small intestine. Then they will get into the lamina propria but, in contrast to the other types of *Salmonella* involved in enteric and typhoid fevers, the organisms usually do not progress beyond the lamina propria. They stay in that area and multiply where they cause an inflammatory response. Unlike *S. typhi* and the paratyphis, these organisms generally do not progress any further, so usually there is no septicemia or systemic infection. The infection remains localized in the intestinal area.

The usual treatment for this type of salmonellosis is none. Antibiotic therapy is usually not given unless septicemia develops. The reason is that antibiotics clear out much of the normal microflora of the intestinal tract and make one more likely to develop other infections. Also, the treatment of such illnesses with antibiotics can select organisms resistant to the antibiotic.

Studies have been done to determine how long the organism resides in the intestinal tract in individuals who have *Salmonella* infections. About 50% of individuals will still excrete the *Salmonella* 2–4 weeks after experiencing the illness. About 10–20% of individuals continue to shed *Salmonella* in the feces 4–8 weeks after they experience illness. Very few individuals shed detectable *Salmonella* in their feces 3 months after they have recovered from the illness, and it is extremely rare to have anyone continue to shed the organism in the feces 6 months after. The 1-month period is quite long, so an individual who is a food handler has to be careful in handling foods after having had an infection.

B.   Infectious Dose

An infectious dose of *Salmonella,* according to Bergey's Manual, is 10^8 to 10^9 cells, but that is misleading. Several retrospective studies have demonstrated much lower doses, depending on the type of food, the strain of *Salmonella,* and other factors. It is difficult to establish an infectious dose because one cannot experiment with the individuals who are most susceptible to infection. There have been several studies done on feeding *Salmonella* to human volunteers, but these volunteers have all been adults who had no underlying illness and hence were less susceptible to infection than would be the elderly or young children.

Another factor is that the virulence of *Salmonella* is strain dependent. Some strains are much more virulent than others. For example, certain strains of *S. dublin* appear to be highly virulent.

There are differences in individual tolerances or susceptibility. Some individuals may have been exposed to *Salmonella* in the past and have high levels of antibody against the organism; they would be more likely to resist infection than those who have low levels. The individual's state of health is also quite important. That is, someone who is immunosuppressed because of cancer therapy, cirrhosis, or underlying disease is much more likely to be sensitive to *Salmonella* infection than an individual who is not.

Stomach contents are also an important factor. Normally when food is eaten the pyloric valve closes, thus retaining the food in the stomach. The food is exposed to gastric acidity—the pH of the stomach is quite low due to the production of hydrochloric acid. The HCl is effective in killing off many bacteria, such as *Salmo-*

nella, that may be present in food. A study done in the Netherlands found that if an individual did not eat for many hours and then drank water, the water would go directly through the stomach to the duodenum, and not really be exposed to the gastric acidity. Under such conditions, very small numbers of *Salmonella* may produce infection.

Two principal types of studies have been done to estimate the infectious dose of *Salmonella.* Feeding studies have been done with normal, healthy adult volunteers, principally prisoners. One of the limitations of such studies is that they deal with a nonsensitive population. These studies revealed that there was a difference between individuals' susceptibility to infection by the same strain of *Salmonella,* likely because of differences in immunocompetence and antibody titers to salmonellae.

A second observation was that the fewest organisms causing illness was 1.3×10^5 cells. This was a strain of *S. bareilly.* For *S. pullorum* the infectious dose was about 10^{10}, so even in this type of population, some strains are more virulent than others.

More valid data have been derived from *retrospective* studies. If after an outbreak of salmonellosis some of the implicated food is still at hand, its *Salmonella* content can be determined. Then, calculating the average amount of food eaten by each person enables an estimate of how many *Salmonella* cells were actually consumed. This has been possible in several instances. For example, from an outbreak linked to imitation ice cream, it was calculated that 11,000 *S. typhimurium* were consumed by those who became ill. Carmine dye has been used in diagnostic tests in infants. An infant was given carmine dye that contained 15,000 cells of *Salmonella,* and this resulted in the death of that infant. As few as 15,000 cells of, in this case, *S. cubana* would kill an individual in a high-risk group. Pancreatin containing about 200 cells of *Salmonella* and fed to pediatric patients with cystic fibrosis produced illness in 31% of the group.

A major outbreak of salmonellosis came from eating ground beef. Some cooks may lick the spoon when preparing hamburger. This particular ground beef was contaminated with a highly virulent strain of *S. newport* at an estimated level of 60–2300 cells per gram.

Several recent outbreaks of salmonellosis have involved chocolate candy. In an outbreak caused by *S. napoli* that occurred in the United Kingdom, it was determined that about 50 cells produced illness. Some investigators suggest that certain foods, of which chocolate is an example, may be exceptionally protective of *Salmonella.* Several outbreaks have involved chocolate with very low numbers of *Salmonella.* Apparently the organisms are entrapped in fat, which protects them from the acidity of the stomach so that smaller numbers cause illness.

C. Sources of Infection

The primary reservoir of *Salmonella* is the intestinal tract of infected domestic and wild animals and humans. *Salmonella* is excreted in the feces and can remain viable in fecal material for several years outside the host. This organism can survive in the dry state, so persistence can be long lasting if the feces dry out.

The principal source of *Salmonella* infection is the ingestion of contaminated food and water. Foods of animal origin such as poultry, beef, and pork are principal sources. Studies suggest that more than 30% of retail poultry in the United States is contaminated with *Salmonella*. That doesn't mean that millions of *Salmonella* are present on each poultry carcass; there are usually a few hundred cells or less.

Studies suggest that about 15% of retail fresh pork and 3% or less of fresh beef is contaminated with *Salmonella*. More cases of salmonellosis are linked to beef than pork, probably because concern for *Trichinella* in pork leads to more thorough cooking.

Another source of infection is person-to-person contact. Individuals recovering from salmonellosis may continue to shed the organism in their feces. Some are long-term carriers and shed the organism for weeks to months. Unsanitary practices by carriers can spread the illness.

Salmonella is also spread through contact with animals. This is a frequently neglected source, but animals, both domestic and wild, are reservoirs of *Salmonella*. The incidence varies; however, to be on the safe side, one must assume that all animals are carriers of *Salmonella*.

Many pets have been shown to be carriers. Studies in the mid-1960s by the Centers for Disease Control (CDC) showed that certain serotypes of *Salmonella* were commonly associated with salmonellosis in young children. These serotypes of *Salmonella* were also principally associated with turtles. The CDC estimated that 280,000 cases of *Salmonella* each year were linked to pet turtles. As a result of the CDC study, many state and local governments began to require that pet shops certify that the turtles they sold were *Salmonella* free. Later, the CDC tested a variety of turtles from many different pet shops and found that about 38% of the turtles tested were in fact contaminated with *Salmonella*, even though they were certified as being *Salmonella* free. In 1975 the Food and Drug Administration (FDA) banned the interstate shipment of pet turtles, which is why one almost never sees pet turtles in stores. The result of this action was an 18% reduction in the frequency of salmonellosis in children aged 1–9 years which corresponded to a 77% reduction in the frequency of turtle-associated serotypes (*S. urbana, S. litchfield,* and *S. java*).

Salmonella can also be transmitted through aerosols, but this is a very minor source. Transmission by this means occurs only in unusual circumstances.

D. Epidemiology

Figure 1 illustrates the magnitude of the salmonellosis problem in the United States. In 1963 about 20,000 cases of *Salmonella* were reported yearly in this country. There has been a continual increase, to more than 48,000 reported cases in 1988. It is estimated that from 30 to as many as 100 cases go unreported for each case that is reported; so if 48,000 were cases reported, the true recent total may be as high as 4.8 million annually.

There appears to be a seasonal variation in the occurrence of salmonellosis; the peak incidence is during the summer months (Fig. 2). There is no certain explanation for this, but increased temperature abuse of foods during the summer may be at least one reason for the increase in salmonellosis.

Another important point is that certain populations are more susceptible to *Salmonella* infections. Susceptibility is greatest among infants (Fig. 3). The highest rates of reported infection are in infants from <1 to 6 months old. About 40% of

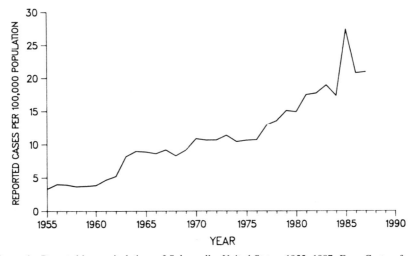

Figure 1 Reported human isolations of *Salmonella,* United States, 1955–1987. From Centers for Disease Control (1988). Summary of notifiable diseases United States, 1987. *Morbid. Mortal. Wkly. Rep.* No. 36 (54), p. 38.

reported cases of salmonellosis occur in children less than 5 years of age. Then there is another peak in adults over 60, due principally to individuals with reduced immune response to *Salmonella.*

Certain serotypes of *Salmonella* are more commonly associated than others with human infection (Table I). *Salmonella typhimurium* leads the way. About 25–30% of human cases of salmonellosis in the United States are attributed to this species. *Salmonella typhimurium* is also a leader among the serotypes that are found in animals.

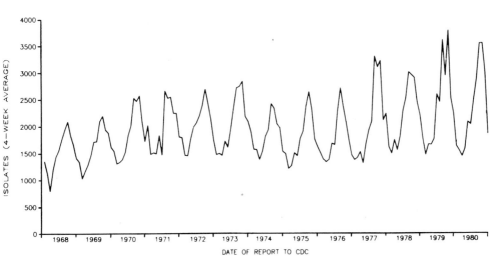

Figure 2 Seasonal pattern of reported isolations of *Salmonella* in the United States from 1968 through 1980. From Centers for Disease Control (1982). "*Salmonella* Surveillance Annual Summary, 1980." CDC, Atlanta.

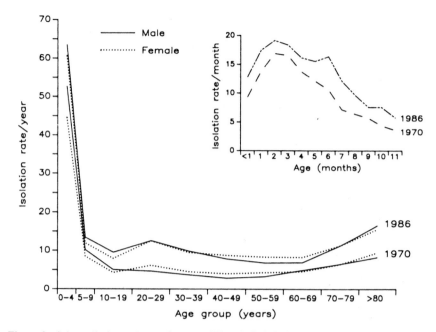

Figure 3 Salmonellosis attack rates by age, 1970 and 1986. Isolation rate is per 100,000 population. From Centers for Disease Control (1988). *Morbid. Mortal. Wkly.* Rep. No. 37 (SS-2), p. 30.

Table I

Salmonella Serotypes Most Frequently Isolated from Humans, United States, 1986[a]

Serotype	1986 isolates		Rank	
	Number	Percentage	1985	1986
S. typhimurium[b]	10,888	26	1	1
S. enteritidis	5,967	14	2	2
S. heidelberg	5,595	13	3	3
S. newport	2,431	6	4	4
S. hadar	1,552	4	5	5
S. infantis	1,104	3	7	6
S. agona	912	2	6	7
S. montevideo	775	2	8	8
S. muenchen	694	2	9	9
S. braenderup	616	1	15	10
S. oranienburg	484	1	10	14
S. saint paul	558	1	13	11
Subtotal	31,576	75		
Other	10,452	25		
Total	42,028	100		

[a]From Centers for Disease Control (1988). *Morbid. Mortal. Wkly.* Rep. No. 37 (SS-2), p. 28.
[b]Includes *S. typhimurium* var. *copenhagen*.

Within the past 5 years, there has been a large increase in the incidence of salmonellosis due to *S. enteritidis*. This species has been an unusual problem in the northeastern United States where there have been a large number of *S. enteritidis* infections from eggs that have been temperature abused in some way or under-cooked. This organism is unusual among salmonellae in that it will colonize the ovaries of laying hens and then be deposited within the yolk. The increased incidence of *S. enteritidis* infections is being seen not only in the United States but also in many other countries.

III. Characteristics of *Salmonella*

A. Classification and Biochemical Characteristics

Salmonella are gram-negative, nonsporeforming rods. Most *Salmonella* are motile by peritrichous flagella. *Salmonella pullorum* and *S. gallinarum* and a type of *S. arizonae* are nonmotile. However, the vast majority of the 2300 serotypes of *Salmonella* now known are motile.

Members of the genus *Salmonella* possess several common properties. Citrate is usually utilized as a sole carbon source. They rarely ferment lactose or sucrose. With the exception of *S. typhi*, salmonellae regularly ferment glucose with the evolution of gas, so they are aerogenic. Additionally, *Salmonella* can grow both aerobically and anaerobically.

The scheme of Kauffmann is often used to group the genus *Salmonella* into subgenera. These subgenera include Subgenus I, which contains most of the *Salmonella* species; Subgenus II, which is *S. salamae;* Subgenus III, which is *S. arizonae;* Subgenus IV, which is *S. houtenae;* and Subgenus V, which is *S. bongor.* Several biochemical characteristics are used to differentiate these various subgenera. Besides grouping on the basis of subgenera, the salmonellae are also classified into species on the basis of serology. This is the most important means of classification. The Kauffman–White scheme is generally used to categorize *Salmonella* species. Serology is based on the O or somatic antigen, the H or flagellar antigen, and the Vi or capsular antigen.

Currently there are over 2300 species of *Salmonella* and new species are being identified each year. Species have common somatic antigens which classify them into groups. "Bergey's Manual of Determinative Bacteriology" classifies *Salmonella* into 50 groups, each of which is given an alphabetic letter, for example, A, B, C_1, C_2, and D. These groups are based on the composition of the O antigen. For example, the dominant somatic antigen of organisms in group A is designated 2. Some strains will also have the 1 or the 12 antigen. Strains in group B principally contain the 4 and 12 somatic antigens and may or may not contain the 1 and 5 antigens. Group C_1 organisms have the 6 and 7 somatic antigens. Group C_2 has 6 and 8, and Group D has 9, 12, and possibly 1. Over 98% of salmonellae that are commonly isolated fall into the first 12 of the 50 groups. Many less commonly isolated types of salmonellae fall into some of the other groups.

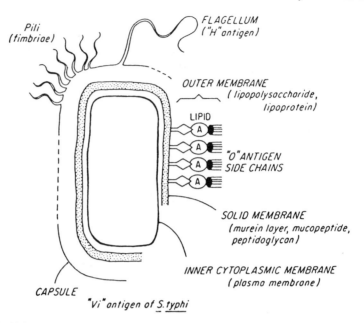

Figure 4   Major surface antigens of *Salmonella*. Reproduced, with permission, from L. S. Young, W. J. Martin, R. D. Meyer, R. J. Weinstein, and E. T. Anderson (1977). Gram-negative rod bacteremia: Microbiologic, immunologic, and therapeutic considerations. *Ann. Intern. Med.* **86,** 456–471.

In epidemiologic investigations and some other situations, it may be necessary to identify the salmonellae to a level of precision beyond the serotype or species. Various means are used: biotyping based on the ability to ferment different sugars, resistance to antibiotics, production of or sensitivity to bacteriocins, resistance to transfer factors, phage types, plasmid profiles, and restriction nuclease profiles of plasmids.

A good example is *S. typhimurium,* a species comprising about 25–30% of United States isolates of *Salmonella.* Phage typing has been developed as a means of differentiating strains of *S. typhimurium,* but even further subdivision is needed for some of the common phage types. This is done by plasmid profiling. Plasmids are isolated from the different strains of bacteria and identified by their molecular weights; then sometimes a restriction nuclease digest and separation of fragments by electrophoresis are done to see if there is a commonality in their DNA composition.

The surface antigens of *Salmonella* are used for serotyping. Major surface antigens of *Salmonella* are shown in Fig. 4. Part of the cell outer membrane contains the somatic antigen (O). The flagellar antigens that extend beyond the cell wall and are responsible for the motility of the cell are the H antigens. Some strains of *Salmonella,* such as *S. typhi,* have a capsular material (the Vi antigen). There are also antigens called fimbriae that are proteinaceous material emanating from the cell's surface. These are also called F antigens or type 1 pili; they are not important in the speciation of *Salmonella* because they are commonly present on the salmonellae and are antigenically similar, so one is not able to use them in differentiation. The F antigen is generally produced in greater amounts when the organism is grown aerobically. Some investigators suggest that the fimbriae are adhesion factors that allow the organism to adhere to surfaces.

The Vi or the capsular antigen is an acidic polysaccharide. *Salmonella typhi, S. dublin,* and *S. hirschfeldii* are the only three species known to express this antigen, so it is not at all common among the salmonellae.

The somatic antigen is very important. It is part of the cell wall which has four layers: the lipopolysaccharide layer (LPS), a phospholipid layer, a lipoprotein layer, and a peptidoglycan layer (Fig. 5). The somatic antigen is part of the LPS layer, which comprises three portions. The outer portion is the O antigen side chains, the middle portion is the core polysaccharide, and the third portion is called lipid A. The LPS layer contains endotoxin, which produces fever in a host when the toxin gets into the bloodstream. All Enterobacteriaceae are believed to have endotoxins.

The lipid A component of the LPS layer is believed to be responsible for the toxic properties of endotoxin. It has a rather small molecular weight of about 2000. The middle portion of the LPS layer, which is known as the basal core or the core polysaccharide, is common among all salmonellae. This portion of the LPS and the lipid A portion are not specific enough to differentiate species of *Salmonella*. The core polysaccharide is composed of a variety of polysaccharides, among which is KDO—2-keto-3-deoxyoctanate. The component of the LPS layer that is used to differentiate species of *Salmonella* is the O antigen side chains. These antigens consist of two to six repeating units of sequences of sugars. For example, a sequence like Glu-Man-Rha-Gal may repeat several times, and the whole would be attached to the core polysaccharide.

This O antigen side chain is the portion of the LPS which is very specific for the different *Salmonella* species. A *Salmonella* organism that is missing these O antigen side chains, when grown on an agar plate, produces a colony with coarse, irregular,

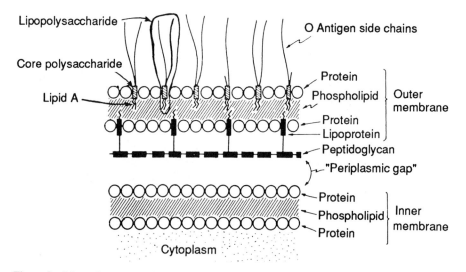

Figure 5 Schematic representation of *Salmonella* cell envelope containing the somatic (O) antigen. Adapted, with permission, from C. A. Schnaitman (1971). *J. Bacteriol.* **108,** 553–563.

rough-appearing edges. Colonies with rounded, smooth-appearing edges after the cells are grown on an agar plate have a full complement of O antigen side chains. Rough strains of *Salmonella* cannot be serotyped because their O antigen side chains are not expressed and, hence, are unknown. When rough strains lose the ability to produce these O-specific sugars, they will not revert and are therefore untypable.

The other antigen of major interest is the flagellar or H antigen. This is a proteinaceous material, and it too is highly specific for species in the genus *Salmonella*. Usually, but not always, two different types of flagellar antigens can be expressed by an organism within the same cell. This is called phase variation; the two different antigens are designated phase 1 and phase 2. A single cell and a *Salmonella* colony resulting from the growth of this cell will express only phase 1 or phase 2.

A *Salmonella* culture will produce colonies representing both phases of flagellar antigens. In order to identify the two phases of the flagellar antigen, which is required to speciate the organism definitively, several approaches are possible. One could subculture several colonies and find one that expresses phase 1 and one that expresses phase 2. However, this may not be a very direct approach nor is it very time efficient if one phase greatly predominates over the other. An alternative procedure is to change the phase of the culture after the dominant phase has been identified. A length of glass tubing with open ends is placed into a tube culture of motility medium which contains antibody against the dominant-phase flagellar antigen that has already been identified. When the unknown *Salmonella* strain is inoculated, cells in the dominant phase are immobilized by the antiserum, but cells in the other phase are free to migrate into the glass tubing, from which they can be subcultured and serotyped.

To prepare antiserum that is going to be used to determine the somatic (O) serotype of *Salmonella,* a broth culture is heated at 100°C for 2 hours. The cell-wall antigen is very resistant to this heat treatment, which will destroy all the flagella because the flagellar protein is heat sensitive. Rabbits are injected repeatedly with the heat-treated cell suspension, and their blood is tested for level of antibody against the O antigen.

In order to produce flagellar antiserum, the flagellar antigen must be preserved. The culture is treated with formalin, and the formaldehyde fixes the protein. The flagellar antigen is fixed in a rigid system such that, when these cells are injected into rabbits, the antibodies evoked react principally with the flagellar antigens. There will also be some antibodies against the somatic antigens. To remove those antibodies, heated cells (somatic antigen) are added to the antiserum. The antibodies in the antiserum that will react with the cell-wall antigens are removed with the cells by centrifugation. What should be left are antibodies that react with the flagellar antigen. Serotyping is an important concept for workers in a laboratory that must classify and identify *Salmonella*.

B. Survival and Growth Characteristics

A portion of *Salmonella* in a food will be killed by freezing and thawing. In terms of reducing the population, generally one can achieve about $1-2 \log_{10}$ reduction in one treatment cycle. By doing this repeatedly, *Salmonella* can be eliminated from poultry meat, but unfortunately quality is reduced to the point that the meat may no longer be edible.

Heat is another means of killing *Salmonella* in foods. Several factors affect the rate at which heat will inactivate *Salmonella*. One of these is the strain of *Salmonella* that is present. For example, unusually heat-resistant strain *S. senftenberg* 775W is about 10–20 times more resistant than an average strain of *Salmonella* sp. This strain of *Salmonella* is unique and, hence, a laboratory curiosity—time–temperature treatments for inactivating *Salmonella* in foods such as eggs cannot be based on such an atypical organism. Another factor that affects the rates at which heat can inactivate *Salmonella* in foods is the composition of the food or the heating menstruum. When sucrose is added to a food substrate, it increases the heat resistance of the organism. For example, in whole eggs contaminated with *S. typhimurium,* the *D* value at 60°C is about 0.27 minutes. By adding 10% sucrose to these eggs, the *D* value is doubled to about 0.6 minutes. A third factor that influences the rate at which *Salmonella* will be inactivated by heat is the water activity in the food or the humidity of the environment. For example, the organism is much more tolerant of heat applied in a dry environment than in a moist environment. *Salmonella* in dried egg whites is about 650 times more heat resistant at an equivalent temperature than in eggs in a liquid state, so there is a tremendous difference between dry heating and moist heating.

Growth temperatures for *Salmonella* range from 5–45°C, or perhaps 47°C. Growth is very slow at the extremes and more rapid in the optimal range of 35–37°C.

Another factor that influences the growth and survival of *Salmonella* is pH. The range in which *Salmonella* will grow is about pH 4–9. Some studies with certain types of apples have shown that the organism can grow at a pH as low as 3.7, but this is fairly unusual, and additional studies are needed to verify these observations. The minimum pH at which the organism will grow depends on several factors, one of which is the strain of the organism. Some strains are slightly more acid tolerant than others. The temperature of incubation is also important. The more nearly optimal the temperature is for growth, the more tolerant the organism is to adverse pH conditions.

The type of acid present is also very important. Permissive acids are generally the inorganic acids, such as HCl, and citric acid. When these acids are used to adjust the pH, the organisms can usually grow at about pH 4. Restrictive acids are more bacteriostatic. An example is acetic acid. When acetic acid is used to adjust the pH of foods—such as when vinegar is added in preparing mayonnaise—salmonellae generally will not grow below pH 5. Other restrictive acids include propionic and butyric acid.

Water activity is another important factor relative to determining the pH range in which an organism can grow. As the water activity gets farther and farther away from the optimum for *Salmonella* growth, the organism will not grow under less permissive conditions and cannot grow at lower pH values. Most *Salmonella* can grow in foods in a water activity range of 0.945–0.999.

The number of organisms present can also be a factor. Growth at a low pH is more likely if the initial level is 10^7 *Salmonella* per gram than with only 10 cells per gram. The composition of food as a growth medium is very important too. With more nutrients present, making the medium more optimal in terms of conditions for growth, the organism can grow at a lower pH than it might otherwise.

Generally if the pH of the food is below 4 or above 9, *Salmonella* will die off. The closer the pH to 4 or 9, the slower the rate of growth; the rate of death becomes very rapid as the pH approaches 2.

Oxidation–reduction (OR) potential is another important factor. Although *Salmonella* can grow under aerobic as well as anaerobic conditions, growth can be inhibited by OR potential below -30 mV. Nutrients can also be an important factor, although salmonellae are not fastidious organisms, that is, they don't have complex nutritional requirements. They can grow in simple glucose–salts medium, but they generally grow more rapidly in complex, highly supplemented media.

IV. Foodborne Transmission of *Salmonella*

A. Causes

Four factors are major contributors to outbreaks of salmonellosis. These include temperature abuse, inadequate cooking, using contaminated raw ingredients, and cross-contamination. There are several other less frequently implicated factors.

B. Prevention

There are many approaches to controlling *Salmonella* in foods. The first way is to prevent entrance of the organism through contaminated raw materials. This is particularly important in ingredients, especially in foods of animal origin or those that may be contaminated by fecal excrement that do not receive a heat treatment that will kill *Salmonella*. For example, a cookie manufacturer must be concerned about ingredients on cookies that do not receive a heat treatment, such as marshmallow cookies that have coconut on top—coconut contaminated with *Salmonella* has been involved in foodborne outbreaks. Therefore, food processors need to have specifications for raw materials that will not receive a further heat treatment to kill *Salmonella*.

An additional measure in controlling *Salmonella* in foods is to apply a heat treatment that would kill *Salmonella* during processing. The pasteurization used in processing liquid eggs is a good example.

Preventing postprocessing contamination is another important measure in controlling *Salmonella*. Several approaches must be considered. First, ensure that plant workers practice proper hygiene and food handling by educating and monitoring these people to make sure that they do not recontaminate products that have been heated. Second, make sure that the utensils in use are properly cleaned and sanitized, and monitor the effectiveness of the sanitation program used to treat these utensils. It is essential to separate equipment used with raw foods from those used with foods that are heat treated or cooked, to avoid cross-contaminating the foods. This can occur in kitchens where a cook cuts up chicken that is raw, cooks the chicken, and then uses that same knife without cleaning it to cut up the cooked chicken.

Another way to prevent contamination of products after thermal treatment is physical separation of areas within a plant. There should be a separate facility or well-enclosed area for handling raw materials and one for processed foods, so that there is no potential for cross-contamination from the raw materials. A further precaution is to monitor the environment, the product during processing, and the finished product for salmonellae.

Another measure that can be used to control salmonellae is to inhibit their growth during storage of food. This can be done through proper refrigeration. Ideally food should be rapidly cooled to <7°C and then refrigerated at <4°C; otherwise the food should held above 60°C.

For many years there has been a myth that *Salmonella* can grow and thrive well in the presence of mayonnaise, but this is untrue. Mayonnaise as it is commercially produced has a pH below 4. About 0.3–0.5% acetic acid is added as vinegar. Mayonnaise is an oil-in-water emulsion, so the concentration of vinegar in the water phase is even more than 0.5%, and the organism cannot survive.

After mayonnaise has been formulated, it should be held at room temperature (18–22°C) for 72 hours before use. The reason is that mayonnaise may contain raw eggs and raw eggs may carry *Salmonella*. In the presence of the acetic acid the organism is killed off in a few days. Hence, commercially prepared mayonnaise is indeed a safe product. If you mix mayonnaise with meat salad, the mayonnaise will retard the growth of *Salmonella*. If the product is temperature abused, *Salmonella* can still grow but mayonnaise will slow the growth.

C. Measures for Control in Poultry

One of the principal reservoirs of salmonellae is poultry. One of the reasons for focusing on poultry is that about one-third of reported foodborne outbreaks of salmonellosis for which a vehicle was identified have been linked to poultry, so poultry is an important vehicle for disseminating salmonellae.

There are many sources from which salmonellae are cycled through poultry. The organism is sometimes carried in the breeder and multiplier flocks. Hatcheries in the United States generally obtain fertile eggs from breeder and multiplier flocks. As many as 40% of these breeder flocks may be infected with salmonellae. When the breeders lay eggs, they contaminate the eggs on the surface. A good example of how *Salmonella* has been spread through these breeder flocks is the *S. hadar* situation in England. There were relatively few cases in 1970, but from 1971 to 1980 there was a continual increase of this species in human cases, and it has continued since (Fig. 6). About 5 years later, 1975 to 1976, there was an increase in *S. hadar* isolates in Canada, and a few years later the increase spread to the United States. When England first saw an increase in human cases of *S. hadar* in 1971, the organism had already become established in their turkey breeder flocks. Then many of these turkeys were brought from England to Canada and subsequently the same increase in *S. hadar* occurred in the United States.

Salmonella pullorum and *S. gallinarum* are known to colonize poultry ovaries and are present within eggs. Their transmission through poultry has been a problem.

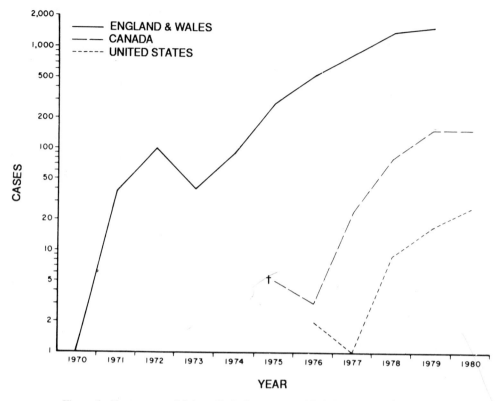

Figure 6 Human cases of *Salmonella hadar* gastroenteritis in England, Canáda, and the United States, 1970+ to 1980. From Centers for Disease Control (1980). *Morbid. Mortal. Wkly.* Rep. No. 29, p. 507.

These two organisms have largely been eliminated in the poultry industry because they caused economic hardship, that is, death of birds. Because of the elimination of these organisms from poultry, until recently it was considered to be a rare event that the interior of the egg would be infected. However, within the last 4–5 years, a problem with *Salmonella* contamination of egg contents has arisen again. However, this problem is caused by *S. enteritidis* strains that can colonize poultry ovaries and are transmitted in the yolk of eggs.

Another source from which eggs become contaminated with *Salmonella* is the intestinal tract or feces. *Salmonella* may contaminate the egg contents from the shell surface if there is adequate moisture on the shell and if there is a significant temperature differential between the egg contents and the environment. The warm egg and the cold air create a vacuum and aspirate *Salmonella* organisms into the egg, ultimately contaminating the yolk. Cracked eggs are more susceptible to *Salmonella* contamination than eggs with intact shells.

If a yolk becomes infected with *Salmonella,* there are three things that can happen. First, the chick may die before hatching. Second, it may hatch into a weak chick that dies or is culled. Third, it may develop into a healthy chick that excretes up to 10^8 salmonellae per gram of feces—this is the largest source of contamination. Poultry also feed on their litter mates' manure, so feces from one contaminated chick are sufficient to spread *Salmonella* to a large portion of the rest of the flock.

Contaminated feed is another source of *Salmonella*. Some type of rendered inedible by-product that is rich in protein, for example, poultry, beef, or fish waste, may be fed to poultry. Generally when this feed is rendered, it is heat treated in a way that would kill *Salmonella,* but through the interactive process that feed is recontaminated. A good example of the spread of *Salmonella* through poultry feed is the *S. agona* situation. Until 1970, this serotype had only been isolated twice from humans in the United States, so it was very rare in this country. In 1970, *S. agona* was isolated from a consignment of Peruvian fish meal that was shipped to the United States. After that, there was an increase in the incidence of *S. agona* isolated from nonhuman sources, particularly from poultry, and to a lesser extent from pigs. Several months later, there was also an increase in the number of cases of human salmonellosis due to *S. agona*. In 1976 *S. agona* ranked third among the most frequently isolated serotypes of *Salmonella* involved in human infection.

The environment is also a source from which *Salmonella* can be spread to poultry. Many studies have been done showing that salmonellae are often present on the cages that are used to bring birds to slaughterhouses. Surveys have revealed *Salmonella* on the surfaces of barns and poultry housing. Rodents and wild birds can carry *Salmonella* in their intestinal tracts and their droppings can infect poultry that feed on them.

Finally, another very important means by which finished poultry products are contaminated is through processing. When poultry is processed, the animals are decapitated, bled out, and then scalded to loosen the feathers. From there they go into a defeathering unit. The defeathering unit has hundreds of rubber fingers that spin around and pull off the feathers. As the animals go through the defeathering unit, the feces often come out and contaminate the rubber fingers. The fingers are not easily cleaned; in fact they crack with time and the *Salmonella* establishes a residence within the crevices. As the birds come through they are contaminated. Then the animals go through an evisceration unit where the entrails are removed. From there the poultry go into cooling tanks. These cooling tanks are also a potential source of cross-contamination. The water is chlorinated, but depending on the flow rate of the water, it will often accumulate large amounts of blood. Chlorine is inactivated in the presence of all this organic matter, so the *Salmonella* can survive.

Several approaches have been taken to eradicate *Salmonella* from poultry. In Denmark they seem to have a fairly good control over the incidence of *Salmonella* in poultry. They go to great extremes to identify flocks that are carrying the organism. Poultry in Europe, where they do have low incidences of *Salmonella* and go to great extremes to control it, is very expensive—four to five times the price of poultry in the United States. There is no simple solution: reduction of levels of *Salmonella* in poultry comes at a very high cost. In fact, in Denmark they have not been able to eradicate *Salmonella* from poultry; they still have an incidence of 3–4%.

One of the principal areas that needs to be addressed is breeder flocks. The Danes have good control over their breeder flocks, which are monitored by testing the animals' blood for antibody against *Salmonella*. If infected flocks are found, they are destroyed. Also it is very difficult to get new breeder hens into Denmark because they have to be quarantined for several months and test negative for *Salmonella* during this quarantine period before being allowed to function as breeders.

Another important approach is to control *Salmonella* in feed. In Denmark, feed must be certified free of *Salmonella,* and they routinely test the feed for *Salmonella.* Feed can be heat treated to kill *Salmonella* but one has to be careful to avoid postprocessing contamination. Killing *Salmonella* by irradiation has been investigated in many countries but it not yet legal in the United States.

Competitive exclusion is another approach taken to control *Salmonella.* This practice was developed by Professor Nurmi, a veterinarian in Finland who had a problem with salmonellosis in poultry in the early 1970s. He found that if feces from adult birds proven to be free of *Salmonella* are fed to day-old chicks, the chicks are protected from future colonization by *Salmonella.* It is a matter of giving the young birds a protective flora because it is believed that if there is relatively little microbial flora in the gut, as few as one *Salmonella* cell could colonize the young birds. If these young birds are made resistant to *Salmonella,* they should continue to be resistant to *Salmonella* infection when they become older birds, because of the indigenous flora that they develop. This process is not really understood and, in fact, is not entirely effective. Even with the inoculation, there may be some chicks that will ultimately become colonized with *Salmonella.* However, they usually are colonized at lower levels; they don't excrete 10^6 to 10^8 salmonellae per gram of feces.

What are the proposed mechanisms by which this process works? It has been suggested that the competitive flora that develops in the cecum may produce volatile organic acids and these organic acids prevent the growth of the *Salmonella* just as organic acids in foods would prevent the growth of *Salmonella.* That mechanism is not as well accepted as the second proposed mechanism, which is that the bacteria fed to the chicks actually colonize specific sites within the cecum and the intestinal tract which are required by *Salmonella* for colonization. These bacteria may be binding to the same receptor sites in the gut as *Salmonella* would, thus preventing *Salmonella* from binding there, colonizing, and invading.

The principal limitation of the Nurmi concept is that only a portion, perhaps 75%, of the chicks may be protected. Hence it may not eliminate all *Salmonella* in flocks. Nonetheless, it is a step in the right direction and any approach that will reduce the incidence of *Salmonella* in these birds is beneficial.

Another approach that has been considered for eliminating *Salmonella* from poultry carcasses is irradiation. Currently this is not an approved practice in the United States; however, it may be in the near future. One has to be careful in adopting this as a solution, however, because United States consumers are not very accepting of the idea of irradiating foods at present. When they see the label "irradiated" (which is required by law in the United States), they may be reluctant to buy. Hence it is likely that even if the irradiation of poultry is approved in the near future, it is not going to be readily accepted by the industry and the consumer for some years. An educational process needs to be instituted so that the consumer is made aware that irradiation levels, 5–7 kGy, that are needed to eliminate *Salmonella* from poultry are safe and do not produce a food that is unwholesome.

V.   Isolation and Identification of *Salmonella*

Five steps are common to most culture procedures for isolating and identifying *Salmonella* in foods. These include (1) preenrichment of a food sample in a nutritious, nonselective broth; (2) selective enrichment in a broth that allows salmonellae to grow but suppresses the growth of competing bacteria; (3) isolation of *Salmonella* by streaking onto selective plating agar; (4) biochemical characterization of isolates; and (5) serological confirmation of biochemically screened isolates.

The initial step of preenrichment is designed to restore injured salmonellae to a stable physiological condition—they then grow on the nutrients present in the medium. Generally, preenrichment media are nutritionally complex and may include Trypticase soy broth, nutrient broth, reconstituted nonfat dry milk, or lactose broth. Preenrichment requires incubating cultures at 35–37°C for 16–24 hours.

Following preenrichment, a portion of the preenrichment culture is transferred to selective enrichment media. Two media commonly used for selective enrichment are selenite cystine broth and tetrathionate broth. These media allow salmonellae to grow but restrict the growth of competing bacteria. Selective enrichment cultures are incubated for 16–24 hours at 35–37 or 43°C.

To isolate *Salmonella*, selective enrichment cultures are plated onto selective agar plates. Examples of selective plating agars include Hektoen enteric, xylose–lysine–desoxycholate (XLD), bismuth sulfite, and MacConkey agars. None of these media is ideal for all situations, hence the use of two or three media is usually recommended. These plates are held at 35–37°C for 24 and sometimes 48 hours and then are examined for colonies typical of *Salmonella*.

Salmonella-like colonies are selected and identified by biochemical tests. Two differential agars, that is, triple sugar iron agar (TSI) [salmonellae typically produce alkaline (red) slant and acid (yellow) butt, with or without production of H_2S (blackening of agar)] and lysine iron agar (LIA [salmonellae typically produce an alkaline (purple) reaction in the butt, with or without production of H_2S], are commonly used in combination to provide initial biochemical data about the isolates. Cultures typical of *Salmonella* in these media are then tested by a complete battery of biochemical tests to confirm the isolates. Biochemical tests typically used include urease (negative), lysine decarboxylase (positive), fermentation of dulcitol (positive), growth in KCN broth (negative), utilization of sodium malonate (negative), and production of indole (negative). Other tests occasionally used include fermentation of lactose and sucrose (both negative), Voges–Proskauer test (negative), and methyl red test (positive). Several commercially available miniaturized diagnostic kits which employ most of the above biochemical reagents are widely used and provide rapid, reliable results.

The final step in the identification of *Salmonella* isolates is serological testing. Cultures are tested by agglutination assays with antisera specific for somatic (O), flagellar (H), and capsular (Vi) antigens.

Several innovative procedures have been developed for detecting salmonellae in foods more rapidly than traditional isolation procedures. Examples include enzyme immunoassay procedures, DNA–DNA hybridization (gene probe) test, hydrophobic grid membrane filtration technique, latex agglutination assays, and flagellar agglutination technique. Although these tests are shorter than conventional isolation procedures, all require preenrichment and usually selective enrichment of samples before being applied. Additionally, not all of these procedures are as accurate in detecting salmonellae in foods as are conventional procedures.

Bibliography

Anonymous (1988). "Salmonellosis Control: The Role of Animal and Product Hygiene," WHO Tech. Rep. Ser., No. 774, pp. 1–83. World Health Organ., Geneva.

Blaser, M. J., and Newman, L. S. (1982). A review of human salmonellosis. I. Infective dose. *Rev. Infect. Dis.* **4,** 1096–1106.

Centers for Disease Control (1982). "*Salmonella* Surveillance Annual Summary, 1980," pp. 1–22. CDC, Atlanta.

D'Aoust, J.-Y. (1989). *Salmonella. In* "Foodborne Bacterial Pathogens" (M. P. Doyle, ed.), pp. 327–445. Dekker, New York.

Hargrett-Bean, N. T., Pavia, A. T., and Tauxe, R. V. (1988). *Salmonella* isolates from humans in the United States, 1984–1986. *Morbid. Mortal. Wkly.* Rep. No. 37 (SS-2), pp. 25–31.

Linton, A. H., ed. (1983). "Guidelines on Prevention and Control of Salmonellosis," WHO VPH/ 83.42, pp. 1–128. World Health Organ., Geneva.

CHAPTER 12

SHIGELLA

Michael P. Doyle

I. Introduction

Shigella causes human diarrheal disease sometimes termed bacillary dysentery or, more frequently, shigellosis. Bacteria of this genus are host adapted to humans and higher primates. Transmission of shigellosis is usually by person-to-person contact by the fecal–oral route but also can occur by fecal contamination of water and food. Foodborne transmission of the disease is usually the result of improper hygienic practices by a food handler infected with *Shigella*.

II. Shigellosis

Shigellosis is an important problem in developing countries where insanitary conditions exist. The illness is also a problem in developed countries where crowded living conditions occur, such as in day-care schools and custodial institutions. About 15,000 to 20,000 cases of shigellosis are reported in the United States each year, mostly in children less than 4 years of age.

Symptoms of shigellosis vary from an asymptomatic infection to mild diarrhea to fulminating dysentery. In severe cases symptoms may include bloody stools with mucus and pus, dehydration, fever, chills, toxemia, tenesmus, and vomiting. The time to onset of symptoms ranges from 1–7 days but is usually less than 4 days. Illness generally persists from a few days to 2 weeks.

Shigella is a highly infectious organism. As few as 10 cells of *Shigella dysenteriae* given orally to adult volunteers caused illness. In studies with other species of *Shigella*, ingestion of $10^2–10^4$ cells caused illness.

The principal sites of infection for *Shigella* are the terminal ileum and colon. Shigellae penetrate the epithelium and multiply within the epithelial cells; then the organisms spread laterally to adjacent cells, producing necrosis and death of patches of cells. This leads to ulcers which exude blood that is present in diarrheal stools. Shiga toxin produced by shigellae may be responsible for the dramatic inflammatory response and necrosis of the surface epithelium of the mucosal layer. This toxin is a protein that has enterotoxic, neurotoxic, and cytotoxic activities. The organism rarely penetrates beyond the lamina propria so it seldom causes a bacteremia.

In most cases, shigellosis is self-limited and resolves within 1–2 weeks after onset of illness, hence antibiotic therapy is unnecessary. However, with infections of the very young or for cases with severe diarrhea, treatment with antibiotics may be needed. Ampicillin is often used because *Shigella* are resistant to many of the other antibiotics used for treating enteric infections.

III. Characteristics of *Shigella*

A. Classification and Biochemical Characteristics

The genus *Shigella* is a member of the family Enterobacteriaceae. Cells stain gram-negative, appear as straight rods, and are nonmotile. The organism is facultatively anaerobic, ferments many carbohydrates (but usually not lactose) with the production of acid but usually not gas, and lacks lysine decarboxylase, phenylalanine deaminase, and urease. DNA–DNA homology studies revealed that *Shigella* and *Escherichia coli* are closely related genetically and could be considered to be in the same genus.

The genus *Shigella* is composed of four species, each consisting of a different serogroup. These include *S. dysenteriae* (serogroup A), *S. flexneri* (serogroup B), *S. boydii* (serogroup C), and *S. sonnei* (serogroup D). *Shigella dysenteriae* has a higher case-fatality rate than the other *Shigella* spp.; however, this species accounts for the smallest number (approximately 1%) of *Shigella* isolations from patients in the United States. *Shigella sonnei* is responsible for most (70–80%) cases of shigellosis reported in the United States annually.

B. Survival and Growth Characteristics

Shigella species generally are not hardy organisms and are not particularly resistant to environmental stresses. Most strains of *Shigella* are killed at 63°C in 5 minutes. Some strains of *Shigella* can grow at temperatures ranging from 7–46°C, but not at 49°C. The optimal temperature for growth is 37°C. *Shigella* can survive for 4 hours in nutrient medium poised at pH 4.0 or 4.5, but can only survive for 30 minutes at pH 3.5. The pH range for growth is about 5–8, with formic and acetic acids preventing growth at pH 6.0. Studies in foods revealed that shigellae at temperatures of $\leq$25°C could survive for more than 50 days in flour, milk, eggs, shrimp, oysters, and clams. Survival in acidic products like orange juice, tomato juice, and carbonated soft drinks was much less, ranging from 5–10 days. Shigellae may grow well in foods with few microbial competitors. For example, *S. sonnei* injected into watermelon held at 22°C for 2 days increased by 10^7 CFU/g.

IV. Foodborne Transmission of *Shigella*

Infected humans and higher primates are the known reservoirs of *Shigella* spp. These organisms are present in the lower gastrointestinal tract and are excreted in feces. Convalescent carriers are an important reservoir of *Shigella* and, hence, an important source for spreading shigellosis. Shigellae are usually shed in feces of convalescent carriers for 3–5 weeks after symptoms of illness subside, although some individuals may continue to excrete the organism for more than 5 months. Additionally, many cases of shigellosis go unrecognized because symptoms are mild. Individuals with mild infections may serve as asymptomatic carriers in transmitting the organism.

Food handlers who practice poor personal hygiene, that is, fail to wash hands properly after defecating and subsequently handle food, are the principal factor contributing to foodborne outbreaks of shigellosis. Improper refrigeration of contaminated foods also often contributes to outbreaks. Although likely infrequent, flies may also serve as a vector for transmitting shigellae from feces to food. Most recognized outbreaks result from food prepared and mishandled in food service establishments.

The type of food most often implicated as the vehicle of foodborne shigellosis is salads. About two-thirds of foodborne outbreaks have been associated with eating salads, especially those made with potatoes, chicken, tuna, or shrimp. Other foods implicated in outbreaks include lettuce, raw oysters, watermelon, spaghetti, beans, apple cider, cream puffs, hamburger, and shrimp. In most instances, *Shigella*-infected food handlers were responsible for contaminating the foods.

V. Isolation and Identification of *Shigella*

Procedures for isolating shigellae from foods are not highly sensitive. Food samples are normally enriched in a broth such as gram-negative (GN) broth which is then plated onto differential selective agar such as xylose–lysine–deoxycholate (XLD) agar and MacConkey agar. Shigellae may be characterized and identified by biochemical reactions. Shigellae are less active than *Escherichia coli* in fermenting carbohydrates. Isolates generally do not utilize acetate, mucate, or citrate; do not ferment lactose; do not produce gas from glucose fermentation; do not possess lysine decarboxylase, arginine dihydrolase, ornithine decarboxylase, or urease activities; and are not motile.

Bibliography

Smith, J. L. (1987). *Shigella* as a foodborne pathogen. *J. Food Prot.* **50**, 788.
Wachsmuth, I. K., and Morris, G. K. (1989). *Shigella. In* "Foodborne Bacterial Pathogens" (M. P. Doyle, ed.), pp. 448–461. Dekker, New York.

CHAPTER 13

ESCHERICHIA COLI

Michael P. Doyle
and Dean O. Cliver

I. Introduction

Escherichia coli is considered to be a part of the normal microflora of the intestinal tract of humans and most other warm-blooded animals. Hence, it is generally present in feces. Most strains of *E. coli* are harmless, but a few are pathogenic.

II. *Escherichia coli*

Organisms of this species are generally lactose fermenters, but sometimes the lactose fermentation is delayed. They are gram-negative, nonsporeforming rods and are generally motile by peritrichous flagella, but there are some nonmotile strains. Many strains produce capsules. They are usually aerogenic—they produce gas from glucose.

The three principal antigens used for serology are the somatic antigen, the capsular antigen, and the flagellar antigen. Presently about 171 O antigens are known; however, there are still many untypable strains of *E. coli*, so there are other O antigens that have not been identified. There are 90 known capsular antigens and to date 56 known flagellar antigens for serotyping *E. coli*. The O antigens are not characterized into single factors as with the *Salmonella*. These O antigens are polysaccharides, but their composition is not completely known. The K antigens are the envelope or capsular antigens, of which different forms are known. Unlike the flagellar antigens of *Salmonella*, the flagellar antigens of *E. coli* are monophasic—they do not express two different antigenic types of flagella.

Several tests may be used to determine if an organism is an enteropathogen, that is, if it has virulence potential and possesses enteropathogenicity. One of the classic tests is the ligated ileal loop test. The animal most often used in this test is the rabbit. The ileal (most distant) portion of the small intestine is tied into 5- to 6-cm segments, and each segment is inoculated with a different material. The inoculum might be whole cells of an organism, a lysate or culture filtrate of the organism, and also appropriate controls, such as PBS or whatever the carrier is for the substance being tested. The small intestine is put back into the animal, left for a certain period, taken out, and examined for fluid accumulation. The accumulation of fluid in a segment is indicative of a diarrheal-type response. The ileal loop test is often used to determine if an organism produces enterotoxins. Fluid accumulation in an ileal segment injected with culture filtrate indicates that enterotoxin was present in the inoculum. Also, if whole cells are inoculated into an ileal segment, one can examine not only for fluid accumulation, but can determine by histopathology whether the organism has invaded the intestinal lining.

Another test that is sometimes used is called the Sereny test. The Sereny test was first developed for *Shigella*. If a large number of cells, usually 10^9 or more, is applied to the the conjunctical lining of the eye of a guinea pig, those organisms that are invasive will ultimately cause a clouding and an ulceration of the eye. This test is indicative of an organism's ability to penetrate epithelial tissue. A positive response indicates that the organism is invasive.

The infant mouse assay is used to determine if an organism can produce heat-stable enterotoxin. Culture filtrates are injected into 2- to 4-day-old mice. After 3 hours, the entire intestine is removed, and the rest of the carcass is weighed separately. If the ratio of the intestinal weight to the carcass weight is greater than 0.083, this indicates that there was fluid accumulation and that heat-stable enterotoxin is present in the culture filtrate. This infant mouse assay is principally used for determining the presence of heat-stable enterotoxin of *E. coli* and also of *Yersinia enterocolitica*.

Various tissue culture assays have been developed, principally for detecting cholera toxin and also *E. coli* heat-labile enterotoxin. These are very similar toxins and produce the same response in certain cells, the Y-1 mouse adrenal cell line, for example. Culture filtrates are simply added to the Y-1 cell line; if the cells are rounded 20 hours later, this indicates that a heat-labile enterotoxin was present in the inoculum. Another cell line that is commonly used to detect heat-labile enterotoxin is the Chinese hamster ovary (CHO) line.

Another procedure that has been used is the vascular permeability assay. This involves injecting culture filtrates intradermally into the skin of an adult rabbit. Six to eighteen hours later, depending on the type of toxin sought, a blue dye is injected into the rabbit's vein. After 2 hours the skin will show a blue area around the original site of injection if vascular permeation has occurred. This assay has been used for detecting cholera toxin, the choleralike toxin of *Salmonella,* and heat-labile enterotoxin of *E. coli.*

Immunologic tests have also been developed to determine the presence of *E. coli* toxins. These tests are based on antibodies to specific toxins. Included are enzyme immunoassays, radioimmunoassays, and other *in vitro* tests.

III.   Enteropathogenic *Escherichia coli*

There are principally four different groups of *E. coli* that have been implicated in foodborne disease outbreaks. The first are the enteropathogenic *E. coli* (EPEC). This organism is prominently known as a cause of outbreaks of neonatal diarrhea which often occur in hospital nurseries. The organism is a serious problem in some developing countries and was a major problem in the United States in the 1940s and 1950s, but has not been as great a problem in recent years. Many adults are carriers of EPEC but they seldom express symptoms of illness. It is believed that adults acquire immunity to this organism so they can carry it and not become ill. However, a few food-related outbreaks of EPEC diarrhea have occurred in adults.

IV.   Enteroinvasive *Escherichia coli*

Another group of pathogenic *E. coli* are the enteroinvasive *E. coli* (EIEC). The EIEC have a pathological behavior very similar to the *Shigella*. Symptoms are chills, fever, abdominal cramps, and dysentery. Studies with adult human volunteers have shown that the infectious dose is quite high, generally 10^6–10^8 organisms. The incubation period usually ranges from 8–24 hours, with an average of 11 hours. The duration of the illness is usually several days. The course of infection is very similar to shigellosis. The organisms invade the colonic epithelial cells, multiply within these epithelial cells, and invade adjacent epithelial cells, causing ulcerations of the colon and ultimately resulting in bloody diarrhea.

About 11 serotypes are primarily responsible for EIEC infections. The most common of these is **O**:124. The EIEC are biochemically similar to *Shigella*. Generally they ferment lactose, but late. Many of the strains are anaerogenic: they do not produce gas from glucose. They often are similar to *Shigella* serologically. For example, *E. coli* **O**:124 is the same somatic antigen as *Shigella* **O**:3. Because of this similarity between the enteroinvasive types of *E. coli* and *Shigella*, it is thought that many cases and perhaps outbreaks of shigellosis that are reported may actually be due to enteroinvasive types of *E. coli*.

V. Enterotoxigenic *Escherichia coli*

The enterotoxigenic *E. coli* (ETEC) is generally more commonly associated with traveler's diarrhea than it is with foodborne disease in the United States. The symptoms of ETEC are similar to those of cholera—a watery diarrhea, dehydration, possible shock, and sometimes vomiting. What little is known about the infectious dose is based on one study done with adult human volunteers in which the infectious dose was determined to be between 10^8 and 10^{10} cells, so it was quite high. The incubation period is in the range of 8–44 hours, averaging 26 hours. The duration of illness is short—about 24–30 hours.

The course of infection is quite different than that described for other *E. coli*. This organism colonizes the epithelial surface of the small intestine and elaborates one or more toxins that act on the small intestine, inducing an outpouring of fluid. The organism does not invade nor does it damage the epithelial layer of the small intestine. It simply colonizes the surface, elaborates the toxin, and induces an outpouring of fluid.

Three requirements must be fulfilled for the ETEC to produce a diarrheal response in a host. First, the organism must be toxigenic—it must have the plasmid that codes for one or two toxins. The second requirement is that the host must ingest a sufficient number of the organism to produce illness. According to present knowledge, ingesting a few hundred cells will not cause illness, but 10^6 or more may be sufficient. Third, the organism must be in contact with the mucosa of the small intestine. This is accomplished through colonization factors.

Enterotoxigenic *E. coli* organisms can produce one of two types of toxin, or perhaps even both toxins, depending on their plasmid content. One toxin is known to be heat labile—it is inactivated in 30 minutes at 60°C. This toxin is very similar to cholera toxin, the toxin produced by *Vibrio cholerae*. This heat-labile toxin can be neutralized with antitoxin to cholera toxin because it is immunologically related.

The second type of enterotoxin expressed by some types of ETEC is heat stable. It withstands 100°C for 30 minutes. There are different types of heat-stable enterotoxins. "STa" toxin is detected by an infant mouse test and is negative in the ileal loop test. "STb" toxin is the reverse—infant mouse assay negative but ileal loop positive. Besides being quite stable to heat treatment, this toxin withstands other treatment with proteolytic enzymes, nucleases, lipases, and organic solvents.

Another very important component of the ETEC are colonization factors. These colonization factors are very specific fimbriae, which are the proteinaceous, hairlike structures—not flagellar, but simply filamentous appendages—on the surface of the cell wall that allow the ETEC to adhere to the intestinal epithelial cells. A variety of types of colonization factors have been identified and shown to be very species specific. K88 is specific for swine and does not colonize other animals. ETEC with K88 are an important cause of diarrhea and mortality in piglets. K99 is specific for calves, lambs, and swine but evidently does not colonize humans. Another colonization factor that is specific for pigs is 987P. Colonization factor antigens I (CFA/I) and II (CFA/II) are specific for humans; they do not colonize other animals.

VI.   Enterohemorrhagic *Escherichia coli*

The fourth type of *E. coli* is **O157:H7**. Among pathogenic groups of *E. coli*, this is probably the most important in terms of foodborne disease. This type of *E. coli* is also known as enterohemorrhagic *E. coli*.

Three principal syndromes have been linked to *E. coli* **O157:H7**. The first is hemorrhagic colitis, in which the stools contain frank (red) blood. The second is hemolytic uremic syndrome (HUS) and is the leading cause of renal failure in children. In HUS, blood clots plug the convoluted tubules in the kidney which results in accumulation of waste products in the blood. The patient may require dialysis treatment and may be permanently debilitated. In some instances the child will go into a coma and die. This syndrome has killed elderly people as well as children. The third syndrome is called thrombotic thrombocytopenic purpura (TTP). It is similar to HUS but also involves brain damage, so the mortality rate is very high; it is very infrequent. *Escherichia coli* **O157:H7** presents a very serious threat, particularly as related to undercooked ground beef and raw milk, which have been identified as vehicles of food-related outbreaks. Surveys have shown that 1–3% of fresh beef, pork, poultry, and lamb samples from grocery stores are contaminated with *E. coli* **O157:H7**, so it does not seem to be present only in beef.

At least three different "verotoxins," one of which is very similar to Shiga toxin, are known virulence factors. Verotoxins are substances that are cytotoxic to Vero tissue culture cells, a line established from the kidneys of an African Green monkey. These toxins have been shown to be very specific for the colon. When injected intravenously or intraperitoneally into mice, toxin goes to the colon, ulcerates the epithelial layer, and ultimately causes bleeding in the gut, so we believe these toxins are probably important in the pathology of hemorrhagic colitis.

VII. Foodborne Transmission of *Escherichia coli*

Enteropathogenic *E. coli* caused an outbreak in the United States in 1968 due to drinking of unchlorinated well water apparently contaminated by human sewage. Several food-associated outbreaks occurred in England. One in 1967 was linked to eating cold, previously cooked pork and another in 1973 was attributed to eating contaminated meat pie. However, this organism is a rather infrequent cause of foodborne disease.

Infected humans are the principal reservoir of EIEC. The organism can be spread by water and food and by person-to-person contact. Not many foodborne outbreaks have been linked to this group, but salmon, poultry, milk, and Camembert cheese have been vehicles. The most prominent of these was the Camembert cheese incident that occurred in late 1971. About 380 persons in the United States became ill. The outbreak was traced to some French-made Camembert cheese that contained *E. coli* O:124 at levels of 10^5–10^7 per gram. A retrospective study of the plant where the cheese was made revealed that its water purification system was not working properly, so improperly treated river water was being used to clean equipment and wash cheese. It is likely that the river water was contaminated with human feces containing *E. coli* O:124.

Enterotoxigenic *E. coli* is the most common cause of "traveler's diarrhea." This is the type of diarrhea one may experience when going from a developed country to a developing country, where the sanitary practices may not be as good and where the water supply is sometimes contaminated. This diarrhea begins within 12 hours to a few weeks of entering a developing country. Enterotoxigenic *E. coli* accounts for 60–70% of cases of traveler's diarrhea. A study was done by members of the American Medical Association in conjunction with a meeting in Mexico City in the mid-1970s. Knowing that one often experiences traveler's diarrhea when one goes to Mexico, they decided to do a prospective study and record what foods they had eaten. Then when they got back to the United States they would pool their data and see if they could make an association between foods that were consumed and diarrhea due to ETEC. The apparent "common denominator" was salads containing raw vegetables, so it appears that raw vegetables can be an important source of ETEC in developing countries.

There have been several foodborne outbreaks due to ETEC. One occurred in northern Wisconsin in 1980. Food from a Mexican-style restaurant made more than 400 people ill. It was determined that food was likely contaminated by a food handler who had had diarrheal illness during the 2-week period before the outbreak. Several food-related outbreaks have occurred on cruise ships. A more recent outbreak occurred in 1983 and it was linked to eating French Brie cheese. It was a multistate outbreak and 169 people became ill; the cause was determined to be ETEC. Illness was associated with cheese from two different lots manufactured 46 days apart, indicating that the plant's products were contaminated at least intermittently during that time. The source of contamination at the plant was not determined.

These types of *E. coli* are also transmitted through water. There was a major outbreak of ETEC at Crater Lake National Park. More than 2000 individuals became ill because the park's water supply was contaminated with raw sewage. Enterotoxigenic *E. coli* was isolated from both the water supply and the patients.

A third means by which ETEC can be transmitted is through person-to-person contact. However, there is little evidence for this except for outbreaks that have occurred at hospital nurseries.

The principal reservoir for ETEC is asymptomatic human carriers. A person who recovers from an ETEC infection may continue to excrete the organism for several months, so there is fecal excretion of this organism and it can ultimately be spread by that individual. Studies in developing countries revealed that ETEC is often present in feces of asymptomatic human carriers.

Until 1982, *E. coli* **O**157:**H**7 had only been isolated once in the United States. This isolation was from a California woman with bloody diarrhea in 1975. In 1982 there were two food-associated outbreaks due to *E. coli* **O**157: **H**7, one in Oregon and one in Michigan. Symptoms included frank or pure blood in the stools, very severe abdominal pain, some vomiting, but no fever. The time onset of illness was 3–4 days and the duration was 2–9 days, with an average of about 4 days. Many of these individuals with bloody diarrhea were hospitalized. Investigators from the Centers for Disease Control were able to link the outbreaks epidemiologically to ground beef patties prepared at specific restaurants. There have since been several more foodborne outbreaks due to *E. coli* **O**157:**H**7. The principal foods linked to transmission of the organism have been ground beef (insufficiently cooked) and raw milk.

The enteropathogenic, enteroinvasive, and enterotoxigenic types of *E. coli* principally come from human feces—that is, humans are the principal reservoir. These infected humans excrete the organism with feces, which ultimately contaminate food. The contamination generally occurs via contaminated water or from contact with infected food handlers. Serious problems with these three types of *E. coli* occur in developing countries, where unsanitary conditions exist and where untreated human sewage may contaminate water that is used for drinking or irrigation of food crops, rather than in the United States.

The situation differs for *E. coli* **O**157:**H**7. It appears that cattle are a reservoir of the organism, which can be found in the intestinal tract of dairy cattle. Hence, meat can be contaminated by this organism during processing. This *E. coli* type is likely to be more widespread in the United States food supply than would the other types of pathogenic *E. coli*. Proper heat treatment of foods of animal origin, such as meats and raw milk, to inactivate pathogens such as *E. coli* **O**157:**H**7, is imperative.

Bibliography

Doyle, M. P. (1985). Food-borne pathogens of recent concern. *Annu. Rev. Nutr.* **5,**24–42.

Doyle, M. P., and Padhye, V. V. (1989). *Escherichia coli*. *In* "Foodborne Bacterial Pathogens" (M. P. Doyle, ed.), pp. 235–281. Dekker, New York.

Gross, R. J., and Rowe, B. (1985). *Escherichia coli* diarrhoea. *J. Hyg.* **95,**531–550.

Robins-Browne, R. M. (1987). Traditional enteropathogenic *Escherichia coli* of infantile diarrhea. *Rev. Infect. Dis.* **9,** 28–53.

WHO Scientific Working Group (1980). *Escherichia coli* diarrhoea. *Bull. W.H.O.* **58,** 23–36.

CHAPTER 14

CAMPYLOBACTER JEJUNI

Michael P. Doyle

217

I. Introduction

Within the past decade *Campylobacter jejuni* has become recognized as the leading cause of acute bacterial gastroenteritis in many developed countries, including the United States. The organism is commonly carried as a commensal in the intestinal tract of warmblooded animals and is often present on foods of animal origin through fecal contamination during processing. *Campylobacter jejuni* does not grow well in foods and does not survive well outside the host's internal environment; however, ingesting relatively small numbers of the organism can produce human illness. Foods, especially those derived from animals, are thought to be the principal vehicle for transmission of *Campylobacter* enteritis.

II. *Campylobacter* Enteritis

Campylobacter jejuni is responsible for one of the most frequently occurring forms of acute bacterial gastroenteritis in humans. A study at eight hospitals in different parts of the United States revealed that *C. jejuni* was isolated from fecal specimens of patients more often than *Salmonella* and *Shigella* combined. The symptoms and signs of *Campylobacter* enteritis are not readily distinguishable from gastrointestinal illness caused by other enteric pathogens. The features of illness may vary from a mild, brief enteritis to a fulminant illness that mimics ulcerative colitis with grossly bloody stools. The predominant symptoms of individuals who seek medical attention include diarrhea, abdominal pain, malaise, fever, nausea, and vomiting. Grossly bloody stools are common, and abdominal pain may mimic acute appendicitis. Time to onset of illness may range from 1–10 days, but is usually within 3–5 days. Illness may persist from 1 day to a few weeks, but most patients recover in less than a week.

Studies in which adult volunteers have been challenged orally with *C. jejuni* have revealed that the infectious dose is low. Ingestion of only a few hundred cells produced infection and, in many instances, illness in several individuals.

In most cases, *Campylobacter* enteritis is mild and self-limited and resolves within a few days of onset of symptoms. Hence, antibiotic therapy is unnecessary. However, when symptoms have been prolonged, or when high fever is present, treatment with antibiotics may be needed—erythromycin is the drug of choice.

III. Characteristics of *Campylobacter jejuni*

A. Classification and Biochemical Characteristics

Campylobacter jejuni, originally classified as *Vibrio fetus*, is a member of the family Spirillaceae. Cells stain gram-negative, are very slender (0.2–0.5 μm wide by 0.5–5 μm long), spirally curved rods, and are motile with a single polar flagellum (at one or both ends) that is two to three times the length of the cell. Motility appears as a unique darting, corkscrewlike movement that is characteristic of campylobacters. When cells form short chains, they appear as S-shaped or gull-winged. Cells in old cultures become coccoid and cells of this type are largely nonviable. The organism is catalase- and oxidase-positive but cannot ferment or oxidize carbohydrates.

Two other species of *Campylobacter, C. coli* and *C. laridis,* are very closely related to *C. jejuni* but differ by their inability to hydrolyze hippurate and ability to grow in the presence of 30 μg nalidixic acid, respectively. Both organisms are recognized causes of gastroenteritis, but occur substantially less frequently than *C. jejuni.* Because these organisms share many clinical and epidemiologic characteristics, they are considered collectively and referred to as *C. jejuni* in this chapter.

B. Survival and Growth Characteristics

Unlike other recognized foodborne pathogens, *C. jejuni* is a strict microaerophile that requires low levels of oxygen for growth; growth is retarded or inhibited at oxygen concentrations less than 3% and greater than 10–15%—5% is best. Additionally, *C. jejuni* is a capnophile (carbon dioxide lover) that grows well in the presence of 10% CO_2, but not well, if at all, in less than 5% CO_2.

The organism grows only within a narrow temperature range, that is, between 30 and 47°C. The optimal temperature for growth is 42–45°C, with growth at 42–45°C approximately twice as rapid as that at 35–37°C. Holding *C. jejuni* at refrigeration temperature (4°C) greatly enhances survival of the organism. Depending on the environment, medium, and initial number of *C. jejuni,* the organism may survive in a nongrowth environment (e.g., pH 4.5) for several weeks at 4°C, several days at 25°C, and only a day or two at 42°C with conditions other than temperature being equivalent.

The organism is sensitive to freezing at temperatures (−20 to −5°C) commonly used for frozen foods. Studies revealed 2–5 $\log_{10}$ *C. jejuni* per gram decreases in meat held at −20°C for 1–3 months. However, although *C. jejuni* is sensitive to frozen storage, the organism can be isolated from a comparatively low percentage of meats and poultry that have been held frozen for several months.

Thermal inactivation studies have revealed that the organism is quite sensitive to heat. The *D* value for *C. jejuni* in skim milk at 55°C is about 1.0 minute. The organism is about 10-fold more sensitive to thermal stress under similar conditions than the typical strain of *Salmonella* spp. Heating foods sufficiently to kill salmonellae will also inactivate *C. jejuni.*

Survival of *C. jejuni* is also influenced by environmental concentrations of oxygen. Reduction products of oxygen, including superoxide anions and hydrogen peroxide which may be generated during cellular metabolism or during autooxidation or photochemical oxidation in the medium, are toxic to microorganisms. *Campylobacter jejuni* is thought to be more sensitive to exogenous superoxide anions and hydrogen peroxide than aerotolerant bacteria, even though the organism possesses superoxide dismutase and catalase activities. Survival of *C. jejuni,* especially at 4°C, is greatly enhanced when oxygen is removed from the environment. Increasing the oxygen concentration concomitantly increases the rate at which *C. jejuni* is inactivated.

The response of *C. jejuni* to pH is influenced by the temperature and type of acid used to adjust the pH. The minimum pH (adjusted with HCl) for growth at 42°C is about 4.9–5.0 or higher, depending on the strain. At an equivalent pH, lactic acid is more inhibitory than HCl to *C. jejuni*. Survival below the pH limit of growth is temperature dependent. For example, the time required to inactivate 99% of *C. jejuni* in a medium adjusted to pH 4.5 with HCl was 8 hours at 42°C, greater than 24 hours but less than 48 hours at 25°C, and 4 days at 4°C.

Campylobacter jejuni is quite sensitive to NaCl and generally will not grow in medium with more than 2.0%. The organism grows best in medium containing 0.5% NaCl. *Campylobacter jejuni* is also quite sensitive to dehydration, especially when drying occurs at room temperature or above. Large numbers of *Campylobacter* in skim milk generally are inactivated ($>10^4$ $\log_{10}$ reduction) within 24 hours when held in an anhydrous environment at 25°C. In contrast, when dehydration occurs at refrigeration temperature, large numbers of *C. jejuni* may survive and remain viable for several weeks if continuously held refrigerated.

Survival of *C. jejuni* in uncooked foods held at 4°C differs greatly depending on the food. In unpasteurized milk there is a substantial reduction (>3 $\log_{10}$/ml) in cell number within 4 days, probably due largely to the lactoperoxidase activity in milk. In contrast, in fresh ground beef there is generally little change (<0.5 $\log_{10}$/g) in cell number within 14 days of refrigerated storage.

IV.   Foodborne Transmission of *Campylobacter jejuni*

A wide variety of wild and domestic warmblooded animals are reservoirs of *C. jejuni*. The organism associates as a commensal with the intestinal tract and is excreted in feces, often at levels of $\geq 10^6$ *C. jejuni* per gram. Cattle, swine, sheep, goats, chickens, turkeys, ducks, cats, and dogs are recognized carriers of *C. jejuni*. Some of the highest rates of *C. jejuni* carriage have been associated with poultry; surveys frequently reveal *C. jejuni* in feces of 30–100% of poultry tested.

Food is the likely source of many *Campylobacter* infections and has been identified as the vehicle of transmission of many outbreaks of *Campylobacter* enteritis. Unpasteurized milk is the most frequently implicated vehicle in foodborne outbreaks, many of which have been quite large. In a single outbreak, 2500 schoolchildren were ill. Outbreaks also have been associated with eating undercooked chicken, processed turkey, raw clams, and raw hamburger. Most outbreaks have been linked to eating foods of animal origin; however, an outbreak has also resulted from eating cake likely contaminated with *C. jejuni* by a food handler. Hence, it appears that asymptomatic human carriers of *C. jejuni* may also transmit *Campylobacter* infections. Convalescent carriers in developed countries may excrete *C. jejuni* in their feces for 6 weeks after illness. Several major waterborne outbreaks resulting from drinking improperly treated surface water have also been reported.

Campylobacter jejuni is associated principally with raw foods of animal origin and is seldom found in processed foods. A large survey of retail uncooked red meats and chicken in the United States revealed *C. jejuni* contamination in about 5% of red meats and 30% of chicken obtained from grocery stores. About 1–1.5% of the raw milk sampled from farm bulk tanks contained *C. jejuni*. Interestingly, the organism also has been isolated from 1.5% of 200 retail packages of fresh mushrooms. Although mushrooms are not of animal origin, they are grown on composted horse and/or chicken manure and are harvested by hand by individuals who may not use acceptable hygienic practices. A large prospective study of the flow of *C. jejuni* from foods to humans revealed there was an increased risk of developing *Campylobacter* enteritis after eating mushrooms. Considering how mushrooms are grown and harvested and that *C. jejuni* has been isolated from retail packages of mushrooms, it is probable that fresh mushrooms are a vehicle of *Campylobacter* enteritis.

Although raw milk is the leading vehicle of outbreaks in *Campylobacter* enteritis, poultry appears to be the principal vehicle of transmission for sporadic cases of *Campylobacter* infection. This has been demonstrated by prospective studies designed to identify risk factors for *Campylobacter* enteritis. Attention of the food handler should be focused on thoroughly cooking poultry and avoiding cross-contamination of contact surfaces of raw poultry with cooked poultry and other foods to avoid transmission of *C. jejuni*.

V.   Isolation and Identification of *Campylobacter jejuni*

The sensitivity of *C. jejuni* to environmental stress, which includes storage at room temperature (20–25°C), exposure to normal atmospheric concentrations of oxygen, and dehydration, necessitates that food specimens to be tested for the organism be properly handled and assayed as soon as possible. If foods are to be transported or stored before analysis, they should be held refrigerated (not frozen) and, when possible, under anaerobic conditions, such as an atmosphere of 100% N_2, or in the presence of an oxygen scavenger such as 0.15% sodium thioglycollate and 0.01% sodium bisulfite.

Isolation of *C. jejuni* from foods usually necessitates enrichment in a selective medium that contains blood and several antibiotics and is held under microaerobic conditions at 42 or 37°C. Enrichment culture is plated onto selective agar, such as Campy BAP, Skirrow's agar, or Preston blood-free agar, that is also incubated under microaerobic conditions at 42 or 37°C.

Campylobacter jejuni is identified by its characteristic darting, corkscrewlike motility with a phase-contrast microscope, by its common S-, gull-, and spiral-shaped cellular morphology, and by several biochemical tests. These include inability to ferment or oxidize glucose, ability to grow at 37 or 42°C but not at 25°C, ability to hydrolyze hippurate, inability to grow in 3.5% NaCl, ability to reduce nitrate, production of H_2S in cysteine medium as detected by a lead acetate paper strip, and possession of catalase and oxidase activity.

Bibliography

Blaser, M. J., Taylor, D. N., and Feldman, R. A. (1983). Epidemiology of *Campylobacter* infections. *Epidemiol. Rev.* **5,** 157–176.

Doyle, M. P. (1984). *Campylobacter* in foods. *In* "Campylobacter Infection in Man and Animals" (J.-P. Butzler, ed.), pp. 163–180. CRC Press, Boca Raton, Florida.

Doyle, M. P. (1985). Food-borne pathogens of recent concern. *Annu. Rev. Nutr.* **5,** 25–41.

Shane, S. M., and Montrose, M. S. (1985). The occurrence and significance of *Campylobacter jejuni* in man and animals. *Vet. Res. Commun.* **9,** 167–198.

Stern, N. J., and Kazmi, S. U. (1989). *Campylobacter jejuni. In* "Foodborne Bacterial Pathogens" (M. P. Doyle, ed.), pp. 71–110. Dekker, New York.

CHAPTER 15

YERSINIA ENTEROCOLITICA

Michael P. Doyle

and Dean O. Cliver

I. Introduction

Yersinia enterocolitica used to be classified in the genus *Pasteurella,* along with *Pasteurella pestis,* the cause of bubonic plague. The latter, too, is now called *Yersinia* (i.e., *Yersinia pestis*) and is classified in the family Enterobacteriaceae. *Yersinia enterocolitica* is gram-negative; microscopically the cells appear pleomorphic—sometimes ovoid and sometimes rod-shaped. It is a facultative anaerobe. The organism is not motile when grown at 37°C, but it is motile and produces peritrichous flagella when it is grown at less than 30°C.

Yersinia enterocolitica once comprised a very heterogeneous group of organisms, but the most recent issue of "Bergey's Manual of Determinative Bacteriology" divides it into several different species, including *Y. enterocolitica, Y. intermedia, Y. fredriksenii,* and *Y. kristensenii.* Therefore, older allusions to "*Y. enterocolitica*-like organisms" usually refer to the *intermedia, fredriksenii,* or *kristensenii* species, which are generally not considered pathogenic.

II. Yersiniosis

The disease caused by *Y. enterocolitica* is called yersiniosis. Symptoms of yersiniosis include severe abdominal pain that suggests an appendicitis-like attack, fever, diarrhea, headache, and vomiting. Symptoms are much more severe in younger children. The incubation period for yersiniosis is 24–36 hours, sometimes longer. The duration of illness is usually 1–3 days. Children and young adults are the most susceptible to yersiniosis. Symptoms are more severe in this population.

Yersiniosis does not appear to be as great a problem in the United States as in Europe and Canada. From 1966 to 1977, there were 1,000 reported cases in Canada, 300 in the United States, 2,000 in Belgium, and—in 1 year in Denmark—200,000 cases. Few countries report illnesses as does the United States and *Y. enterocolitica* is not one of the most frequently sought agents.

Significant food-associated outbreaks of yersiniosis have occurred in the United States. The first occurred in 1976 in upstate New York. More than 220 schoolchildren became ill. Thirty-six of them were hospitalized with what was thought to be appendicitis. Of these, 16 children had their appendices removed; the surgeons observed that their appendices were normal, but the lymph nodes surrounding the appendices were swollen. It was later confirmed that *Y. enterocolitica* had caused the problem and that chocolate milk was the vehicle of infection. This milk was prepared at a small dairy by vat pasteurization; the chocolate was added after pasteurization and mixed in with a paddle, so there was plenty of potential for postprocessing contamination.

From December, 1981, through February, 1982, an outbreak of yersiniosis occurred in the Seattle, Washington area. The vehicle was tofu that had been packaged in untreated spring water contaminated with *Y. enterocolitica.*

In 1982 there was a three-state outbreak in Tennessee, Arkansas, and Mississippi linked to drinking pasteurized milk. There were more than 170 confirmed cases, but epidemiologic studies showed that more than 1000 people were ill. A very unusual serotype of *Yersinia* was identified as the causative agent. Investigators from the Food and Drug Administration (FDA) determined that this particular type of *Yersinia* could also be isolated from the plastic carrying cases used to carry the milk after it was bottled. What had happened was that outdated milk was brought to a pig farm in carrying cases. The cases were set down in mud and manure, the milk was poured into troughs for the pigs, and then the carrying cases were brought back to the plant and superficially washed. The FDA isolated the *Yersinia* from the carrying crates and showed that the pig farm was the source of the organism. However no one was able to demonstrate how the organism got from the carrying cases into the milk.

III. Characteristics of *Yersinia*

A. Classification and Biochemical Characteristics

There are several factors that affect the pathogenicity of *Yersinia*. One is the strain. The "atypical" *Yersinia enterocolitica*-like organisms, that is the *intermedia, fredriksenii,* or *kristensenii* species, are believed to be avirulent. However, certain types of *Y. enterocolitica* are more prominent and pathogenic than others. For example, in Europe **O**:3 and **O**:9 are the predominant serovars of *Y. enterocolitica* that produce illness; in Canada it was the **O**:3, and in the United States it appears to be the **O**:8 and more recently the **O**:5,27 serovar. When foods are surveyed for *Y. enterocolitica* the organism is often present, but it is rarely a pathogenic type. Most types of *Yersinia* in foods and in the environment are avirulent.

Certain factors are linked to virulence in *Y. enterocolitica*. One that is a virulence factor for *Escherichia coli*, but perhaps not for *Y. enterocolitica*, is ability to produce a heat-stable enterotoxin. Both virulent and avirulent strains of *Yersinia* can produce such a toxin, but some virulent strains cannot. This toxin is somewhat unusual in that it is produced at 25°C and below, but not at body temperature (37°C), so it is not thought to be a major factor in terms of pathogenicity.

A more significant factor is the presence of a virulence-associated plasmid. Those strains that are virulent have a 40- to 48-MDa plasmid, regardless of serovar. The plasmid has been associated with the expression of virulence antigens at 37°C but not at 26°C. The V antigen is a protein with a molecular weight of 38,000, and the W antigen is a lipoprotein with a molecular weight of 145,000. These antigens are also expressed by *Y. pestis*, in which they were first recognized and defined. It is believed that these V and W antigens are important in providing protection for *Yersinia* and allowing it to grow, rather than be killed, after phagocytosis by macrophages. Thus virulent *Y. enterocolitica* is considered an intracellular parasite.

A significant property of the virulent strains of *Y. enterocolitica* is that these cells have the ability to autoagglutinate. In liquid culture, the cells drop out of suspension, sink to the bottom of the medium, and agglutinate when they are grown at 37°C but not at 25°C. Unfortunately this property is not totally consistent among all virulent strains of *Yersinia,* so it cannot be used as a definitive test for pathogenicity.

Another significant property is that virulent strains of *Y. enterocolitica* require calcium for growth at 37°C. Magnesium oxalate agar is used to differentiate virulent from avirulent strains. The oxalate in the medium binds the available calcium and the added magnesium is needed to allow growth of the organism. When these plates are held at 37°C, virulent strains will not grow, or they form pinpoint colonies. Virulent strains held at 25°C on magnesium oxalate agar do grow as larger colonies. Avirulent strains will grow as larger colonies at both 25 and 37°C on this type of medium. Of all the tests the most reliable is that for the 40- to 48-MDa plasmid— the ability of the cells to autoagglutinate and the calcium-dependent relationship are not always seen. Even the plasmid test is not foolproof—there are some strains with a 40- to 48-MDa plasmid that are not virulent.

The plasmid in the virulent strains is rather unstable. It is often lost if the organism is grown at 37°C on a selective medium containing bile salts. The cells that do not express the plasmid will often outgrow those that do and will alter the characteristics of the culture.

There are differences in pathogenicity among different strains or serovars of *Y. enterocolitica.* Serovar **O:8, O:4,32,** and **O:21** strains tend to be more virulent and will kill orally dosed mice. These strains also produce a Sereny-positive test; that is, when applied to the cornea of a guinea pig they produce an ulceration or cloudiness of the eye. In contrast, the serovar **O:3, O:9,** and **O:5,27** strains, which are also known to be pathogenic, are not as severe; orally dosed mice show diarrhea but do not die. Second, these strains are generally Sereny test negative.

Another means used to differentiate virulent from avirulent strains is the HeLa cell test. HeLa cells are tissue culture cells. Most clinical isolates of *Y. enterocolitica* demonstrate greater adherence to and penetration of HeLa cells than most of the atypical strains of *Y. enterocolitica,* that is, those that are avirulent.

It has been shown that the virulent strains of *Y. enterocolitica* express unique outer-membrane polypeptides. Some antisera to these outer-membrane polypeptides are very specific for virulent strains of *Yersinia.* There have been a few additional tests. For example, virulent strains may erratically take up Congo red dye, whereas avirulent strains do not. The reason for this is unknown.

B. Survival and Growth Characteristics

Temperature affects the growth of *Yersinia. Yersinia enterocolitica* is a psychrotroph. It can grow in temperatures as low as 0°C and as high as 44°C. The optimum temperature range for growth is 32–34°C. *Yersinia enterocolitica* inoculated into raw pork or raw beef at 300 cells/g and held at 7°C reach 10^9–10^{10} cells/g within 10 days.

The pH range for growth is 4.6–9.0, with an optimum pH of 7–8. The organism can grow in the presence of 5% but not 7% NaCl.

IV.   Foodborne Transmission of *Yersinia*

A principal source or reservoir of virulent *Y. enterocolitica* is pigs. Virulent strains of *Y. enterocolitica* often reside in the oral cavity and the gastrointestinal tract of pigs. They colonize the tonsillar area and are often on the tongue. Foods surveyed for *Y. enterocolitica* show that the organism is quite widely distributed—beef, lamb, pork, oysters, shrimp, crabs, and water. By far, most of these isolates are avirulent, and seldom does a virulent strain occur in any of these foods. Studies in Japan have examined the fecal droppings of rats near slaughterhouses. These rodents carried virulent *Y. enterocolitica*, probably picked up from the pork that was being processed in the slaughterhouses.

V.   Isolation and Identification of *Yersinia*

Several approaches have been taken to isolate this organism from food. One old standby is the cold enrichment procedure. The ability of *Y. enterocolitica* to grow at 4°C is used as a means for selecting for the organism; food is simply macerated in PBS, held at 4°C, and sampled at 2–4 weeks. Another selective treatment used in the isolation of *Y. enterocolitica* involves putting the enrichment culture into some dilute KOH, generally about 0.5% for about 15 seconds. It is then streaked onto selective agar. The purpose of this is to reduce the level of background flora that is sensitive to KOH—*Y. enterocolitica* is slightly more tolerant and will survive. Both alkali-treated and untreated cultures are plated on selective agars. The two types of agar often used are MacConkey, which is less selective, and cefsulodin–Irgasan–novobiocin (CIN) medium. The CIN medium appears to be the best available for the selective isolation of *Y. enterocolitica*. Colonies of *Y. enterocolitica* on CIN look like a bull's eye, red in the middle and white in the periphery. This makes it easy to distinguish the *Yersinia* from the background bacteria. On MacConkey agar, the colonies appear a translucent pink color like many other kinds of bacteria, so it is not as easy to recognize the *Yersinia*. MacConkey agar is useful when the CIN medium is too selective.

For biochemical characterization, typical isolates of *Y. enterocolitica* from the selective agar go to triple sugar iron agar (TSI) slants. A *Y. enterocolitica* strain should appear as an acid slant, an acid butt, with no gas and no blackening of the butt. The organism is motile at 25°C but not at 37°C, so one should also do a test for motility. *Yersinia* is urease positive. Isolates characteristic of *Y. enterocolitica* by these tests are then biotyped. Biotyping schemes that have been developed include the Wauters and the Nilehn; the Wauters scheme is more often used. Serotyping of *Y. enterocolitica* is based principally on the O antigen, of which more than 57 types have been recognized. However, only a few laboratories in the world can serotype

Y. enterocolitica, so if it is isolated in a food laboratory, the most that can be determined is if it is virulent. If serotyping is essential, the isolate must be sent to a reference laboratory.

Bibliography

Bottone, E. J. (1977). *Yersinia enterocolitica:* A panoramic view of a charismatic organism. *CRC Crit. Rev. Microbiol.* **5,** 211–241.

Doyle, M. P. (1985). Foodborne pathogens of recent concern. *Annu. Rev. Nutr.* **5,** 211–241.

Schiemann, D. A. (1989). *Yersinia enterocolitica* and *Yersinia pseudotuberculosis. In* "Foodborne Bacterial Pathogens" (M. P. Doyle, ed.), pp. 601–672. Dekker, New York.

Swaminathan, B., Harmon, M. C., and Mehlman, I. J. (1982). A review—*Yersinia enterocolitica. J. Appl. Bacteriol.* **52,** 151–183.

CHAPTER 16

CLOSTRIDIUM PERFRINGENS FOOD POISONING

Eric A. Johnson

I.   Introduction

Clostridium perfringens type A is a sporeforming, anaerobic bacterium that is widespread in soils and is a normal resident of the intestinal tracts of humans and certain animals. The organism is distinct from many other clostridia in being non-motile, reducing nitrate to nitrite, and carrying out a stormy fermentation of lactose in milk. It is the cause of a common type of food poisoning in the United States and the United Kingdom and in several other countries where surveillance has been conducted. The principal biological factors that contribute to *C. perfringens'* ability to cause foodborne illness include its formation of resistant endospores that survive cooking of foods, its extremely rapid growth rate in warm foods, and its synthesis of enterotoxins in the human intestine.

II.   Historical Background

In the 1890s two bacteriologists, F. W. Andrewes and E. Klein, independently associated the consumption in foods of *"Clostridium welchii" (Clostridium perfringens)* with several outbreaks of food poisoning characterized by mild to severe diarrhea and abdominal pain. Klein suggested that the consumption of rice pudding was the source of the illness in two epidemics in a hospital involving 59 and 144 cases, and he showed that the incubation period of illness following consumption of the food was approximately 12 hours. The stools from the sickened patients were watery, brownish-yellow in color, and contained considerable mucus and bacterial spores. In the worst cases, streaks of blood were also present in the stools. Vomiting was rare and fever did not occur in any of the cases examined. Recovery usually occurred in about 12 hours. Simonds in 1915 claimed that sporulation of *C. perfringens* in the intestinal tract was connected with intestinal disturbances. In summary, early workers in Europe around the turn of the century and up to the 1930s provided evidence suggesting that entry of *C. perfringens* cells into the intestine and sporulation were involved in generating a gaseous diarrheal condition. However, several scientists were skeptical of these claims because of the well-recognized facts that *C. perfringens* is commonly found in human stools and in foods and is spread widely in the environment. Furthermore, numerous attempts were made to produce diarrhea experimentally by feeding cultures of *C. perfringens*, but usually with little success. Therefore, the connection between *C. perfringens* and diarrheal epidemics was suggested but remained largely unproven.

In 1933 in England, *C. perfringens* was implicated in a diarrheal outbreak in infants and children and in three food poisoning outbreaks. The classical studies of Hobbs *et al.* of these epidemics provided the most critical evidence for *C. perfringens* as a food poisoning agent. Her bacteriological investigations of the outbreaks showed that foods heavily contaminated with *C. perfringens* could result in diarrheal food poisoning when the contaminated foods were eaten. The growth of

C. perfringens to levels that caused illness was especially common in foods that were recooked or kept warm for long periods of time, for example, during the war years when meat was in short supply.

The first proven outbreak in the United States took place in 1945 and was investigated by McClung. He examined four outbreaks of diarrhea connected to the consumption of chicken steamed 24 hours prior to consumption. Shortly following McClung's investigations filtrates of *C. perfringens* cultures were given orally to volunteers, but the incubation time before cramps and diarrhea occurred in some of the individuals was 45–88 minutes, typically short compared to food poisoning outbreaks. Feeding living vegetative cells produced cramps and bloating in approximately 4 hours and diarrhea several hours thereafter. These results suggested that food poisoning occurred through the ingestion of live organisms in heavily infested foods. The positive volunteer findings with live cells were decisively confirmed by Hobbs *et al.*

Hobbs and her co-workers noticed that spores of *C. perfringens* could be differentiated into two broad classes: heat-sensitive or heat-resistant. The food poisoning outbreaks were thought to be caused by the heat-resistant strains; however, in the 1960s several investigators showed that heat-sensitive strains could also cause food poisoning. Conclusive evidence accumulated in the 1960s and 1970s that *C. perfringens* food poisoning is caused by the release of toxin during sporulation of the bacterium in the intestine of victims who have eaten foods heavily infected with the clostridium. Detailed investigations of the strains involved have demonstrated that organisms of toxin type A are solely responsible for the human illnesses.

Another discovery that sparked interest in *C. perfringens* was the occurrence of a large outbreak of a severe and sometimes lethal intestinal disease called enteritis necroticans or Darmbrand that struck approximately 400 victims in postwar Germany. The outbreaks resembled the "pig-bel" syndrome that later occurred in New Guinea, and both illnesses were due to consumption of large numbers of *C. perfringens* in pigs which were roasted and feasted upon for several days.

III.   Nature of *Clostridium perfringens* Foodborne Illness

A.   Incidence

In the 5-year period 1972 to 1978, *C. perfringens* accounted for 70 outbreaks (9.7% of confirmed bacterial food poisoning outbreaks) and 4573 cases (11.3%) in the United States. In 1982 (the most recent statistics available from the Centers for Disease Control) the organism caused 22 outbreaks (10.0%) and 1189 cases (10.8%). Generally, in recent years the confirmed number of cases ranks third behind enteric infections and staphylococcal food poisonings. Similar frequencies have been reported from England and Wales. In common with many other foodborne pathogens, however, the diagnosed and confirmed cases certainly represent less than 5% of those that actually occur. In 1966 and 1968, *C. perfringens* caused more cases of food poisoning than any other recognized bacterial etiologic agent.

This leading statistic has changed probably because of increased attention to food-handling practices, changes in supplies of foods and consumption trends, and recognition of newer pathogens.

Numbers of cases are typically high in outbreaks of *C. perfringens* food poisonings. The median number of individuals affected per outbreak is usually relatively constant at 40 to 70. These figures are biased somewhat since smaller outbreaks are often not reported. Outbreaks are most frequently investigated and reported from institutions such as schools or prisons or from large social gatherings where foods are cooked in large quantities. Food poisonings on these occasions are caused by the necessity of cooking foods in large quantities. The foods are not properly cooled after preparation, which enables *C. perfringens* to grow to very large vegetative cell populations.

Due to the wide distribution of *C. perfringens,* outbreaks do not generally occur in specific geographic locations. Persons of both sexes are equally susceptible and the poisonings are not age dependent beyond the infant stage. For unknown reasons, most cases of *C. perfringens* food poisoning occur in fall and winter. This seasonal occurrence is strikingly different from the common outbreaks of salmonellosis and staphylococcal food poisonings in the summer months.

B. Description of the Illness

Clostridium perfringens illness is relatively mild and consists of profuse diarrhea and acute abdominal pain. Fever, nausea, and other signs of infection are relatively rare. Especially if carbohydrates such as lactose (in milk) are eaten, the persons may suffer from gas liberated by *C. perfringens* during its strong saccharolytic fermentations. The incubation period of most cases ranges from 6–24 hours with a median of about 12 hours. Onset has been reported to occur as soon as 2 hours and as late as 26 hours after consumption of contaminated food. The symptoms generally subside in 12–24 hours. Fatalities occur rarely, among elderly or hospitalized persons with underlying complications.

The lack of signs of infection such as fever and the relatively rapid onset of symptoms suggest that *C. perfringens* food poisoning is an intoxication. It required several years following the identification of *C. perfringens* as an etiologic agent to understand the mechanism of the disease. The difficulty in identifying the mechanism of pathogenesis was mainly due to a puzzling aspect of the poisoning; several investigators failed to produce typical symptoms on feeding of culture filtrates or dead bacterial cells to volunteers. Eventually it was revealed that sickness occurred only when large numbers of live vegetative cells were ingested by the victims. Extremely large numbers ($>10^8$) of live cells were found necessary to obtain an attack rate of 50% in human volunteers. Upon ingestion, the bacteria grow in the intestine, sporulate, and produce an enterotoxin during the sporulation process. When spores are produced in the intestine, enterotoxin can be detected approximately 3 hours after the sporulation process begins. The use of specially designed culture media that encourage sporulation has confirmed the release of enterotoxin during sporulation. Formation of the enterotoxin correlates with the release of the free spores from the mother sporangia. Toxin formation in the intestine causes a number of pathologic effects including salt and water secretion into the lumen and rapid intestinal motility. Mouse and rat models have demonstrated extensive damage to ileal tissue.

C.   Foods Involved in Outbreaks

Most outbreaks of *C. perfringens* food poisoning occur through the ingestion of meat or poultry products that have been boiled, stewed, or casseroled. These cooked foods are held for several hours at room temperature, in a warm oven, or refrigerated in large masses that do not drop to a temperature cool enough to prevent growth. The foods most often involved in *C. perfringens* food poisonings are protein staples including beef, chicken, and turkey. The spores of *C. perfringens* are commonly present on the surfaces of these foods or are introduced in ingredients such as dried spices. The spores present in the raw foods survive cooking and may be "heat shocked" for germination. On the other hand, cooking kills much of the vegetative flora of other organisms and therefore provides near-virgin territory for growth of *C. perfringens*. Growth properties of *C. perfringens*, including its ability to produce hydrolytic enzymes to scavenge nutrients, its rapid growth rate, and the tolerance of temperatures to 50°C (122°F, see below), contribute to its ability to rapidly grow to high cell concentrations (10^5–10^6 cells per gram of food).

Insufficient, slow cooling of foods to temperatures that prevent growth of *C. perfringens* is probably the most common handling error that leads to illness. The contaminated food also is often not reheated sufficiently to kill the population of *C. perfringens* that may have accumulated. Outbreaks of food poisoning do not occur when foods are eaten hot soon after cooking, are stored with proper and rapid refrigeration (<7°C; <45°F), or are reheated to an internal temperature of 74–100°C (165–212°F) before serving.

D.   Enteritis Necroticans

The so-called "pig-bel" illness in New Guinea and the Darmbrand epidemics in Germany that occurred in the postwar period involved large numbers of individuals that suffered from a severe necrotizing gastroenteritis of the small bowel. Outbreaks of pig-bel are closely correlated to oral consumption of pigs in feasts. The pig is insufficiently cooked and large quantities are orgiastically eaten during a celebration lasting several days. In contrast to usual food poisonings that are caused by *C. perfringens* type A, the pig-bel syndrome is inflicted by toxin type C, perhaps through zoonotic transfer from the pigs. The *C. perfringens* species also causes necrotic enteritis in lambs, severe enterotoxemia in cattle and sheep, and approximately 80% of the gas gangrene cases in humans.

IV.   Biological Properties of *Clostridium perfringens*

A.   Reservoirs

Smith and Holdemann have claimed that *C. perfringens* is more widely spread in nature than any other pathogenic organism. It has been detected in nearly every soil or mud sample examined and occurs free-living in these habitats. Its wide distribution may largely be due to dispersal of dormant and environmentally resistant endospores. The organism is scattered by abiotic vectors such as dust and also is distributed by insects that contact soil or feces. The organism's success in habitation is mostly due to several important attributes: its relatively high tolerance to oxygen, its extremely rapid growth rate on a number of substrates (especially substrates high in protein), and its survival through dormancy which is broken for rapid vegetative growth when conditions are suitable. In addition to its free-living distribution, it is also found in the intestinal contents of most animals but especially in carnivores including wolves, seals, badgers, humans, whales, and many other species. *Clostridium perfringens* has also been detected in herbivorous animals including rats, elephants, camels, chickens, and turkeys. The factors that control its competitive colonization of the intestine are not currently understood. The number of *C. perfringens* in the intestinal tracts varies greatly from animal to animal and among individuals of the same species.

Because *C. perfringens* is present in soils and forms resistant endospores, it is probably on nearly every surface exposed to dust contamination. Many foods contain viable *C. perfringens* or its dormant spores. The organism is common on foods of animal origin because the carcasses become contaminated during slaughtering. Dried foods such as spices are also a common source of *C. perfringens* (see Bryan for tables showing its numbers on various raw foods).

B. Vegetative Growth

The cells in rich media are gram-positive, nonmotile rods that usually occur singly or in pairs, rarely in chains. They are usually 2–4 μm long and 0.8–1.5 μm wide, with blunt ends. In young, rapidly growing cultures the cells nearly resemble cocci in their morphology. Some of the rods may become quite large (up to 15–20 μm long), similar to the anthrax bacillus, especially in older cultures. The transformation of vegetative cells to spores is sporadic and rarely occurs in laboratory media. Several investigators have studied the requirements for sporulation in culture media. The carbohydrate source and a pH greater than neutrality seem to be especially important. When spores do occur they are large, oval, centrally or subterminally located, and swell the cells.

On sheep's-blood agar colonies grow overnight which are circular, 1–3 mm in diameter, semiopaque, gray to grayish-yellow, with a glossy appearance. After longer incubation the colonies may appear dome-shaped with a raised center and flattened periphery. Pure cultures of the organism may give rise to several other colony morphologies including dwarfs, rough irregular colonies, and flat colonies with a filamentous periphery. Mucoid colonies are also encountered where the individual cells are surrounded by a thick capsule. A characteristic double zone of hemolysis is observed with most strains on human, rabbit, or cow-blood agar. An inner zone of complete hemolysis due to θ toxin is surrounded by a larger incomplete hemolysis caused by α toxin. On egg-yolk agar, colonies of *C. perfringens* are smooth, raised, yellow, and surrounded by wide zones of precipitate indicating lecithinase activity. Cultures in peptone–yeast extract–glucose broth are frequently surrounded by a capsule easily demonstrated with the addition of India ink to a wet mount of the organism. Capsules have been found to be common in cultures recovered from intestinal infections. The capsules are composed mainly of polysaccharides that contain rhamnose, galactose, and glucose as the principal sugars.

Clostridium perfringens grows well in complex media containing protein digests or peptones as a source of amino acids, a fermentable carbohydrate, and a complex source of vitamins and nucleotides such as yeast extract. The organism is quite demanding in its nutritional needs and probably requires 14 amino acids, 5 vitamins, and uracil and adenine as essential nutrients. Since *C. perfringens* produces a wide variety of extracellular hydrolytic enzymes including hemolysins, urease, lecithinase, collagenase, hyaluronidase, and deoxyribonuclease, it can scavenge many of its required nutrients from polymeric sources such as gelatin or starch. Some strains produce proteases that hydrolyze gelatin and casein. Foods supporting growth of *C. perfringens* are often rich in protein and other required nutrients. The organism is a vigorous fermenter of sugars and uses fructose, galactose, glucose, inositol, lactose, maltose, mannose, starch, and sucrose. Some strains will also ferment cellobiose, glycerol, inulin, raffinose, or salicin. It does not use arabinose, erythritol, mannitol, rhamnose, ribose, sorbitol, sorbose, trehalose, or xylose. Lactose fermentation is useful as a diagnostic test for *C. perfringens*. During fermentations it frequently produces considerable gas (H_2 and CO_2) and acidic and alcoholic end products. The gas formation in milk is so vigorous that the clotted protein blows to the top of the fermentation tube in 4–6 hours after inoculation. *Clostridium perfringens* has the unusual property among the clostridia of reducing nitrate to nitrite and sulfite to sulfide, thereby ridding the cell of hydrogen equivalents in the process. The organism does not require stringent anaerobic conditions in order to initiate growth. The optimum E_h is approximately -200 mV. The lag period for growth is extended at higher redox values. The ability to initiate growth in a food, of course, depends on interrelated factors including initial cell density, pH of the food, and so forth.

Several strains of *C. perfringens* are able to deconjugate bile acids and to convert 3-α-hydroxy bile acids to 3-β-hydroxy and 3-oxo bile acids. Others have been observed to dehydrogenate steroids or cause cyclization of steroids. These transformations have been postulated to be involved in the generation of carcinogens in the gut.

The optimum temperature of most strains is about 45°C (109.4–116.6°F). Growth will take place up to 50°C (ca. 122°F). *Clostridium perfringens* does not generally grow significantly below 20°C (68°F), although a few doublings of healthy cultures may occur at temperatures as low as 6°C (42.8°F). True psychrophilic strains of the organism have not been isolated. At the optimum temperature for growth (45°C; 113°F) and in rich media doubling times as short as 8–10 minutes have been observed. These extraordinary growth rates give *C. perfringens* the distinction of being the fastest growing bacterium known.

Clostridium perfringens will grow over the pH range 5.5–8.0 or 8.5. At temperatures below 45°C (113°F) certain strains will grow at pH 5. The optimum pH for growth is about 6.5. Growth rate of cultures is not affected by salt concentrations less than 3%. The organism has been observed to grow in up to 8% NaCl, but most strains are inhibited by 5–6.5% salt. Spores of *C. perfringens* were reported to germinate in 5% salt and to outgrow into a vegetative cell population, but this did not occur in 10% NaCl. The maximum concentration of brine that will allow growth is dependent on various factors including temperature, availability of nutrients, and pH. Growth has been reported in media containing 10,000 mg/liter $NaNO_3$ or 400 mg/liter $NaNO_2$.

Many strains of *C. perfringens* are found to be sensitive to bacteriocins produced extracellularly by certain unrelated species of bacteria, especially enterococci. *Streptococcus faecium* in particular produces proteins active against *C. perfringens*. Contrastingly, *C. perfringens* has been reported to produce inhibitors active against *Clostridium botulinum* types A, B, E, and F. As expected, cultures of *C. perfringens* produce bacteriocins that are active against other closely related strains of *C. perfringens*. The antagonistic factors may be borne on plasmids, and recent investigations have shown promiscuity in transfer of plasmids among strains in the species *C. perfringens*.

Since the late 1940s, *C. perfringens* has been recognized to harbor a number of bacteriophages. Certain phages are lysogenic and upon induction the liberated viruses may infect rough but not generally smooth (encapsulated) strains. Phage infection has been reported to be involved in the proportion of heat-resistant versus heat-sensitive spores produced by cultures of *C. perfringens*.

C.   Spores and Survival

Clostridium perfringens rarely sporulates in laboratory culture media. When sporulation is observed, the spores are oval in shape, subterminal in position, and swell the sporangium of the mother cell. The spores do not have appendages or an exosporium as do spores of many other clostridia. The heat resistance of spores varies considerably from strain to strain. In general, two classes of heat sensitivity are common. The heat-resistant spores have D_{90} (90°C or 194°F) values of 15–145 minutes and Z values of 9–16°C (16–29°F) compared with the heat-sensitive spores that have D_{90} of 3–5 minutes and Z values of 6–8°C (11–14°F). The spores of the heat-resistant class generally require a heat shock of 75–100°C (167–212°F) for 5–20 minutes in order to germinate. The basis of the wide variation in heat resistance is not currently understood. The spores of both classes may survive cooking of foods and may be stimulated for germination during the heating procedures. It is evident that the more heat-resistant strains will survive longer heating periods and are probably responsible for food poisoning in well-cooked foods.

Injury of *C. perfringens* spores during heating is a relatively common occurrence. Injured spores may appear to be killed but can germinate if given a suitable environment and enough time. One of the most frequent heat injuries occurs in the lytic enzyme system that breaks down the outer layers of peptidoglycan during germination. Consequently, cells may be stimulated to germinate and outgrow by adding lysozme to the media or by using egg-yolk agar that naturally contains lysozyme.

D.   Classification of Cultures

The species *C. perfringens* is divided into five groups (types) depending on the production of four major extracellular toxins (α, β, ϵ, ι). Only type A cultures occur

Table I

Classification of *Clostridium perfringens*
by Toxin Type

| *Clostridium* | Toxin produced | | | |
perfringens type	α	β	ε	ι
A	+	−	−	−
B	+	+	+	−
C	+	+	−	−
D	+	−	+	−
E	+	−	−	+

free-living in the soil and also in the intestinal tracts of animals. The remaining types, B, C, D, and E, seem to be obligate intestinal parasites of animals. The type A strains are responsible for human food poisonings.

Laboratory discrimination among the principal toxin types is easily done: (1) the strain is purified by single-colony isolation; (2) it is grown overnight at 35°C (95°F) in cooked meat broth + 1% soluble starch; (3) the culture is subcultured in the morning to fresh medium and grown 4–6 hours; (4) it is chilled and centrifuged; and (5) the supernatant is divided into two equal quantities. One portion is treated with trypsin, [0.1% for 45 minutes at 37°C (98.6°F)]; this procedure activates certain of the toxins. One-milliliter quantities are then treated with antiserum raised against the respective purified toxins. Additionally, nonimmunized serum is used as a control. The neutralized toxin solutions are injected (0.3 ml intravenously or 0.5 ml intraperitoneally) into mice and the mice are observed carefully for typical signs of death. An antitoxin prepared against a given toxin type will neutralize all the toxic factors associated with that specific toxin.

As summarized in Table I, type A antiserum will protect only type A strains. Type B will protect against serotypes A, B, C, and D; type C against A and C; type D against A and D; and type E against A and E. Often, strains of type A will not produce lethal quantities of toxin. The various toxins have a variety of pathologic effects on mice. Experienced personnel can evaluate the symptoms and judge which toxins are active. The book by L. D. S. Smith cited in the bibliography is an excellent reference for description of the characteristic symptoms.

V.   Characteristics of the Enterotoxin

Food poisoning by *C. perfringens* occurs when large numbers of the pathogen ($>10^8$) grow in foods and are eaten by unsuspecting victims. Generally, the foods do not seem spoiled, especially if served in gravy. In the intestine, the organism sporulates and releases the enterotoxin responsible for the diarrheal symptoms. The sporulation-specific gene product is produced during stage II to III of sporulation. It is a major protein product of *C. perfringens* spores, accounting for $>5\%$ of the total spore protein. Variable quantities are produced depending on the strain. The enterotoxin is probably located in the spore coat. Its role in sporulation is not clear and cultures that sporulate well do not necessarily produce increased quantities of the enterotoxin.

In common with several other food poisoning toxins, its study has been hampered by the absence of a convenient and sensitive biological assay of activity. Early workers showed that the enterotoxin caused fluid accumulation in ileal loops of rabbits and lambs. Later it was noticed that application of the toxin to guinea pig skin caused erythema and increased permeability in the skin of guinea pigs. The determination of erythemal activity is one of the most sensitive biological assays and can detect 1.25–2.5 μg/ml of enterotoxin. Serological methods based on antibody reactions including reversed passive hemagglutination, radioimmunoassay, or enzyme-linked immunosorbent assay (ELISA) methods can detect 0.001 μg/ml of enterotoxin protein. Even though the immunological procedures do not necessarily detect biologically active toxin, they are useful in confirming *C. perfringens* outbreaks. The oral dose of purified enterotoxin that is required to produce diarrhea in a normal human is 8–10 mg, which is quite high compared with other food poisoning toxins such as staphylococcal enterotoxin, where only approximately 1 μg is needed to inflict illness.

The type A enterotoxin has been purified and characterized. It is a single-chain polypeptide that has a molecular weight of 34,000 to 36,000. It is acidic, bearing an isoelectric point (pI) of 4.3. The protein from the anaerobic clostridium contains a single cysteine (—SH) residue and no disulfide bonds. This property correlates with the anaerobic nature of the organism, where redox potential may not encourage the formation of disulfide bonds. Trypsin treatment of the molecule has been demonstrated in some cases to increase biological activity about 2.5-fold. The toxin may have two domains or regions that have different functions in the molecule. One domain is hydrophobic and probably binds to apolar surfaces such as membranes. The second region in the protein is acidic and is probably the actual toxic portion that enters the intestinal ileum, where it stimulates fluid secretion, electrolyte loss, and rapid bowel movement, thus culminating in the diarrheal symptoms. Electron micrographs of intestinal ileal tissue have shown that the enterotoxin necrotizes and kills the intestinal ileal cells, causing gross damage.

The *C. perfringens* enterotoxin is heat labile and is destroyed by heating for 10 minutes at 60°C (140°F). It is stable to freezing at −21°C (−5.8°F).

VI. Diagnosis of *Clostridium perfringens* Foodborne Illness

A. Investigation of a Food Poisoning Outbreak

Outbreaks of *C. perfringens* food poisoning are suspected when examination reveals the characteristic symptoms, incubation period, methods used in food preparation, and time of consumption of the meal. Confirmation of *C. perfringens* poisoning depends on the isolation of large numbers ($>10^5$ organisms per gram of implicated food) and also the isolation of $>10^6$ spores per gram of feces. The detection of large numbers of cells in the implicated food is probably the most important criterion since the organism is commonly found in the intestine. *Clostridium perfringens* type A can be further distinguished by determining the serotype of polysaccharide antigens in the capsule. Investigations of the relation of capsular serotypes to outbreaks have shown that of >75 serotypes known, <10 are associated with the majority of outbreaks. Most investigators in the United States do not serotype the capsular antigens, although this procedure is very common in the United Kingdom.

B. Isolation and Enumeration

The aerotolerance and rapid growth rate of *C. perfringens* make it one of the easiest clostridia to isolate. Its relative resistance to several antibiotics and inhibitory agents, including polymyxin, neomycin, kanamycin, sulfadiazine, cycloserine, and sodium sulfite, have enabled the development of several selective media. When *C. perfringens* is required from a source where it is outnumbered by other bacteria, it can generally be enriched by incubation for 4–6 hours at 45°C (113°F) in cooked-meat medium with glucose. The organism is then subcultured to a tube of iron–milk medium incubated at 37°C until clotting occurs. The culture is then streaked to egg-yolk or blood agar and incubated overnight at 37°C. Characteristic double zones of hemolysis and a strong lecithinase indicate that *C. perfringens* is the major isolate.

The resistance of *C. perfringens* to inhibitory agents including antibiotics and sulfite has facilitated the construction of selective media, some of which are recommended for isolation from foods (see Bibliography). Certain of these media contain sulfite and iron; when reduced to sulfide the iron forms a black precipitate, turning the colonies black. Recommended media for isolation from foods include TSN (tryptose–sulfite–neomycin), SPS (sulfite–polymyxin–sulfadiazine), and TSC (tryptose–sulfite–cycloserine). In a direct comparison TSC was found to work most satisfactorily. It is recommended that pour plates instead of surface inoculation be used. Identification of *C. perfringens* is then carried out on the basis of morphology, toxin production, and cultural characteristics. To prevent killing of the vegetative cells, most samples of food containing *C. perfringens* should not be refrigerated or frozen. The food samples should be analyzed immediately or as soon as possible since populations of the organisms in contaminated foods tend to die off rapidly. Food samples that require more than 2-day storage should be mixed with buffered glycerol salts solution to give a 10% final concentration of glycerol and frozen as rapidly as possible to <−50°C (e.g., on dry ice). On reaching the laboratory, the samples are blended in buffered peptone and plated onto selective agar. The plates are incubated anaerobically at 37°C for 20–24 hours. The black colonies on TSC surrounded by a zone of precipitation are enumerated as presumptive *C. perfringens* colonies.

For confirmation of the species, 10 or more purified colonies are picked and inoculated to motility–nitrate agar, iron–milk medium, lactose–gelatin medium, and carbohydrate diagnostic broths. The principal diagnostic characteristics have been described above: *C. perfringens* is obligately anaerobic, nonmotile, reduces nitrate, hydrolyzes gelatin, and vigorously ferments lactose. Further tests are described in diagnostic manuals published by the Food and Drug Administration and the American Public Health Association. Serotyping of capsular antigens has been useful for epidemiological characterization.

VII.   Treatment and Prevention

Acute cases of *C. perfringens* type A food poisoning are generally rather mild and self-limited. Antibiotic therapy is not recommended in most instances. Attention to dehydration is the most important concern.

Nearly all food poisonings caused by *C. perfringens* could be avoided if the food-handling practices of rapidly chilling foods and thoroughly reheating before consumption were strictly adhered to. The objective in prevention is to limit the multiplication of vegetative cells in the food. Since the spores are widespread and are resistant to heat they will often survive the cooking procedure. It is not generally practical to eliminate spore contamination of the food, although monitoring spore levels is a good practice in the quality control of raw food ingredients. When possible, foods should be prepared and eaten immediately after cooking. Hot foods should be held at 60°C (140°F) or higher. Foods that must be stored should be cooled to 7°C (45°F) as rapidly as possible and reheated to 71–100°C (160–212°F) to kill vegetative cells before consumption.

Bibliography

Bryan, F. L. (1969). What the sanitarian should know about *Clostridium perfringens* foodborne illness. *J. Milk Food Technol.* **32**, 381–389.

Cato, E. P., George, L. W., and Finegold, S. M. (1986). Genus *Clostridium* Prazmowski 1880. *In* "Bergey's Manual of Systematic Bacteriology" (P. H. A. Sneath, ed.), Vol. 2, pp. 1141–1200. Williams & Wilkins, Baltimore, Maryland.

Harmon, S. M., and Duncan, C. L. (1984). *Clostridium perfringens*. *In* "Compendium of Methods for the Microbiological Examination of Foods" (M. L. Speck, ed.), 2nd Ed., pp. 483–495. Am. Public Health Assoc., Washington, D.C.

Hobbs, B. C. (1983). *Clostridium perfringens* food poisoning. *IN* "CRC Handbook of Foodborne Diseases of Bacterial Origin" (M. Rechcigl, Jr., ed.), pp. 295–322. CRC Press, Boca Raton, Florida.

Hobbs, B. C., Smith, M. E., Oakley, C. L., Warrack, G. H., and Cruickshank, J. C. (1953). *Clostridium welchii* food poisoning. *J. Hyg.* **51**, 75–101.

Murrell, T. G. C., Roth, L., Samuels, J., and Walker, P. D. (1966). Pig-Bel: Enteritis necroticans. *Lancet* **1**, 217–222.

Simonds, J. P. (1916). "Studies in *Bacillus welchii*, with Special Reference to Classification and Its Relation to Diarrhea," Monogr. Vol. 50 Rockefeller Inst. Med. Res., New York.

Smith, L. D. S., and Williams, B. L. (1984). *Clostridium perfringens*. *In* "The Pathogenic Anaerobic Bacteria" 3 Ed., pp. 101–136. Thomas, Springfield, Illinois.

CHAPTER 17

VIBRIO

Michael P. Doyle
and Dean O. Cliver

I. Introduction

The genus *Vibrio*, of which *Vibrio cholerae* is the type species, belongs to the family Vibrionaceae. *Vibrio cholerae* cells are short and comma shaped. They are motile by a single polar flagellum and are facultative anaerobes. Their metabolism is both oxidative and fermentative. Other *Vibrio* species will be described below.

II. *Vibrio cholerae*

Vibrio cholerae can grow in a temperature range of 15–42°C, ideally between 30 and 37°C. It grows between pH 6 and 10. It has a high alkaline tolerance, so alkaline conditions are often used to select for the organism in isolation procedures. It dies off rapidly in the presence of acid, however. *Vibrio cholerae* is not an obligate halophile, as are some of the other vibrios. It will grow in the presence of up to 6% sodium chloride but not more.

A. Serological Classification

The *V. cholerae* are classified on the basis of serology into three primary groups—serogroup **O**:1, atypical serogroup **O**:1, and nonserogroup **O**:1. *Vibrio cholerae* serogroup **O**:1 comprises epidemic strains that, by definition, agglutinate with the poly **O**:1 antiserum and produce cholera toxin. Atypical serogroup **O**:1 strains do not produce the cholera toxin. Typical strains belonging to serogroup **O**:1 are the most important. They are often involved in the epidemics of cholera that occur in developing countries. Serogroup **O**:1 is subdivided into two biotypes—*cholerae* and *El Tor*—based on such properties as hemolysis of sheep red blood cells, agglutination of chicken red blood cells, polymyxin B sensitivity, and Group IV phage sensitivity (Table I). These biotypes are further serotyped as Ogawa, Inaba, or Hikojima, based on some somatic antigen factors designated AB, AC, and ABC (very rare), respectively. The other major group of *V. cholerae* are the nonserogroup **O**:1 strains, which are sometimes called the nonagglutinating **O**:1 *V. cholerae* (NAG) and sometimes the non-*Vibrio cholerae* (NVC).

Table I
Properties that Differentiate the Major Biotypes of *Vibrio cholerae* Serogroup **O**:1

Biotype	Hemolysis of sheep (RBCs)[a]	Agglutinate chicken (RBCs)	Polymyxin B sensitivity (50 mg)	Group IV phage sensitivity
cholerae (classical)	−	−	+	+
El Tor	±	+	−	−

[a]RBC, red blood cell.

B. Serogroup *O*:1 and Cholera

The disease caused by *V. cholerae* **O**:1 is cholera. The symptoms are quite different than those caused by some of the other enteric pathogens. There is a profuse, watery diarrhea, sometimes described by physicians as "rice water stool." Also included are abdominal pain and very rapid, severe dehydration, which results in intense thirst and very cold and clammy skin. An individual at the height of illness will often lose several liters of fluid in a day. The onset time for cholera is generally 2–3 days. The infectious dose has been estimated at 10^8–10^9 cells; however, more recent studies have shown that certain strains are more virulent. For example, ingestion of as few as 10^3 cells of some *El Tor* strains after the stomach acidity was neutralized with bicarbonate has been known to produce illness.

This organism colonizes the gut as does enterotoxigenic *Escherichia coli*, although the colonization factors of *V. cholerae* are not totally defined. *Vibrio cholerae* does not invade the intestinal tract. The organism produces a toxin known as choleragen that causes an outpouring of fluid into the gut and dehydration of the host.

Vibrio cholerae is quite widely distributed in marine environments. There was a cholera outbreak in Louisiana in 1978, the first in the United States since one in 1911 in New York. Investigation revealed that the organism was in crabs that had been improperly cooked. The crabs came from the Gulf of Mexico and had been steamed to an extent that the organism survived. More recently, there have been cases and outbreaks of cholera in this country from eating raw oysters. *Vibrio cholerae* **O**:1 appears to be present in our marine environments, but to a lesser degree than are non-**O**:1 strains.

The epidemic types of *V. cholerae* are believed to be principally transmitted through humans. The organism resides in the intestinal tract of symptomatic and some asymptomatic individuals and is present in their feces, often at levels of 10^2–10^9 vibrios per gram. Fecal contamination of water or food results in transmission of these types of vibrios. Water is implicated more often than food as a vehicle of cholera infection, but recent studies have shown that infected shellfish can also be reservoirs of epidemic-type *V. cholerae*. The organism can survive in shellfish for long periods of time and has been isolated from moist portions of mussels, crabs, shrimp, and clams.

C. Atypical Serogroup *O*:1

The second group of *V. cholerae* are the atypical *V. cholerae* serogroup **O**:1. By definition, these strains agglutinate with polyvalent **O**:1 antiserum but they do not produce cholera toxin. These organisms are primarily present in marine environments. They have been isolated from a variety of seafoods, water, and sewage. These organisms have never been associated with diarrheal disease—sometimes extraintestinal or wound infections, but not diarrheal disease. Therefore they are not generally considered to be enteric pathogens.

D. Nonserogroup *O*:1

The remaining group are the nonserogroup **O**:1 *V. cholerae* (NAG). These have the same biochemical and morphological characteristics as *V. cholerae* but do not agglutinate with polyvalent **O**:1 antiserum. There have been a few sporadic cases and a few foodborne outbreaks linked to these organisms. General symptoms are diarrhea and vomiting, which are relatively mild. Illness generally lasts less than 3 days. There was an outbreak of *V. cholerae* non-**O**:1 that occurred in Florida in 1979 resulting from eating raw oysters. These organisms appear to have worldwide distribution. There does appear to be some seasonality—most infections occur during the late summer and early fall. The organism is primarily transmitted through food and water. Relative to pathogenicity, some strains produce cholera toxin and some produce a heat-stable toxin. Some strains cause enteritis in infant rabbits without any evidence of toxin production, but not much is known of the mode of pathogenesis.

III. *Vibrio parahaemolyticus*

Vibrio parahaemolyticus has the same cell morphology as *V. cholerae* but is an obligate halophile (i.e., it requires NaCl for growth). It is the leading cause of foodborne disease in Japan and has caused several outbreaks in the United States. A watery diarrhea is the most common syndrome that it produces, with an incubation period of 4–96 hours (average 15 hours) and a duration of 3 days. It can also produce a dysentery syndrome with mucus and blood in the stool. The incubation period is very short—20 minutes to 9 hours—with a duration of about 2-1/2 days. The infectious dose is usually high, requiring ingestion of more than 10^5 cells. Most cases occur in the summer to early fall months. *Vibrio parahaemolyticus* has worldwide distribution; it is part of the normal flora of estuarine and coastal waters. It is believed to be primarily transmitted through seafood. It grows very rapidly in seafood that is temperature abused; for example, in raw squid at 30°C a generation time of 15–18 minutes has been reported. It is quite sensitive to cold storage and dies off during refrigerated (4°C) or frozen (-10°C) storage.

Mechanisms of pathogenicity of *V. parahaemolyticus* are not well understood but most strains that are clinical isolates are positive for the Kanagawa phenomenon. That is, these isolates hemolyze rabbit or human red blood cells when grown on "Wagatsuma agar," comprising peptone, 1.0 g; yeast extract, 0.3 g; NaCl, 7.0 g; mannitol, 1.0 g; K_2HPO_4, 0.5 g; crystal violet, 0.001 g; agar, 1.5 g (pH 7.5; do not autoclave but steam to melt agar); and 5% rabbit or human defibrinated blood. A thermostable hemolysin is responsible for the Kanagawa phenomenon. In contrast, most food isolates are Kanagawa phenomenon negative.

IV. *Vibrio vulnificus*

Vibrio vulnificus is a halophile, ferments lactose but usually not sucrose, and is salicin positive. Among marine bacteria, it is unusually virulent for humans, often causing septicemia and death in more than 40% of cases. Persons who have chronic liver disease or other dysfunction that increases serum iron levels are uniquely susceptible. However, extraintestinal illnesses can occur in normal, previously healthy persons who wound themselves while cleaning shellfish or harvesting crabs or oysters in such a way that the lesion becomes contaminated with sea water.

In a survey of 80 locations along the Eastern seacoast of the United States from Miami to Portland, Maine, *V. vulnificus* was detected in 4.2% (163 of 3887) of samples of sea water, sediment, plankton, and animals. Clams and oysters were the source of most of the isolates. It was detected in low numbers (<10 CFU/ml) in sea water, but in high numbers (average 6×10^4 CFU/g) in oysters.

In persons with preexisting liver disease characterized by high serum levels of iron, the organism causes a fulminating septicemia that produces severe hypotension and shock. The organism apparently infects these people via the digestive tract. Eating raw oysters is a common means of infection. Previously healthy individuals, infected via sea-water contamination of cuts, are likely to undergo a rapidly progressive cellulitis (inflammation of cellular or connective tissue) that often necessitates amputation of the affected limb.

Other species of the genus *Vibrio* are being recognized as associated with foods in ways that may threaten human health. However, none of the others appears to be as significant as the three that have been discussed.

Bibliography

Blake, P. A., Weaver, R. E., and Hollis, D. G. (1980). Diseases of humans (other than cholera) caused by vibrios. *Annu. Rev. Microbiol.* **34,** 341–367.

Joseph, S. W., Colwell, R. R., and Kaper, J. B. (1982). *Vibrio parahaemolyticus* and related halophilic vibrios. *CRC Crit. Rev. Microbiol.* **10,** 77–124.

Madden, J. M., McCardell, B. A., and Morris, J. G., Jr. (1989). *Vibrio cholerae. In* "Foodborne Bacterial Pathogens" (M. P. Doyle, ed.), pp. 525–542. Dekker, New York.

Oliver, J. D. (1989). *Vibrio vulnificus. In* "Foodborne Bacterial Pathogens" (M. P. Doyle, ed.), pp. 569–600. Dekker, New York.

Twedt, R. M. (1989). *Vibrio parahaemolyticus. In* "Foodborne Bacterial Pathogens" (M. P. Doyle, ed.), pp. 543–568. Dekker, New York.

WHO Scientific Working Group (1980). Cholera and other vibrio-associated diarrhoeas. *Bull. W. H. O.* **58,** 353–374.

CHAPTER 18

LISTERIOSIS AND *LISTERIA MONOCYTOGENES*

Jaerim Bahk

and Elmer H. Marth

I. Introduction

Listeriosis was recognized years ago, but it is among the least understood bacterial infections of humans, animals, and wildlife. More than six decades have passed since the organism known today as *Listeria monocytogenes* was described. Meanwhile, we have learned that the host range of the organism includes at least 42 kinds of domestic and wild animals, 22 avian species, fish, ticks, flies, and crustacea. The organism's wide distribution contrasts with the sporadic occurrence of specific forms of listeriosis, suggesting that infection is restricted by unknown factors.

This chapter will deal with (1) the history of *Listeria* and listeriosis, (2) *L. monocytogenes,* (3) outbreaks of listeriosis and pathogenicity of *L. monocytogenes,* (4) transmission of *L. monocytogenes* via food, and (5) control of *L. monocytogenes* and listeriosis.

II. History of *Listeria*

An organism closely resembling *L. monocytogenes* was described as early as 1891 and 1911. In 1926, the organism was isolated from the livers of sick rabbits and guinea pigs and was named *Bacterium monocytogenes.* The following year, the identical bacterium was isolated from the livers of several gerbils and was called *Listeria hepatolytica.* The disease now known as listeriosis was seen in sheep in Germany as early as 1925 and an outbreak of encephalitis of unknown etiology in cattle was reported, which very likely was listeriosis. In 1933, an illness among sheep in Wales was called "circling disease," a name still often applied to listeric encephalitis of ruminants. Two years later a bacterium was isolated from stored brain tissue of the affected animals. However, 6 more years passed before the true identity of the bacterium was determined.

The first confirmed report of listeric infection in humans appeared in 1929. The bacterium was isolated from three patients with an infectious mononucleosis-like disease. Soon after that, *L. monocytogenes* was established as a cause of meningitis and of infection in the perinatal period. Since then, the bacterium has been isolated from various kinds of animals, and it seems to be everywhere.

Listeria monocytogenes was called *Listerella bovine, L. cuniculi, L. gallinarum, L. gallinarium, L. gerbilli,* and *L. suis* by early authors; these names are seldom encountered today. Other names applied to what presumably was *L. monocytogenes* are *Bacterium hepatitis, B. monocytogenes, Corynebacterium infantisepticum, C. parvulum, Erysipelothrix monocytogenes, Listerella hepatolytica, L. monocytogenes hominis, L. ovis,* and *Listeria infantiseptica.* Recent case reports have increased awareness of the importance of listeriosis.

III. *Listeria monocytogenes*

A. Characteristics

Five species of *Listeria* are currently recognized. Three of these, *L. innocua, L. welshimeri,* and *L. seeligeri,* are considered to be avirulent. *Listeria ivanovii* evidently may produce disease under certain conditions. Only *L. monocytogenes* is currently believed to be pathogenic for humans, although a few reports suggest that some of the other species have caused human illness.

Listeria monocytogenes is a small (1.0–2.0 μm × 0.5 μm), gram-positive, nonsporeforming, non-acid-fast, diphtheroidlike rod with round ends. It is aerobic, motile at room temperature, and hemolytic. The bacterium is catalase-positive, Voges–Proskauer-positive, and can produce β-hemolysis on blood agar. Esculin is hydrolyzed. In gram stains of cerebrospinal fluids, *L. monocytogenes* may appear coccoid or in pairs and be mistaken for a gram-positive coccus, especially the pneumococcus. Cells from 24- to 36-hour-old colonies are definitely gram-positive, but older colonies or broth cultures often contain gram-negative cells. On colorless solid media, colonies of *L. monocytogenes* are round, translucent, and slightly raised and are blue-green when viewed with obliquely transmitted light.

There are at least 11 serotypes, but 3 cause 90% of the clinical infections; types Ia, Ib, and IVb. Types Ia and Ib are more common in neonates infected *in utero* (early neonatal onset), whereas type IVb is more common in those assumed to be infected at or after birth (late neonatal onset).

B. Culturing of *Listeria monocytogenes*

Listeria monocytogenes adapts to and usually grows well on most common bacteriological media. Tryptose agar (Difco) is an excellent substrate for cultivation and preservation of the bacterium. *Listeria monocytogenes* grows best in a neutral to slightly alkaline medium and will grow at pH values from 5.2 (in cheese) to 9.6. Growth can occur in broth at pH ≤ 5.0, depending on the type of acid added to the broth. The organism grows better in an atmosphere containing about 5% O_2 and 5–10% CO_2 than in air, although aerobic growth does occur. The organism can survive below pH 5.2 for weeks or months, depending on the acidity of the substrate. Carbohydrates are essential for growth of *L. monocytogenes*. Glucose serves as a source of carbon and energy. The bacterium is very salt tolerant. It can survive for 4 months in a solution of 25.5% NaCl held at 4°C.

Listeria monocytogenes is psychrotrophic. Although it grows best at 30–37°C, the organism thrives at refrigeration temperatures. It grows at temperatures as low as 3°C in tryptose–phosphate broth, 4°C in milk, and 0°C in sterile meat after 16–20 days. It also can withstand freezing, as is evident from its recent discovery in bulk ice cream and ice cream novelties. Although growth is slow at 3–4°C, turbidity in broth or growth on a solid medium can be observed in 5–8 days. At 6°C, the log phase is reached in 5–11 days.

The D value (time for 90% destruction) at 71.7°C is about 1 second, so about 10^{15} freely suspended *Listeria* per milliliter of raw milk are needed for the organism to survive 71.7°C for 15 seconds. The organism can occur and grow within leukocytes in milk. Under such circumstances the D value increases to about 5 seconds, and survival after 15 seconds at 71.7°C is possible provided the initial number of *L. monocytogenes* exceeds 10^3/ml.

Three methods to isolate and identify *L. monocytogenes* are currently being used, although others have been suggested. The oldest and simplest is the cold enrichment method. Material thought to contain the pathogen is macerated and added to tryptose broth, followed by incubation at 4°C. Storage at this temperature retards growth of many organisms but allows growth of the psychrotrophic *L. monocytogenes*. Furthermore, it is thought that incubation at 4°C increases recovery of the organism by enhancing repair of stressed or injured cells. The culture is sampled at intervals for 4–8 weeks and plated on McBride Listeria Agar, a medium that contains the selective agents glycine anhydride and lithium chloride, which inhibit many gram-positive bacteria. The phenylethanol agar base of the McBride Listeria Agar inhibits many gram-negative organisms. Sheep blood is added to the medium to demonstrate β-hemolysis. Plates are incubated 48 hours at 35°C. An atmosphere of 10% CO_2, 5% O_2, and 85% N_2 may be used for incubation. However, *L. monocytogenes* produces well-formed colonies with normal aerobic incubation. Colonies may be screened for tumbling motility and biochemically for metabolic profile and catalase reaction. Serological testing also may be done.

The U.S. Food and Drug Administration (FDA) has developed a method for isolating *L. monocytogenes* from foods. Trypticase soy–yeast extract enrichment broth is supplemented with three selective agents: acriflavine hydrochloride, naladixic acid, and cycloheximide. Cultures are stored at 30°C and plated after 24 hours and 7 days on modified McBride Listeria Agar (no blood). Colonies thought to be *L. monocytogenes* are transferred to blood agar to determine hemolysis and later confirmed as for the cold enrichment method. This method has been modified by the FDA. The USDA also has developed a method to detect listeriae in meat and poultry products.

A shortened selective enrichment procedure (SEP) developed at the Food Research Institute, University of Wisconsin–Madison, uses the antibiotic polymyxin B in addition to acriflavine hydrochloride and naladixic acid for selectivity. Cultures are sampled after 24 hours at 37°C.

The cold enrichment method is slightly more sensitive than the SEP and FDA methods for testing cheese. Other suggested methods include a gum-based naladixic acid medium and a modified McBride Listeria Agar with moxalactam, but these are not widely used. Both cultural and rapid (ELISA and DNA-probe) methods for detection of *Listeria* continue to evolve as research progresses.

Listeria monocytogenes produces a soluble, filterable hemolysin capable of attacking most mammalian erythrocytes. It is most pronounced in freshly isolated cultures and may be completely absent in old laboratory-maintained strains. No increase in hemolysin production occurs by increasing the CO_2 content of cultures incubated at 37°C or room temperature. The proteinaceous hemolysin can be precipitated from culture filtrates at 5°C by 60% saturated $(NH_4)_2SO_4$.

IV. Outbreaks of Listeriosis and Pathogenicity of *Listeria monocytogenes*

Listeria monocytogenes is widespread in the environment, so humans can be exposed to the bacterium in various ways. The organism has been isolated from soil, dust, animal feed, water, sewage, and almost every type of animal cultured, including asymptomatic humans. Animals from which positive cultures have been obtained include 42 domestic and wild mammalian species, 22 avian species, and others. The bacterium also has been isolated from an assortment of plants including corn, cereals, soybeans, clover, weeds, and cabbage. In Western Canada cattle graze on Ponderosa pine needles and frequently suffer abortion; mice fed such pine needles develop listeriosis. Limited evidence suggests that the bacterium harbored in dust and dirt can become airborne, be inhaled by humans, and cause the pneumonic form of listeriosis.

Transmission of *L. monocytogenes* from one human to another certainly occurs. Persons suffering from listeriosis may spread the causative bacterium through nasal and throat secretions, urine, feces, conjunctival secretions, epidermal pus, and blood. From 1 to 10% of healthy humans excrete the organism in their feces. The bacterium has appeared in raw foods such as milk, red meats, poultry, seafood, vegetables, and fruits.

A. Prevalence of Listeriosis

In Denmark, there have been 2.3 cases of listeriosis per million persons per year. Similar reports have come from Holland, Sweden, and Germany. During 34 years (1933–1966), there were 731 bacteriologically confirmed cases in the United States; in the next 3 years (1967–1969), 255 cases were reported to the Centers for Disease Control from only 35 states. These data are fragmentary because listeriosis has not been a reportable disease in the United States. In Denmark and the United States, about one-third of the cases occurred in women during pregnancy or during the neonatal period, while in Sweden and Germany, two-thirds of the cases occurred in women during these periods. The fecal excretion rate of the bacterium from normal persons is estimated at a minimum of 1%, whereas it is 26% from symptomatic patients, and 4.8% from workers in slaughterhouses. Although the infection has been regarded as a zoonosis, most cases in the United States occur in urban areas in persons without a history of animal contact. Seasonally, the incidence is higher in humans in summer and in animals in winter.

The first major reported outbreak of listeriosis in North America occurred in Canada in 1981. Coleslaw was implicated as the source of *L. monocytogenes* type IVb in this outbreak of 41 cases of listeriosis. The second, associated with pasteurized whole or 2% fat milk processed by a certain dairy, occurred in Massachusetts in 1983. Of 49 confirmed cases, 7 were newborns and 42 were adults; 14 died. The third major outbreak occurred in 1985 in Los Angeles County, California, from Mexican-style cheese made in California. There were more than 100 confirmed cases, of which more than 90 were infants; at least 40 died. These outbreaks are discussed in greater detail later in this chapter.

B. Pathogenicity of *Listeria monocytogenes*

Listeria monocytogenes can invade the eye and skin of humans after direct exposure. This has been observed in laboratory accidents and by veterinarians. During maternal bacteremia, the bacterium can infect the placenta, the amniotic fluid, and the fetus. In most human cases, however, the portal of entry is not evident. If the portal of entry is the gastrointestinal tract and more than 1 person in 100 is at least a transient carrier, then why are only certain people affected? Many patients with listeriosis are immunosuppressed, either by a basic disease such as a lymphoma or by administration of various agents, usually including adrenocorticosteroids. From clinical observations of infected humans, and from studies in laboratory animals and *in vitro,* it is apparent that the mononuclear phagocyte is very important in the response of the host to *L. monocytogenes.* In mice, resistance is correlated with development of a delayed hypersensitivity skin reaction and inactivation of bacilli by macrophages (mononuclear phagocytes).

The cell wall of *L. monocytogenes* also is involved in its pathogenicity, although a variety of constituents seems to contribute to the total effect. A water-soluble toxic polysaccharide from the cell wall is able to induce lymphopenia and granulocytosis. Protein and carbohydrates appear in extracts that are antigenic, pyrogenic, or able to induce lymphopenia and granulocytosis. A fractionated glycine lysate, which increased virulence of the bacterium, also was pyrogenic and caused granulocytosis. Lipids from the cell, possibly phospholipids, produce marked monocytosis and depression of lymphocyte activities. Hemolysin (listeriolysin) also is thought to be involved in the pathogenicity of *L. monocytogenes.*

C. Symptoms of Listeriosis

Infection with *L. monocytogenes* can cause several different forms of listeriosis, which can be divided into five categories. They are pregnancy infections, granulomatosis infantiseptica, sepsis, meningoencephalitis, and focal infections. However, the most common result of contact with the organism appears to be a transient, asymptomatic carrier state.

Infections during pregnancy may occur any time, but they appear most often in the third trimester. The patient usually complains of chills, fever, back pain, headache, and discolored urine. In some instances, pharyngitis, diarrhea, and pyelitis have been noted. When the flu-like symptoms are evident, *L. monocytogenes* can be isolated from blood, umbilical cord blood, lochia, tissue obtained by curettage, vaginal mucus, urine, and placental tissue. Infection of the pregnant woman leads to infection of the fetus either via the transplacental route or during delivery.

Transplacental infection of the fetus is likely to produce bacteremia, which can lead to presence of *L. monocytogenes* in fetal urine. The fetal urine is discharged into the amniotic fluid, which is then aspirated by the fetus, leading to widespread involvement of the respiratory and gastrointestinal tracts. Symptoms of listeriosis of the newborn commonly include respiratory distress, heart failure, difficult and forced respiration, cyanosis, refusal to drink, vomiting, convulsions, soft whimpering, early discharge of meconium, and mucus in stools. Listeriosis of the newborn is characterized by involvement of numerous organs, which develop nodules, including the liver, spleen, adrenal gland, lung, esophagus, posterior pharyngeal wall, and tonsils. Granulomas may be found subepithelially and in lymph nodes, thymus, bone marrow, myocardium, testes, and skeletal muscles.

The third category is sepsis. Patients are adults or neonates and have chills, fever, severe pharyngitis, and a leukocytosis accompanied by mononucleosis. Adults in most instances are immunosuppressed; the neonates become symptomatic after 3 days of age, and the infection likely is contracted during or after birth rather than *in utero*. The mother is almost always asymptomatic.

Fourth, meningitis and meningoencephalitis develop in newborns and in older persons, usually men more than 50 years old. The fatality rate is approximately 70% for patients who are either untreated or treated too late. Symptoms in newborn or very young infants include shallow and rapid breathing, slight cyanosis, lethargy, fever, failure to thrive, anorexia, convulsions, irritability, and usually death. Two of eight survivors examined at 16 months of age had neurodevelopmental handicaps. In adults, this form of listeriosis often begins with flu-like symptoms which are followed by headache, pain in the legs, chills, pyrexia, increasing rigidity of the neck, nausea, vomiting, photophobia, and cirrhosis. Victims become increasingly somnolent, have intermittent bouts of convulsions and delirium, and finally die in a coma.

Encephalitis caused by *L. monocytogenes* has two phases; the first lasts about 10 days and includes such symptoms as headache, backache, vomiting, conjunctivitis, and rhinitis. The second phase begins with a high fever, which is followed by disturbances in the central nervous system. Death usually follows in 2–3 days if the patient does not receive appropriate treatment with the antibiotics ampicillin, penicillin, or erythromycin.

Other manifestations of listeriosis include conjunctivitis, the cutaneous form, granulomatosis septica, the cervicoglandular form, and the pneumonic form. Focal infections with *L. monocytogenes* also can result in arthritis, osteomyelitis, spinal or brain abscesses, peritonitis, and cholecystitis.

Mortality varies considerably according to the syndrome. Granulomatosis infantiseptica and meningitis in immunosuppressed patients are associated with the highest mortality, ranging from 33–100% in the former and from 12.5–43% in the latter form of illness. Survival rates of up to 100% in meningitic listeriosis have been associated with a normal glucose level in cerebrospinal fluid.

V. Transmission of *Listeria monocytogenes* and Food

The first recorded outbreak of listeriosis, which probably was milk mediated, occurred in post–World War II Europe when milk was rationed and sold on the black market. The first major foodborne outbreak of listeriosis recorded in North America occurred in 1981. Of 41 confirmed cases, 7 were adults and 34 were perinatal. The mortality rate was about 30%, mostly in infants who died following abortion. The causative organism was *L. monocytogenes* serotype IVb, and the probable vehicle was determined to be coleslaw made from cabbage grown on a field fertilized with manure of listeric sheep.

The second outbreak occurred in 1983 in Massachusetts. There were 49 confirmed cases, of which 7 were newborns, 42 were adults, and 14 died. The causative agent was *L. monocytogenes* serotype IVb and the probable vehicle was pasteurized milk. However, the vehicle was not confirmed at that time.

The most recent major United States outbreak of listeriosis, in 1985 in Los Angeles County, California, comprised more than 100 confirmed cases of which more than 90 were infants. At least 40 patients died. The causative agent was again found to be serotype IVb. The vehicle was determined to be Mexican-style cheese. *Listeria monocytogenes* was isolated from the cheese and from environmental samples from the factory.

Since 1985, *L. monocytogenes* has been found in several dairy products in Texas, in chocolate milk in Michigan, in chocolate milk and ice cream in Wisconsin, in ice cream in Iowa, in ice milk mix and casein in California, in Mexican-style soft cheese in Arizona, and in similar dairy foods from other locations. As this chapter was being written, newspaper accounts appeared which indicated illness and death from listeriosis in some Swiss citizens who had consumed a locally produced surface-ripened specialty soft cheese.

Evidence suggests that improperly fermented silage can harbor *L. monocytogenes*. This and other environmental sources can lead to contamination of raw milk with freely suspended cells of *L. monocytogenes*. Infection of cows' udders is of special concern because the organism is shed in milk from mastitic animals. Occurrence of *L. monocytogenes* in raw milk has been noted in several countries. In Europe, from 0.9 (in Germany) to 45.3% (in Spain) of raw milk samples tested positive. Of 650 samples taken from three areas of the United States that the FDA examined, 27 (4.2%) were positive, and 25 of these were pathogenic according to results of the mouse test.

The ability of *L. monocytogenes* to grow in fluid dairy products (skim milk, whole milk, chocolate milk, and cream) has been determined at several temperatures. After a lag phase of approximately 5 days at 4°C, the bacterium grew at essentially the same rate in all of these fluid products. At 15 days, there were close to 10^6 cells of *L. monocytogenes* per milliliter of the products. Ultimately, after 3–4 weeks, the population of *L. monocytogenes* cells reached nearly 10^7 per milliliter in all of the products except chocolate milk, in which the population reached 10^8–10^9 per milliliter. During the growth phase, doubling times averaged 35 hours at 4°C, 4.5–6 hours at 13°C, 2 hours at 21°C, and 41 minutes at 35°C. It was also noteworthy that there was no apparent decrease in numbers of *L. monocytogenes* after 65 days of storage at 4°C.

With nonfat dry milk, the drying process caused a 90% decrease in numbers of *L. monocytogenes*. During room-temperature storage, the population decreased over time in nonfat dry milk made from concentrated or regular skim milk, but the agent could still be detected for 84–96 days.

In cottage cheese, there was no appreciable growth of *L. monocytogenes* during the lag phase of the starter culture, about 5 hours at 32°C. Results indicate small numbers of the organism survived the cheesemaking process and 28 days of storage at 3°C in creamed or uncreamed cottage cheese. The lack of growth probably resulted from the low pH.

Cheddar cheese was made from pasteurized milk that was inoculated with *L. monocytogenes,* coagulant, and starter culture. The level of *L. monocytogenes* held approximately constant during the manufacturing process. Ripening the cheese at 6 or 13°C caused limited inactivation of the bacterium, but survival exceeded the 60-day period required in the United States when cheese is made from raw or heat-treated milk. In one instance, *L. monocytogenes* survived for more than 434 days.

Camembert cheese made from pasteurized milk inoculated with *L. monocytogenes* was ripened at 6°C after 10 days of storage at 15–16°C to allow proper growth of *Penicillium camemberti*. Numbers of *L. monocytogenes* cells decreased or remained unchanged, depending on the strain, in cheese during the first 18 days of ripening. All strains began multiplying in cheese after 18 days of ripening. Maximum populations of 1×10^6–5×10^7 CFU/g were attained after 65 days of ripening. Generally, numbers of *L. monocytogenes* 10- to 100-fold greater occurred in wedge or surface than in the interior cheese during the latter half of the ripening period.

VI. Control of Listeriosis

Most people exposed to *L. monocytogenes* do not become ill. On the basis of studies in mice, it appears that *L. monocytogenes* in the blood is cleared rapidly by the liver and, to a lesser extent, the spleen. Destruction of the organism in the liver is largely the work of resident tissue macrophages, which are activated by soluble products (lymphokines) of specifically sensitized thymus-derived lymphocytes. Elsewhere in the body, mononuclear phagocytes are especially important, but peritoneal macrophages and polymorphonuclear leukocytes are also active. When antibody against *L. monocytogenes* is present, it promotes phagocytosis—with the assistance of complement. Clearly, people who develop listeriosis are those in whom this normal resistance process has failed.

For those who become ill with listeriosis, survival may depend on prompt diagnosis of the disease and administration of a proper antibiotic. Serologic tests for diagnosis include enzyme-linked immunosorbent assays and microagglutination and complement-fixation methods. The complement-fixation test appears to be the most sensitive and accurate of these. Antibodies of the IgM class are compared for activity against *L. monocytogenes* serotypes IVb and Ia. Penicillin and ampicillin are usually the antibiotics of choice, though penicillin resistance may occur. Most strains of *L. monocytogenes* are also sensitive to tetracycline, erythromycin, chloramphenicol, and cephalothin. Treatment failure may result if the antibiotic is administered too late in the course of the disease.

Persons likely to be susceptible might try to reduce their risk of infection by minimizing exposure to *L. monocytogenes*. The susceptible person should avoid contact with animals that might be shedding *L. monocytogenes,* places in the environment likely to be contaminated with the bacterium, humans suffering from listeriosis, and foods that might contain *L. monocytogenes*.

How can the food industry act to prevent *Listeria* contamination in processing areas, thus reducing the likelihood of offering contaminated foods to the consumer? One basic precaution is to allow no refrigerated return product to come into the factory. Refrigerated storage may have allowed *Listeria* cells to repair the heat damage they suffered during processing. Processing areas should not be entered by truck drivers, raw product handlers, and other unauthorized persons. The milk hauler, in particular, has been in the milk house on the farm and possibly has been in contact with bovine feces which may be brought into the factory on shoes and boots. Handlers of raw foods in a factory should be excluded from areas where finished products are found, but should practice rigorous sanitation in their own work area.

Cleaning should not be relegated to the newest employee in the factory. Workers must be given the needed training and guidance for proper cleaning and sanitizing of equipment. Particular attention should be given to the clean-up of clarifiers and separators because *Listeria* cells tend to localize within somatic cells of milk, which are found in large numbers in material removed from milk by these machines. Cellulose sponges and nylon pads should not be allowed in product contact areas. Cellulose sponges, in particular, tend to be heavily contaminated with micro-organisms. Throwaway paper towels should be routinely used.

Laboratory personnel should collect samples from the filler, first product through, and last product through during a day's operation to determine the sanitary status of the process.

If possible in dairy factory layout, clarifiers and separators should be isolated from the pasteurization area. Wherever possible within a factory, movement of air should be from a zone of positive pressure, particularly in the processing and packaging areas, outward. Traffic coming into the in-house quality control laboratory should be minimized. *Listeria* testing should be done by an outside laboratory.

VII. Summary

Listeria monocytogenes, one of five species in the genus *Listeria* and the only one currently believed to be pathogenic for humans, is a small, gram-positive, non-sporeforming, aerobic, motile, hemolytic, rod-shaped bacterium. The bacterium is widespread in the environment, having been isolated from soil, dust, animal feed, water, sewage, almost every type of animal that has been tested, and asymptomatic humans. *Listeria monocytogenes* causes listeriosis, a disease which most often affects humans whose immune system is compromised. Included are pregnant women, infants, and adults suffering from such diseases as cancer, cirrhosis of the liver, or AIDS, or being treated with drugs such as corticosteroids. Listeriosis is manifested by such syndromes as pregnancy infections, granulomatosis infantiseptica, sepsis, meningoencephalitis, and focal infections. Infections can be treated successfully with penicillin, ampicillin, or erythromycin. However, a mortality rate of about 30% has occurred in outbreaks of listeriosis. Food-associated outbreaks of listeriosis have been attributed to coleslaw (Canada, 1981), pasteurized milk (United States, 1983), and soft cheese (United States, 1985; Switzerland, 1987). Presence of *L. monocytogenes* in various dairy foods has prompted recalls of such products from the United States marketplace. Preventing transmission via milk and dairy products depends on rigorous sanitation in the plant and on proper pasteurization. *Listeria monocytogenes* also has been found in raw meats and seafood.

Bibliography

Brackett, R. E., Marth, E. H., Doyle, M. P., Lovett, J., and Schlech, W. F. (1988). *Listeria monocytogenes:* A foodborne pathogen (symposium). *Food Technol.* **42(4),** 161–178.

Doyle, M. P., Glass, K. A., Beery, J. J., Garcia, G. A., Pollard, D. J., and Schultz, R. D. (1987). Survival of *Listeria monocytogenes* in milk during high-temperature, short-time pasteurization. *Appl. Environ. Microbiol.* **53,** 1433–1438.

Fleming, D. W., Cochi, S. L., MacDonald, K. L., Bronctum, J., Hayes, P. S., Plikaytis, B. D., Holmes, M. B., Audurier, A., Broome, C. V., and Reingold, A. L. (1985). Pasteurized milk as a vehicle of infection in an outbreak of listeriosis. *N. Engl. J. Med.* **312,** 404–407.

Gray, M. L., and Killinger, A. H. (1966). *Listeria monocytogenes* and listeric infections. *Bacteriol. Rev.* **30,** 309–380.

Lovett, J., Francis, D. W., and Hunt, J. M. (1987). *Listeria monocytogenes* in raw milk: Detection, incidence and pathogenicity. *J. Food Prot.* **50,** 188–192.

Marth, E. H., and Ryser, E. T. (1990). Occurrence of *Listeria* in foods: Milk and dairy foods. *In* "Foodborne Listeriosis," (A. J. Miller, J. L. Smith, and G. A. Somkuti, eds.), pp. 151–164. Elsevier, Amsterdam.

Ralovich, B. (1984). "Listeriosis Research—Present Situation and Perspective." Akadémiai Kiadó, Budapest.

Rosenow, E. M., and Marth, E. H. (1987). Growth of *Listeria monocytogenes* in skim, whole and chocolate milk, and in whipping cream at 4, 8, 13, 21 and 35°C. *J. Food Prot.* **50,** 452–459.

Ryser, E. T., and Marth, E. H. (1987). Behavior of *Listeria monocytogenes* during the manufacture and ripening of Cheddar cheese. *J. Food Prot.* **50,** 7–13.

Ryser, E. T., and Marth, E. H. (1987). Fate of *Listeria monocytogenes* during the manufacture and ripening of Camembert cheese. *J. Food Prot.* **50,** 372–378.

Schlech, W. F., Lavinge, P. M., Bortolussi, R. A., Allen, A. C., Haldane, E. V., Wort, A. J., Hightower, A. W., Johnson, S. E., King, S. H., Nicholls, E. S., and Broome, C. V. (1983). Epidemic listeriosis—evidence for transmission by food. *N. Engl. J. Med.* **308,** 203–206.

Seeliger, H. P. R. (1961). "Listeriosis." Hafner, New York.

Seeliger, H. P. R. (1984). Modern taxonomy of the *Listeria* group—relationship to its pathogenicity. *Clin. Invest. Med.* **7,** 217–221.

Tenth International Symposium on Listeriosis (1989). *Int. J. Food Microbiol.* **8,** 181–297.

CHAPTER 19

INFREQUENT MICROBIAL INFECTIONS

Eric A. Johnson

I. Introduction and Historical Background

Surveillance of food poisonings in the United States by government regulatory agencies has shown that the predominant types of foodborne diseases and the patterns and characteristics of outbreaks have changed over the past century. The specific pathogens and patterns of disease continually evolve as a result of changes in food preferences and habits, human ecology, and social change. Factors that have contributed to the rise and eradication of particular food-transmitted diseases include the size and density of human communities, the domestication and intensive farming of food sources, especially animals, and the importation of foodstuffs. Many foodborne diseases that historically caused significant mortality and morbidity have largely been eradicated in developed countries through food processing technologies (e.g., milk pasteurization), increased urbanization, and human or animal vaccinations. Diphtheria, scarlet fever, typhoid fever, tuberculosis, and brucellosis belong to this category. The transmission of these diseases in food may occasionally recur if food is mishandled or if special circumstances lead to food contamination.

Newer forms of microbial pollution are also periodically recognized. The majority of these new human diseases exist initially as zoonotic diseases that become adapted to humans as domestication and human contact with animals becomes frequent. Changes in food preferences such as the current trend in many communities of favoring fish over beef offers newer reservoirs of organisms that gradually may gain the ability to infect the gastrointestinal tract of humans. Their origin may be either terrestrial or marine. Some of these agents have not yet convincingly been proved as causes of foodborne sickness in humans or are so rare that they are neglected by many microbiologists and public health authorities. The purpose of this chapter is to describe the infrequent microbial infections that have occurred historically, are currently infrequent causes of food poisoning, or are not yet recognized as proven sources of foodborne illness.

II. Virulence of Foodborne Pathogens

Several foodborne illnesses historically important in the United States involved highly virulent microorganisms that resulted in frequent mortality. Virulence is a term that describes the infective dose of the pathogenic agent and the severity of the illness produced. Virulence factors are those traits of a pathogen that, when lost (e.g., by mutation), decrease the pathogenicity or toxigenicity but not the viability. The traits that determine the pathogenicity of an organism can be defined by showing the effects of mutations in specific genes. For example, mutations in the *tox* genes of *Corynebacterium diphtheriae* or *Vibrio cholerae* **O**:1 render the organisms nonpathogenic but do not otherwise impair their growth properties. These attenuated organisms can be used to vaccinate human populations and protect them against possible infections.

The two general classes of virulence factors are *toxins* and *surface molecules*.

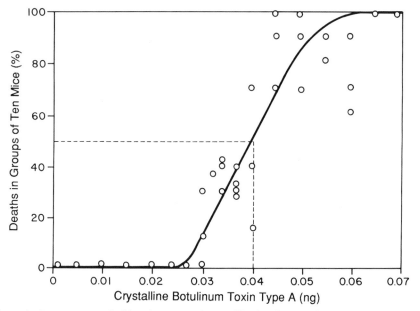

Figure 1   Dose response of white mice to type A crystalline botulinum toxin. Each mouse was challenged intraperitoneally with the dose contained in 0.5 ml of 0.05 M sodium phosphate at pH 6.2 containing 0.2% gelatin. Each point corresponds to a group of 10 mice. Deaths were recorded in a 96-hour time period. From E. J. Schantz and A. B. Scott (1981). Use of crystalline type A botulinum toxin in medical research. *In* "Biomedical Aspects of Botulism" (G. E. Lewis, ed.), pp. 143–148. Academic Press, New York.

These two classes are broad and their expression may be temporal and depend on the environmental conditions since these traits are not ordinarily required for viability of the pathogen.

Virulence is generally quantitatively expressed as the LD_{50} (for a toxin) or ID_{50} (for an infection). These terms define the dose that causes illness in 50% of test animals or humans in a designated period of time. The 50% dose point is used to quantify virulence because of the shape of the dose–response curve (Fig. 1). The sigmoidal shape of the curve indicates that the rate of change in mortality as a function of dose is steepest at the point of 50% survival. Clearly, the dose is most accurately designated at the steepest portion of the curve and is most precisely defined in response curves with the steepest slopes. The sigmoidal shape of the LD_{50} curves is due primarily to the chance occurrence of lethal events in a given test animal. Heterogeneity in the test animal population also contributes to the flattening of the curve at extremes of dose.

III.   Importance of Epidemiological Investigations

Recognition of new foodborne pathogens usually begins with an epidemiological association, where the consumption of a food is shown to be connected with an illness. Foodborne disease surveillance began in the United States in the early 1900s in response to the morbidity caused by milk-transmitted typhoid fever and infantile diarrhea. Surveys by the U.S. Public Health Service demonstrated the importance of foods, especially milk and milk products, in transmitting disease. As a result of the food/disease connection, improved food processing procedures and public health measures greatly helped to reduce the incidence of illness. The surveys by the U.S. Public Health Service and also by the Centers for Disease Control (CDC) beginning in 1966 have been very important in detecting incidences of known diseases and recognizing previously unperceived pathogens.

Disease surveys are particularly useful in detecting outbreaks, which are defined as occurrences where two or more people suffer a similar illness after eating the same food. In recent surveys, approximately 400 outbreaks are reported each year by the CDC. The actual occurrence of foodborne disease is at least 10–200 times higher. Most cases, especially those occurring in homes, are not reported. Certain diseases, particularly those with long incubation periods and nondistinctive symptoms, are not reported and the etiologic agent is not identified. Even in reported outbreaks, the etiologic agent is not identified for over one-half the incidents. Diseases with short incubation times and abrupt onset of symptoms (e.g., staphylococcal food poisoning) or severe morbidity (e.g., botulism) are diagnosed in many occurrences. Diseases that have long incubation times and mild or chronic symptoms are less well reported and characterized. Detection and confirmation of newly recognized pathogens occur at low frequency partly because suitable analytical procedures and understanding of pathogen biology have not been developed. Similarly, certain fastidious pathogens or viruses probably are often not identified because of the difficult procedures necessary for isolation. Following the isolation of a potential pathogen, it is desired that pathogenicity be proved by following Henle–Koch's postulates (see Chapter 7).

IV. Microbial Hazards in Foods of Historical and Contemporary Importance

The bacteria that are known to cause foodborne illness can be taxonomically classified into a few natural groups (Table I). The properties of pathogens that were important historically or that are infrequent and often unproven causes of foodborne illnesses today are discussed in the following section. The more often encountered pathogens are described in other chapters of this text.

A. Facultatively Anaerobic Gram-Negative Rods

1. Enterobacteriaceae

The enteric bacilli comprise the two families Enterobacteriaceae and Vibrionaceae. These families, along with the campylobacters (formerly classified with the Vibrionaceae), are the most common causes of food poisoning in several

Table I
Classification of Known and Emerging Foodborne Pathogens

Major bacterial group	Pathogen genus or species	Importance in the United States	Pathogenesis or disease
Enterobacteriaceae	*Salmonella*	Contemporary	Gastroenteritis
	Escherichia	Contemporary	Gastroenteritis
	Shigella	Contemporary	Gastroenteritis
	Yersinia	Emerging	Gastroenteritis
	Edwardsiella	Emerging	Gastroenteritis
	Arizona	Opportunistic	Gastroenteritis
	Citrobacter	Opportunistic	Gastroenteritis
	Klebsiella	Opportunistic	Gastroenteritis
	Proteus	Opportunistic	Gastroenteritis
	Providencia	Opportunistic	Gastroenteritis
Vibrionaceae	*Vibrio cholerae*	Contemporary	Gastroenteritis
	Vibrio sp.	Emerging	Gastroenteritis
	Aeromonas	Emerging	Gastroenteritis
	Plesiomonas	Emerging	Gastroenteritis
	Campylobacter	Contemporary	Gastroenteritis
Nonfermentative gram-negative bacilli	*Pseudomonas*	Opportunistic	Gastroenteritis
Miscellaneous gram-negative	*Brucella*	Historical	Chronic infection
	Mycobacterium	Historical	Penetration to joints
	Francisella	Historical	Typhoidal tularemia
	Streptobacillus	Historical	Infection with rash and fever
	Coxiella	Historical	Q fever
Gram-positive cocci	*Staphylococcus*	Contemporary	Intoxication
	Streptococcus	Historical	Pharyngitis, scarlet fever
Irregular, nonspore-forming rods	*Erysipelothrix*	Emerging?	Septicemia
	Listeria	Contemporary	Uterine infections, etc.
	Corynebacterium	Historical	Diphtheria
Gram-positive spore-formers	*Clostridium botulinum*	Contemporary	Intoxication
	Clostridium perfringens	Contemporary	Infection
	Clostridium difficile	Contemporary	Gastroenteritis
	Bacillus cereus	Contemporary	Gastroenteritis
	Bacillus anthracis	Historical	Infection

areas of the world, especially in developed countries that consume large quantities of animal meats as sources of protein. The natural habitat of these bacteria is the intestinal tract of animals. The enteric bacilli have held the prominent position for several years of being the most frequent cause of foodborne illness, and statistics show no signs that this trend will change. The natural habitat of these organisms is a huge and varied reservoir of domestic and wild animals, which in developed countries are a major source of nutrition. The presence of the enteric bacilli in animal gastrointestinal tracts has increased over the past two decades as domestic animals become more concentrated on larger farms, processing densities increase, marketing areas expand, and antibiotic use in feed increases.

Several species of enteric bacilli are well-known causes of gastroenteritis including *Salmonella* spp., *Shigella* spp., *Escherichia coli, Campylobacter jejuni, Vibrio* spp., and *Yersinia enterocolitica*. Other related genera are believed also to cause opportunistic gastroenteritis when ingested in large numbers including *Edwardsiella tarda, Klebsiella* spp., and *Proteus* spp. Positive ileal loop activity showing the presence of an enterotoxin has been demonstrated for *K. pneumoniae*. Strains in several genera of Enterobacteriaceae have been suggested to cause foodborne disease but have not been shown as conclusively pathogenic under normal circumstances. Such genera include *Arizona, Citrobacter, Proteus, Providencia, Klebsiella,* and *Enterobacter*. Isolates of these organisms have been obtained from patients with diarrhea but also from healthy patients. To prove that these organisms cause food poisoning, it is desired to show identity of isolates, for example, by serological and phenotypic tests, from food, from food handlers, and from victims' stools. Further evidence of biological activity should be obtained such as enterotoxigenicity in test animals, for example, ileal loop tests, and infectivity in volunteer studies.

In addition to gastroenteritis, *Proteus* spp., some other Enterobacteriaceae, *Achromobacter* spp., and *Clostridium perfringens* can cause histamine poisoning, which is an allergy-like illness characterized by a throbbing headache, nausea, vomiting, cramps, diarrhea, facial swelling and flushing, rash, and itching. The bacteria decarboxylate histidine to produce histamine.

2. Vibrionaceae

The Vibrionaceae consist of facultatively anaerobic, comma-shaped, gram-negative bacilli with polar flagella. All of the vibrios are motile except for *Vibrio cholerae*, which is also the only terrestrial species. The Vibrionaceae, comprising the genera *Vibrio, Aeromonas,* and *Plesiomonas,* have been demonstrated to be closely related to the Enterobacteriaceae by nucleic acid homology studies. The vibrios are commonly found in freshwater and marine environments. Food poisonings caused by *V. cholerae, V. parahaemolyticus,* and *V. vulnificus,* which are frequent causes of illness in certain countries, are discussed in detail in Chapter 17. Many incidents of *Vibrio* infections in the United States are caused by less often encountered species including *V. fluvialis, V. hollisae, V. furnissii,* and *V. mimicus*. These organisms occur free-living in marine and brackish waters. In common with *V. parahaemolyticus, V. mimicus* is an obligate halophile. This group causes acute incidents of gastroenteritis with reported clinical features including diarrhea, vomiting, abdominal pain, dehydration, and sometimes fever. The symptoms typically last for about 3 days. The poisonings are often associated with the consumption of raw or poorly cooked seafoods. Raw oysters, crabs, and other mollusks and crustacea are often implicated as sources of *Vibrio* infections. Food poisonings are most common in the summer months. Many of the *Vibrio* strains tested produce an enterotoxin(s) that is active in ileal loop tests. Some strains also produce a heat-labile toxin that is similar to cholera toxin. The increasing frequency of detection of *Vibrio* gastroenteritis and the recent recognition of several species capable of causing illness suggests that members of this group should be considered emerging pathogens.

Several *Vibrio*-like organisms also have recently been recognized as causes of foodborne gastroenteritis including *Aeromonas hydrophila* and *Plesiomonas shigel-*

loides. Their recognized incidence in human gastroenteritis is steadily increasing and some former infections may have been misdiagnosed as *Escherichia coli*. *Aeromonas hydrophila* occurs widely in fresh and brackish waters and also may be present in stools of healthy persons. Since 1968, *A. hydrophila* has been recognized as an opportunistic pathogen in immunocompromised hosts, but more recently it has also been demonstrated to cause enteritis in normal hosts. The aeromonads produce an enterotoxin similar in structure and mode of action to cholera toxin, and some strains also produce cytotoxins and hemolysins. Therefore, they may produce disease by more than one mechanism, as occurs in *E. coli*. Although *A. hydrophila* is usually transmitted through drinking water, it may also be transmitted in foods that contact contaminated water.

Plesiomonas shigelloides has been implicated as a potential agent of diarrhea in humans, but it has not received the attention given to the vibrios and enterics. The organism produces an enterotoxin(s) which is related immunologically to cholera toxin. Definitive data on incubation periods, infective doses, and so forth are lacking for *P. shigelloides* and *Aeromonas hydrophila*. Epidemiological studies are currently appearing in the literature, which should lead to better understanding of bacteriological and pathogenic aspects of these two species in the Vibrionaceae.

B. Miscellaneous Gram-Negative Bacilli

1. *Brucella*

The brucellae are nonmotile, gram-negative, aerobic, small pleomorphic bacilli about 0.5–1.5 μm in length and 0.5–0.7 μm in breadth. They are well adapted obligate parasites of animals. Isolation of the organisms from their hosts requires special media rich in nutrients. The genus contains four species that are pathogenic to humans. These were originally classified according to their animal hosts: goats and sheep for *Brucella melitensis*, cattle for *B. abortus*, swine for *B. suis*, and dogs for *B. canis*. In the animal hosts the brucellae tend to inhabit the pregnant uterus and are shed in milk or in aborted fetuses. *Brucella*-infected animals do not necessarily show symptoms but pose a continuous threat to humans as chronic carriers and excreters. Brucellae have the ability to survive for long periods in animal products. They last for up to 180 days in goat's cheese and also survive for long periods in other nonpasteurized dairy products. They are killed by pasteurization [62.7°C (145°F) for 30 minutes or 71.6°C (161°F) for 15 seconds] or by low pH. They survive indefinitely at temperatures below 0°C (32°F). Humans can become infected through consumption of fresh goat's or sheep's cheeses made from unpasteurized milk, by consumption of insufficiently cooked infected meats, or by consumption of raw vegetables that come in contact with manure or urine of infected animals. Infection of domestic animals is particularly dependent on the quality of husbandry, the sizes and densities of the herds, and the standards of personal and environmental hygiene.

Human brucellosis has an incubation period varying from a few weeks to several months. In foodborne brucellosis, the organisms probably invade through the mucous membranes of the pharynx and tonsils. After infection the brucellae tend to colonize in bones, joints, nerves, brain, and sexual organs. The symptoms occurring soon after infection are indistinct and include chills, persistent fever, malaise, sweating, headaches, and mental depression. The disease is difficult to diagnose in humans. Patients often have a chronic and unexplained fever. Diagnosis requires isolation of brucellae from blood, bone marrow, liver, or lymph nodes.

Although distribution of brucellosis is worldwide and parallels domestic livestock distribution, vaccination of calves and pasteurization of milk have decreased the incidence greatly in the United States. The Federal–State Cooperative Brucellosis Control Program began in 1945 and has largely eliminated the organism from herds. Strong brucellosis control in herds and milk pasteurization have greatly diminished the incidence from 6000 human cases per year to the current level of about 225 cases per year. The disease recurs periodically, especially through raw milk consumption and in workers, such as meat packers or veterinarians, who handle infected animals. However, these are the diagnosed cases, and the actual frequency is certainly underestimated; it has been reported that approximately 4% are promptly recognized.

2. *Mycobacterium bovis*

Mycobacterium bovis is a slow-growing, acid-fast, pleomorphic bacillus. Colonies develop in 3–8 weeks at 37°C (98.6°F) on egg-yolk media. Acid-fastness is a distinctive property of mycobacteria and involves trapping of intracellular fuchsin in their external cell surface. Mycobacteria have an unusually high lipid content, more than 25% compared to 0.5% in most gram-positive bacteria and 3% in gram-negative bacteria. The high fat content is thought to be responsible for the resistance of the mycobacteria to desiccation, alcohol, acids, alkali, and certain food preservatives. The organism, an obligate parasite, is quite fastidious in its growth requirements.

Mycobacterium bovis causes tuberculosis in cattle and can also be transferred to humans in unpasteurized milk or products derived from unpasteurized milk. The incidence in the United States is presently rare. Most cases occur in persons 60–80 years of age who were infected before tuberculin testing of cattle and pasteurization of milk were introduced. Infections also occasionally occur in rural communities in persons that consume raw milk.

The pathogenic process is unusual and chronic. Virulent mycobacteria do not produce toxins or other extracellular virulence factors. The ingested organisms penetrate the intestinal mucosa and spread to bones and joints. Hunchbacks of earlier times were believed in some cases to have become deformed through infection of vertebrae. Measures to eliminate *M. bovis* from herds and mandatory pasteurization of milk have virtually eliminated human infections.

3. *Streptobacillus moniliformis*

Streptobacillus moniliformis is a pleomorphic, nonmotile, gram-negative bacillus. Pleomorphism results largely from the formation of L forms, which are spontaneous variants that lack a rigid cell wall. *Streptobacillus moniliformis* causes an acute disease in humans called rat-bite fever. Most human infections occur through rat bites and, as such, this organism is a hazard in the laboratories of investigators who use rats. In some cases of rat-bite fever, a bite has apparently not been necessary. In 1926 in Haverhill, Massachusetts, an outbreak of the disease was traced epidemiologically to consumption of raw milk. It was eliminated when the dairy began pasteurization. It was thought that the milk contamination resulted from naso-pharyngeal secretions of infected rats. The disease is characterized by a fever, regional lymphadenitis, upper respiratory symptoms, polyarthritis, and a rash over the palms and soles.

4. *Francisella tularensis*

The species *Francisella tularensis* consists of tiny gram-negative, obligately aero-bic, rod-shaped cells approximately 0.2 by 0.7 μm. Virulent strains are surrounded by a thick capsule that can be removed in the laboratory by washing cells in sodium chloride solution. After this treatment virulence is lost but viability is unaffected. The organism has certain immunological relationships to *Brucella* and *Pasteurella*. *Francisella tularensis* is widely distributed and is found on all continents except Australia and Antarctica. The principal animal reservoirs for the virulent serovars of the organism in the United States and Soviet Union, where most infections occur, are voles and water rats in the Soviet Union and beavers, muskrats, and voles in the United States. Wild rabbits, squirrels, game birds, and the waters frequented by these various animals also harbor the organism.

Francisella tularensis causes an infectious disease in humans. Infection usually occurs during handling of carcasses or ingestion of improperly cooked meats or contaminated waters. *Francisella tularensis* can penetrate unbroken skin. Also the organism invades the regional lymphatics and results in necrotizing inflammation and enlargement of lymph nodes. These lesions are known as buboes. Typhoidal tularemia follows ingestion of the organism. It is similar to typhoid fever, with gastrointestinal symptoms, fever, and toxemia. The incubation period for tularemia ranges from 3–7 days and is manifested as fever, headache, and malaise. The bacteria are killed when heated at 56°C (132.8°F) for 10 minutes. Although the organisms do not usually grow below 10°C (50°F), they may survive for up to 3 months in tap water and 6 months in dry straw.

The incubation time after ingestion of uncooked meat is typically 3–4 days, with a range of 2–10 days. Abrupt onset of chills, headache, vomiting, fever, prostra-tion, and aching are common. Ulcerative tonsillitis or pharyngitis is characteristic, and anginal or typhoidal lesions may also be present in the gastrointestinal tract. The disease usually occurs over a period of 3–4 months but may be chronic in some cases.

5. *Pseudomonas aeruginosa*

The pseudomonads are short (0.5–1 μm × 1.5–4 μm), unicellular, strictly aerobic, gram-negative rods. They are generally motile by polar flagella. *Pseudomonas aeruginosa* secretes proteases and phospholipase C (a hemolysin). *Pseudomonas aeruginosa* is an opportunistic pathogen that can invade mucous membranes not protected by polymorphonuclear leukocytes, as occurs in immunocompromised humans. The organism synthesizes a potent endotoxin or lipopolysaccharide. It also produces an ADP-ribosylating enterotoxin similar in mode of action to diphtheria and cholera toxins. It has been reported that ingestion of large numbers ($>10^6$) of *P. aeruginosa* can cause gastroenteritis. It seems unlikely under most circumstances that food poisoning would be caused by this organism since severe spoilage of food would take place before a large population would be established. Many pseudomonads have the ability to spoil proteinaceous foods at low temperatures.

6. *Coxiella burnetii*

Coxiella burnetii (Rickettsia diasporica, Rickettsia burnetii), the causative agent of Q fever, is an obligate parasite that multiplies only in living cells. It is a pleomorphic, small rod that has a dense outer layer resembling gram-negative peptidoglycan. The organism has tremendous resistance to physical treatments; it survives temperatures of 63°C (145.4°F) for 30–40 minutes. It has been demonstrated to survive in sterile skim milk for 1 year at 4°C (39.2°F).

Coxiella burnetii is enzootic in a broad array of animals including sheep, cattle, goats, rabbits, rodents, and certain birds. Infected animals shed large numbers of *C. burnetii* in their milk, urine, and feces. The organism causes a disease which is frequently transmitted through aerosols or bites by ticks. Sporadic cases have been reported through ingestion of raw milk from infected animals. However, volunteers who have consumed raw infected milk did not become diseased. Therefore, *C. burnetii* may cause food-transmitted disease only under specialized circumstances.

The incubation period for Q fever ranges from 11–26 days, and the illness often begins in 18–20 days. Fever occurs suddenly and rises over 2–4 days to 39–40°C (102.2–104°F). High fever may be accompanied by prostration and delirium. Severe headaches, shivering, sweating, sore throat, and muscle pain also occur. The body temperature generally starts to fall after approximately 1 week and subsides to normal over a course of about 15 days.

Because epidemiological studies have inferred the ingestion of raw milk as a source of infection in humans, prevention of Q fever is accomplished by pasteurization of raw milk at 71.7°C (161°F) for 15 seconds or 62.8°C (145°F) for 30 minutes. Animal hygiene and vaccination also help to control Q fever transmittal.

C. Nonsporeforming Gram-Positive Rods

The gram-positive bacteria that cause food poisoning can be broadly distinguished by their morphology (rods or cocci) and by their capacity to form endospores. The gram-positive pathogens either cause infections or intoxications. Some of the pathogens infect the human pharynx or the gastrointestinal tract, whereas others produce potent toxins extracellularly in foods that result in sickness following consumption of the food. The clostridial and corynebacterial toxins are among the most potent protein toxins known. Several of the gram-positive bacteria have been important historically since they caused devastating diseases such as diphtheria and scarlet fever. Widespread outbreaks with high morbidity and mortality stimulated public health authorities to enact protective measures such as pasteurization of milk. The organisms of historical importance and those which currently cause rare food poisonings are discussed in the following sections.

1. *Corynebacterium diphtheriae*

The genus *Corynebacterium* consists of nonmotile, aerobic, tapered, gram-positive, rod-shaped bacteria. The name corynebacteria refers to the club-shaped morphology of many of these organisms in certain media or from clinical specimens.

Only one century ago diphtheria was a rampant disease in many countries with a case fatality rate of about 8%. The organism produces a highly potent exotoxin; in humans approximately 130 ng/kg is lethal. The toxin is liberated into the culture medium during growth and is therefore called an exotoxin. It is a single polypeptide chain stabilized by two disulfide bonds. The toxin as it is produced in cultures of C. diphtheriae can be considered a proenzyme with two functional domains. The carboxyl terminus binds to sensitive animal cells; this is followed by proteolytic cleavage and reduction of the disulfide bonds, which liberates the amino terminus. This domain enters the mammalian cells and attacks elongation factor 2. The toxin acts by ADP-ribosylating elongation factor 2 and stops protein synthesis in mammalian cells. The genes encoding toxin production (tox) are located in the genome of a bacteriophage. Phage growth and toxin synthesis begin when the bacterial host is starved for iron.

In the late 1800s and early 1900s C. diphtheriae was transmitted to humans in milk. From 1919 to 1948 the outbreaks subsided and only 11 more took place. The organism is transmitted to milk from workers who carry the organism or from cows with mastitis. The bacterium invades the mucous membranes of the throat and produces a tightly adhering pseudomembranous growth that spreads over the tonsils and pharynx and occasionally to the trachea. With the immunization of human populations, diphtheria has become a rare but still occasionally foodborne disease of humans.

2. *Erysipelothrix rhusiopathiae (insidiosa)*

Erysipelothrix rhusiopathiae is a facultatively anaerobic, gram-positive rod that shares properties with *Listeria monocytogenes,* corynebacteria, and certain streptococci. The rods are generally straight and slender (0.2–0.4 μm $\times$ 0.8–2.5 μm) with a tendency to form long filaments and V forms. The organism grows between 4 and 42°C (39.2 and 107.6°F), with an optimum of 30–37°C (86.0–98.6°F). The bacteria are killed by heating at 60°C (148°F) for 15 minutes. The organism is microaerophilic and probably requires CO_2 for growth. It is widely distributed in nature and is parasitic in mammals, birds, and fish. It is most commonly found in swine, where it causes serious infectious erysipelas. Infection in pigs occurs orally. In humans, infections nearly always occur through the skin during handling of infected animals. Rare reports have claimed foodborne transmission. Although the organism is not highly heat tolerant, it survives in salted and pickled foods. It has been isolated from bacon 170 days after pickling or 30 days after salting. The organism should be considered primarily an occupational hazard in handlers of meats and fishes and does not appear at present to be a foodborne disease hazard to consumers.

D.   Gram-Positive Cocci

1. *Streptococcus pyogenes*

The streptococci are gram-positive, nonmotile, spherical or ovoid (<2 μm in diameter) cells that normally grow in chains. They do not form catalase or related heme proteins, and their fermentation of carbohydrates results in mostly lactic acid and little gas (homofermentative). Many species are commensals in animals and humans, whereas others are highly pathogenic. The streptococci have traditionally been differentiated according to their patterns of hemolysis; the virulent strains are strongly hemolytic. The organisms that produce a clear zone of β-hemolysis (as well as nonhemolytic streptococci) are further differentiated into immunologic groups A through O. Many hemolytic streptococci produce a large capsule that contributes to their virulence. The Group A streptococci in particular produce numerous extracellular enzymes and toxins that probably also contribute to virulence.

Most strains of streptococci that cause food poisoning belong to Lancefield Group A; the characteristic species is *Streptococcus pyogenes*. β-hemolytic Group C streptococci may also rarely cause milkborne food poisoning. *Streptococcus pyogenes* causes several diseases in humans including scarlet fever, septic sore throat, rheumatic fever, tonsillitis, and other pyogenic and septicemic infections. Following an infection, individuals may harbor the streptococci in their throats and spread them to foods. For example, a milker with streptococcal sore throat can serve as a carrier and transmit *S. pyogenes* to an udder infection, which then serves as a source for spread of pharyngitis in milk. One of the largest streptococcal outbreaks in history occurred in 1912 in Chicago and involved more than 10,000 cases and 200 deaths. In this incident, several of the workers who handled the milk had pharyngitis and transmitted to milk the causative organism, *S. pyogenes*. Normally the milk in this dairy was pasteurized but during the episode the pasteurization equipment had failed. Besides milk, other foods have recently been involved in the transmittal of streptococci with resulting scarlet fever or septic sore throat outbreaks. Some of these foods included shrimp and lobster salads, tuna salad with eggs, egg salad, potato salad, ice cream, custards, pudding, cheese, and ham and meat sandwiches. Most of these outbreaks took place through the inoculation of the foods by infected workers. Improper storage of foods at nonrefrigerated temperatures also contributed to growth of the organisms in some cases. Two of the outbreaks involved type G streptococci and one reportedly involved type M. In England in 1984 an outbreak occurred from consumption of unpasteurized milk which reportedly involved *S. zooepidemicus* (Lancefield Group C). This organism is a frequent cause of bovine mastitis. Of 11 patients, 7 died, despite antibiotic treatment. Type C streptococci also caused two deaths in 1983 in the United States from the consumption of homemade cheese prepared from unpasteurized milk.

Since the implementation of milk pasteurization and mechanical refrigeration, the incidences of diagnosed streptococcal food poisonings have been uncommon (0.5% of reported outbreaks in the United States from 1978 to 1981). Diseases caused by hemolytic streptococci have historical importance because the large milkborne outbreaks of septic sore throat and scarlet fever early in this century helped to promote the pasteurization of milk. From 1912 to 1926 the quantity of milk pasteurized increased from 34 to 83%, and septic sore throat outbreaks nearly disappeared. When streptococcal sore throat does occur it is characterized by sore throat, fever, chills, and hoarseness. It can be treated with antibiotic therapy.

2. Group D streptococci—*Streptococcus faecium, Streptococcus faecalis*

The enterococci or fecal streptococci inhabit the gastrointestinal tract of healthy humans. Several reports have suggested that the enterococci were involved in food poisoning outbreaks. Since these organisms are normal residents of the gastrointestinal tract, sufficient evidence is sorely needed in many claims but is often lacking. Severe vomiting and diarrhea have been reported in persons who ate cheeses contaminated with enterococci. Bacteriological analysis showed that these organisms were present in the foods at time of consumption but did not necessarily exclude the presence of other pathogens or toxins. In order to convincingly show virulence of fecal streptococci, animal or human volunteer studies should be carried out. Human volunteer experiments have been done but have not provided a definitive answer to the question of enterococcal pathogenicity. Carefully designed studies have mostly been negative. Because the fecal streptococci are relatively heat resistant—for example, they survive milk pasteurization—they occur widely in foods. Their presence, however, merely indicates survival or contamination and probably does not necessarily indicate a threat of food poisoning.

E. Gram-Positive Sporeforming Rods

Of the five genera of endosporeformers, species of *Bacillus* and *Clostridium* are important as food hazards. These two genera are composed of gram-positive rods that have the prominent feature of producing endospores. Spores are dormant structures that have remarkable resistance to environmental forces including heat, desiccation, and adverse chemicals and gases. Some of the more common foodborne sporeforming hazards are discussed in other chapters.

1. Aerobic sporeformers—*Bacillus anthracis*

Although *Bacillus* is one of the most successful and widespread genera of bacteria, only 2 of the more than 34 species are recognized as foodborne pathogens of humans. These two species, *B. anthracis* and *B. cereus,* are closely related compared with other species of *Bacillus. Bacillus anthracis* and *B. cereus* are unusually large rods ($1-1.5$ μm $\times$ $4-10$ μm) that tend to grow in chains. Both species possess lecithinase activity and are serologically related. Some taxonomists have concluded that *B. cereus* is a less virulent form of *B. anthracis. Bacillus anthracis* differs from *B. cereus* by being nonmotile, which is an unusual trait in the aerobic bacilli, and by synthesizing a very potent exotoxin.

The anthrax bacillus was one of the first bacteria demonstrated to be pathogenic. Anthrax probably emerged as a zoonotic disease 10,000 to 12,000 years ago when neolithic man began to domesticate livestock. During the mid-1800s in certain European countries anthrax caused death in 20–30% of the livestock. In the late 1800s the disease spread to Russia; it was also documented in the United States in the mid- to late 1800s. Several pioneering microbiologists including Louis Pasteur and Robert Koch investigated anthrax. Pasteur showed that the supernatant of a broth culture did not inflict disease whereas the sediment did. In 1901 he dramatically showed, by inoculating sheep with an avirulent, nonencapsulated strain, that animals could develop immunity to anthrax. Koch in the late 1870s discovered that mice were susceptible to the pathogen. He infected this animal model, removed the spleens from the perished animals, reisolated *B. anthracis,* and again completed a cycle of infection. The organism isolated from the sick animals on artificial media was identical to the pure, inoculated culture and was repeatedly infectious. These early investigations led to vaccination programs, which have dramatically reduced the once devastating incidence of anthrax in domestic livestock.

Cutaneous anthrax accounts for >90% of the estimated 20,000 to 100,000 human anthrax cases per year. Inhalation of spores can cause pulmonary anthrax that is manifested as severe hemorrhagic mediastinal adenitis and is nearly always fatal. Intestinal anthrax with a high mortality rate can also occur when undercooked meat from diseased animals is consumed. The disease is presently very rare in developed countries. When intestinal anthrax does occur, the disease follows a series of events. The spores germinate in the intestine; vegetative cells multiply and invade submucosal tissue, where they produce their potent toxin. Ulceration occurs due to the synthesis of necrotizing toxins. The lesions in the terminal ileum become severe and may eventually lead to hemorrhaging.

Incubation time after eating contaminated meat is 2–5 days. Initial symptoms include nausea, vomiting, anorexia, and fever. These symptoms are followed by abdominal pain and sometimes by bloody diarrhea. The disease may progress to toxemia, shock, cyanosis, and death. The mortality rate for intestinal anthrax has been reported as 25–50%.

2. Anaerobic sporeformers—*Clostridium difficile*

The clostridia are anaerobic, fermentative, gram-positive rods that form endospores. They do not use inorganic compounds as electron acceptors in metabolism, which distinguishes the genus from *Desulfotomaculum*. Many clostridia are motile, saccharolytic, and/or proteolytic. Of the more than 83 species of *Clostridium* described in the 1986 edition of "Bergey's Manual of Systematic Bacteriology," several are known to cause infectious diseases. However, only two species, *C. botulinum* and *C. perfringens,* are well-known causes of foodborne disease. In developed countries, *C. difficile* is the second most common cause of antibiotic-associated gastroenteritis next to *Salmonella* spp. It is the most important cause of antibiotic-associated diarrhea, especially in hospital environments. The organism has proved difficult to isolate from infected intestines and environmental sources. Most strains produce an enterotoxin that is lethal for hamsters and a toxin that is cytopathic in mammalian cell cultures.

The disease caused by *C. difficile* is characterized by diarrhea that is often associated with mucosal lesions and pseudomembranous colitis. Pseudomembranous colitis is caused by the overgrowth of the organism in the colon, generally about 1 week after the intestinal flora has been disturbed with antibiotics. In some patients diarrhea begins 4–6 weeks after stopping antibiotic treatment. It has been hypothesized that in certain of these delayed infections the organism is acquired after therapy.

Clostridium difficile has not been demonstrated to be food transmitted. Most cases apparently involve increases in numbers of the organism in the gastrointestinal tract after antibiotic treatment. The organism is a normal component of the fecal flora of infants but has been isolated from only about 3% of healthy adults. The clostridium also occurs free-living in soils and sediments and can contaminate food. There is currently controversy regarding the source of *C. difficile* in disease; the clostridium has not been found in foods of sickened victims, which suggests that *C. difficile* is not transmitted by exogenous sources such as foods. Most investigators believe that antibiotics favor endogenous growth of the organism in the gastrointestinal tract, but the roles of exogenous transmission and antibiotic-related endogenous growth remain to be elucidated.

V. Conclusion: Eradication of Known Foodborne Diseases and Emergence of New Pathogens

From the time when bacterial pathogens began to be identified in the late 1800s, epidemiologists have carefully documented the emergence and eradication of food-borne diseases. As a result of the identification and characterization of etiologic agents, it became possible to decrease the incidence of diseases by improved food processing technologies (e.g., milk pasteurization) or by elimination of pathogens from zoonotic or environmental sources. Despite the understanding of long-existing diseases such as salmonellosis, there has been little reduction in its prevalence partly because its zoonotic reservoir is so wide and varied. Increasing sizes of farms, increased densities of animals on farms, and mass processing further contribute to the stability of the disease. In developed countries the desire for meat as a source of protein has also contributed to the maintenance of salmonellosis.

Just as certain diseases are eventually eradicated, still others will be revealed. New diseases arise in part because of changes in food preferences, such as current trends for consumption of marine and freshwater fishes, crustacea, and shellfish. Increased demand necessarily leads to intensive farming and greater densities of animals and their contact with humans. Potential pathogens will be positively selected for by the increased opportunity for colonization in the human ecosystem. Perhaps mutation to drug resistance will first allow colonization in compromised hosts, and eventually variants will arise that will be fit to infect the normal gastrointestinal tract by ingestion in food.

As diseases emerge, it is important that surveillance and epidemiological studies be carefully performed to elucidate connections between food and disease. These connections should be communicated to the bacteriologist, who can then isolate, identify, and characterize the agent. The methods for detection of a new etiologic agent have been outlined by Bryan (see Bibliography). The continual changes in pathogenic organisms will lead to improved expertise in epidemiology and bacteriology for detection. These improved skills will hopefully not only elucidate acute gastrointestinal diseases, but will also reveal subtle foodborne diseases, perhaps chronic in nature. Discovery of new illnesses in humans will provide a basis to continually improve food safety by enacting preventive control measures.

Bibliography

Bryan, F. J. (1979). Infections and Intoxications caused by other bacteria. *In* "Food-Borne Infections and intoxications" (H. Riemann and F. L. Bryan, eds.), 2nd Ed., pp. 211–297. Academic Press, New York.

Bryan, F. L. (1983). Epidemiology of milk-borne diseases. *J. Food Prot.* **46,** 637–649.

Fenner, F. (1971). Infectious disease and social change. *Med. J. Aust.* **12,** 1043–1047.

Steele, J. H., ed. in chief (1983). "CRC Handbook Series in Zoonoses." CRC Press, Boca Raton, Florida.

CHAPTER 20

VIRUSES

Dean O. Cliver

I. Introduction

Viruses are transmitted as particles too small to be seen with a conventional (visible light) microscope. They also cause diseases that cannot be treated successfully with the physician's usual "wonder drugs." As a result, viruses have a rather mysterious reputation and are often blamed for illnesses that do not respond to treatment. Illnesses of unknown etiology probably are caused by viruses much of the time, but viruses ought not always be blamed by default. This chapter is intended to identify the situations in which viruses, as they may be transmitted via foods, are a true threat to human health.

II. The Nature of Viruses

These agents exist alternately as inert particles and as nebulous, replicating, intracellular parasites. Since it is the particle that is transmitted through food, the particle will be discussed first.

A. Particle

The particle form of a virus is produced and occurs inside the host cell, but it is also the form in which the virus is transmitted from host to host.

1. Size

Viral particles are generally 25–250 nm in their smaller dimension. Those that are transmissible through foods are roughly spherical (technically, but not obviously, icosahedral) and range from 25–30 nm, usually, to as large as 75 nm in diameter.

2. Chemical components

Viral particles are simpler chemically than truly living things. They contain either DNA or RNA (almost never both), protein, and sometimes lipid. There is generally no metabolic apparatus, so all of the energy-processing components of the viral replication system must be borrowed from the host cell.

3. Structure

The most important foodborne viruses contain RNA, usually single stranded. The nucleic acid is coated with "structural" protein, and additional proteins (enzymes or other) may be present and function in intracellular replication. Finally, some viruses—though few that are transmitted through foods—are enveloped with a lipid-containing material that usually derives from the plasma membrane of the host cell in which the particle was produced.

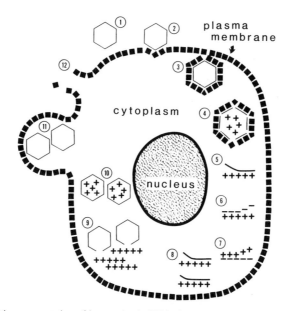

Figure 1   Schematic representation of how a simple RNA virus replicates in a human cell. A virus particle that is free outside the cell (1) contacts a homologous receptor on the cell's plasma membrane and attaches (2). The cell engulfs the entire viral particle (3) and breaks down the coat protein, freeing the viral nucleic acid (4). The viral nucleic acid acts as messenger RNA, which is translated by the cell into virus-specific proteins including an RNA-dependent RNA polymerase (5). This virus-specific polymerase catalyzes transcription of the viral RNA to a complementary ($-$) strand (6). Additional + strands are synthesized by transcription from the $-$ strands (7). These + strands serve as messenger RNA and are translated to produce structural proteins for progeny viral particles (8). Viral RNA and coat protein components accumulate within the host cell (9) and assemble themselves into mature progeny particles (10). Progeny particles are released from the host cell, often in membrane-bound packets (11). A cell that has devoted itself to virus replication may in time lyse and die (12).

4.   Inertness

The viral particle has no metabolism of its own, nor can it carry out any life process autonomously. Each particle is totally inert and can only retain or lose its infectious potential during the time it is outside a host cell.

B.   Replication

Viral replication takes place entirely inside a susceptible cell. The essence of infection at the cell level is that the host cell is induced to synthesize virus components at the expense of its own function and well-being.

1.   Attachment and penetration

The replicative cycle of a virus begins when an infectious particle attaches to the surface of a susceptible cell (Fig. 1). The susceptibility of a cell to a given virus depends primarily on the presence of receptors on the cell's plasma membrane to which the viral particle can attach. Therefore, the presence of these receptors is a principal determinant of virus specificity. Viruses are generally selective about which species they will infect and which route or tissue they can use to begin their invasion. Once the particle has attached to receptors on the host cell, the cell may engulf the particle and at the same time modify the viral coat so that it becomes susceptible to removal that will free the nucleic acid.

When the viral coat protein is removed from the particle by the host cell, the particle loses its identity, and the virus is said to be "in eclipse." This simply means that the infecting particle can no longer be recovered or be located by electron microscopy.

2. Synthesis

The viral nucleic acid that is liberated in the eclipse stage proceeds to direct the host cell in the synthesis of components of progeny virus. Not all of the components need be synthesized at the same site in the cell. Proteins are synthesized using the viral RNA as messenger—assuming that the agent is an RNA virus, as is true of the majority of foodborne viruses (otherwise, the viral nucleic acid must first be transcribed from DNA to RNA). Viruses containing RNA that is transcribed to DNA by means of reverse transcriptase are not known to be transmissible via foods. Some of the virus-specific proteins will make up the coats of progeny viral particles, but others function as enzymes (e.g., RNA-dependent RNA polymerase) that direct syntheses of virus components or modify the metabolism of the host cell (e.g., shutting down DNA-dependent RNA synthesis).

3. Assembly

As the components synthesized according to viral specifications accumulate in the host cell, they assemble spontaneously into progeny viral particles. This capacity to "self-assemble" is apparently inherent in the virus; viral particles will assemble spontaneously from high concentrations of components brought together outside a host cell. The process of assembly of progeny viral particles within the host cell is also called "maturation."

4. Release

Unlike bacterial viruses, progeny of animal viruses can be released without lysing the host cell. Release may take place in a variety of ways, and the host cell may eventually lyse, but the damage caused to the host cell by the viral infection (cytopathic effect or cytopathology) is not a prerequisite to release of the progeny virus. On the other hand, release of animal virus progeny from host cells is sometimes quite inefficient. That is, the total yield of progeny virus may have been synthesized and assembled hours before release occurs, and progeny virus may remain associated with all or part of the host cell indefinitely.

C. Pathogenesis at the Cell Level

Since viruses are obligate intracellular parasites, all of the damage that they may do takes place at the cell level.

1. Cell killing

As was suggested earlier, if death of the host cell occurs, it is not the result of lysis to release progeny virus. In fact, some cells infected *in vivo* survive the viral replicative cycle and return to normal. Alternatively, the host cell may die. One example of why the host cell dies is arrest, by polioviruses, of DNA-dependent RNA synthesis; when this occurs, the host cell is unable to sustain its normal functions and may die and lyse as a result. Other means by which the viral infection kills the host cell exist but will not be considered here. It is perhaps more remarkable that cells infected *in vivo* sometimes recover and regain their normal function.

2. Loss of special function

Cells of the human body have specialized functions to perform in the life of the organism, in addition to sustaining themselves individually. Viral infection may induce the cells to abdicate their specialized function, with the result that they are temporarily not an active part of the parent organism. If enough cells are recruited to produce virus at the expense of their normal, specialized function in the host organism, the organism is likely to suffer abnormality sufficient to be perceived as disease. Furthermore, if the infected cells are part of a vital organ, the host organism may die before any of the virus-infected cells have been killed individually by the virus. Fortunately, death of the host organism is a rare outcome of viral infection.

3. Proliferation

Another result of infection, seen only with certain viruses, is proliferation of the host cells. Sufficient proliferation can produce tumors or cancer in the host organisms.

D. Infection at the Organism Level

In vivo infections involve cells that are part of a host organism, so the impact and progress of the infection must also be viewed at the organism level.

1. Tissue tropisms

The tissue in which virus first replicates in the body is determined by the presence of receptors for the virus on the cells' plasma membranes and by whether virus entering the body can gain access to the cells in question. The site at which virus first begins to replicate is called its primary tropism.

2. Transport

Progeny virus from the primary tropic site is carried, principally via the lymph and blood, to other parts of the body. This exposes the virus to the host's defense mechanisms, but during the first infection with a given virus, these defenses are not very effective.

3. Secondary tropisms

Other cells that have receptors for the virus may be infected at this point, in organs that are not directly accessible from outside the body. The organs involved are often those with which recognized symptoms of viral disease are associated, such as the spinal cord in meningitis and the liver in hepatitis.

4. Specific immunity

The host organism defends itself by producing antibody against the virus, often both systemically (circulating via the bloodstream) and locally (mainly at the site of infection). Circulating antibody is usually of the IgM class and, over longer periods, the IgG class; local antibody tends to be of the IgA class. Protective levels of antibody may take days to weeks to attain, so specific immunity evidently is not the principal means by which some short-duration viral infections are limited. On the other hand, specific immunity against a virus tends to last a long time and is of great value in preventing subsequent infections with the same virus. At best, specific immunity can be induced by vaccination before the host's first exposure to a given virus.

5. Nonspecific immunity

Other host defense mechanisms involve substances such as interferons that are active against viruses in general, rather than just the virus causing the present infection. Nonspecific immunity mechanisms are probably what limit the duration of some short-term viral infections. Although the onset of these defenses is rapid, they do not last long after the infection has ended.

III. Rickettsiae and Chlamydia

These agents are bacteria, not viruses. They are larger than most viruses, have distinct cell walls, contain both DNA and RNA, multiply by binary fission, and are sensitive to antibiotics. They are mentioned along with viruses because they are obligate intracellular parasites, so that the laboratory procedures by which they are studied are similar. Only one rickettsia (*Coxiella burnetii*) and one chlamydia (*Chlamydia psittaci*) are of concern here.

IV. Transmission between Hosts

Since a viral infection only lasts a finite period in a single host before the host becomes immune (or, less likely, dies), it is incumbent on the infecting agent to reach and infect another susceptible host fairly promptly if the parasite is to continue to exist.

A. Routes of Entrance and Shedding

1. Entrance

Entrance of infecting viruses into the susceptible host generally occurs by way of moist tissues, principally mucous membranes. Ingestion or inhalation leads to the mucous membranes of the digestive and respiratory tracts, respectively. Some infecting viruses are injected beneath the skin by sharp objects or by biting insects; otherwise, the skin (cornified epithelium) is not a significant route of entry for viruses.

2. Shedding

Shedding of virus from the infected host is determined by where in the body the virus has been produced. Respiratory infections lead to shedding of the virus by the respiratory route, in conjunction with mucus and the bacteria that inhabit that part of the body. Intestinal infections lead to shedding of the virus in feces, together with fecal solids and a great many bacteria. Superficial infections lead to shedding of virus from skin lesions, together with lymphlike fluid and whatever bacteria are present. A few viruses are shed via the infected kidneys in urine or with milk from the infected, lactating mammary gland. In no case is virus shed from the host in pure form.

B. Passage from Host to Host

1. Direct transmission

Direct transmission (also called contact transmission) is probably the most common way that virus passes from one host to another, even for viruses transmissible via food. Even so, direct transmission seems to have been less studied and is less understood than some alternative modes. Direct transmission of enteric viruses occurs either through anal–oral contact or, more commonly, by way of hands soiled with feces. Respiratory viruses are likely to pass from host to host over short distances in air, by aerosols of droplets from sneezes or coughs. At least in the case of enteric viruses, the frequency of direct transmission is greatly dependent on the level of personal hygiene of the host and, perhaps, the recipient.

2. Indirect transmission

Indirect transmission is the alternative means of passage of viruses between hosts. Of several potential modes of indirect transmission, passage over long distances via aerosols appears to be least likely. Animals serve as "vectors" for some viruses; the animal is called a biological vector if it becomes infected and produces more of the virus (e.g., mosquitoes in the case of yellow fever) or a mechanical vector if it simply carries the virus from place to place as a contaminant on its feet or in its digestive tract (e.g., flies in the case of many enteric viruses). Inanimate objects on which viruses are transported are said to act as "fomites" (singular "fomes"); for example, a fecally soiled diaper might carry an enteric virus from an infected infant to someone else. Finally, foods (including drinking water) by which viruses are transmitted are said to act as "vehicles." Vehicular transmission of viruses is, of course, the principal concern of this chapter.

C. Factors in Transmission

1. Virus stability

Virus stability is apparently a selective factor in the transmission of viruses via vehicles and fomites. Only the more durable viruses (which are, incidentally, usually of intestinal origin) are transmitted by these means with significant frequency. Though the reason for this might seem self-evident, it will be shown later that some of the most common modes of virus transmission via vehicles appear to demand little of the virus with regard to stability.

2. Routes of entrance and shedding

As was just stated, the viruses transmitted via vehicles and fomites are ordinarily those shed from the intestines in feces. These viruses infect after ingestion.

3. Availability of means of indirect transmission

The virus-containing feces must ultimately contaminate the vehicle or fomes, though even the route from the intestines to the food, for example, may be indirect.

4. Population factors

Population factors generally comprise the age and experience of the population in which virus transmission is occurring. Active immunity to intestinal viruses is gained at an earlier age in developing countries than in the United States. Transmission of a virus in an isolated community may eventually cease because almost no susceptible people are left; this is called "herd immunity."

V. Food as a Vehicle in Virus Transmission

A. Human Virus Diseases Associated with Foods

Human virus diseases associated with foods are relatively few in number. During the 5-year period ending in 1982 (the most recent year for which a year-end summary has been issued at this writing), only hepatitis A and Norwalk-type gastroenteritis were reported in the United States. Together, these two viral diseases comprised 50 outbreaks, including 6122 individual illnesses. Among all reported outbreaks, these made up 1.8% of the outbreaks and 8.6% of the cases; these were 4.9% of the outbreaks and 15.3% of the cases if only outbreaks for which etiology was established are considered. It is also possible that viruses such as the Norwalk agent caused some of the nearly 50% of reported food-associated illnesses for which no etiology could be determined.

1. Poliomyelitis

Poliomyelitis was the first reported foodborne viral disease, having been transmitted via raw milk as early as 1914. Raw milk predominated as the vehicle among the 10 outbreaks recorded through 1949, the last year in which foodborne poliomyelitis is known to have occurred in the United States or other reporting, developed countries. Poliovirus transmission by this route ceased before the advent of the poliomyelitis vaccines, perhaps partly because of improved sanitation and the increased use of pasteurization of milk. However, the hepatitis A virus and other related agents (enteroviruses) are still transmitted via foods on occasion.

2. Hepatitis A

Hepatitis A (or infectious hepatitis) is transmitted via an anal–oral cycle. It is characterized by an incubation period of 15–50 days, with a median near 28 days. Viral infection of the liver produces a debilitating, low-mortality disease that some-times includes jaundice. Virus shedding begins 10–14 days before onset of symp-toms. The virus is an enterovirus and cannot yet be detected practically in *in vitro* laboratory host systems.

During the 5-year period ending in 1982, the total reported incidence of hepatitis A in the United States had gone down from nearly 30,000 to about 24,000 per year (but has recently begun to rise again). Included were 45 food-associated outbreaks that comprised 943 individual cases, or 0.68% of the total. The cumulative record shows that shellfish (bivalve mollusks) have most often served as vehicles for hepatitis A, apparently because (1) the waters in which they grow are increasingly subject to human fecal pollution; (2) the shellfish collect the viruses from the water during their filter-feeding activities; (3) though the shellfish are not infected by the virus, we eat the virus-containing digestive tract along with the rest of the animal; (4) shellfish are often eaten raw or nearly so; and (5) shellfish appear to protect virus during heating. Many other foods, including salads, sandwiches, and virtually anything else that may have been handled by an infected person, have served as vehicles for hepatitis A on several occasions.

3. Gastroenteritis caused by "Norwalk-like" viruses

The "Norwalk-like" viruses are called "small, round, structured viruses" in the United Kingdom. They are perhaps 30–35 nm in diameter, show a distinctive surface structure, and probably contain RNA. Because these agents do not replicate in any known cell culture or other laboratory host system, diagnosis is usually based on serological detection of the virus antigen in the stools or of antiviral antibody in the blood of those who are ill. The viruses cause gastroenteritis, typically with diarrhea and vomiting, with an incubation period of 18–36 hours and a duration of 24–48 hours. Attack rates (the percentage of those who, for example, eat a contami-nated food, who become ill) are usually relatively high, often exceeding 50%. These high attack rates may be due in part to the existence of more than one serotype in the group; but it is also noteworthy that volunteers made ill by a single dose of the Norwalk virus became ill again, more than a year later, upon challenge with the same virus. Although those infected and made ill by the virus are known to produce homologous antibody, it appears that they remain susceptible to reinfection and repetition of the illness.

The year 1982 [again, the most recent for which year-end totals for foodborne disease have been issued by the Centers for Disease Control (CDC) at this writing] was exceptional in that the Norwalk virus was the leading cause of reported food-borne disease, with two outbreaks comprising 5000 cases. Both of these outbreaks took place in Minnesota, one (3000 cases) from a worker with diarrhea who contaminated buttercream frosting used on pastries served to many people, and the other (2000 cases) from two workers who prepared salads for social events catered by a hotel. Although no outbreaks this large appear to have occurred since 1982, Minnesota now recognizes the Norwalk-like viruses as a major cause of foodborne illness, with salads the predominant vehicles. These viruses are also a major cause of foodborne illness reported in the state of New York and in the United Kingdom, but in these locales shellfish predominate as vehicles. It seems likely that any vehicle which is known to have transmitted hepatitis A virus could as well have transmitted the Norwalk-like viruses.

4. Other

a. Rotavirus

Rotavirus particles are approximately 75 nm in diameter and contain double-stranded RNA. They typically cause gastroenteritis in infants and in children under 5 years of age, but are sometimes implicated in outbreaks associated with water and, occasionally, food. The victims in these vehicle-associated outbreaks include adults as well as children.

b. Tick-borne encephalitis

"Tick-borne" encephalitis is caused by an enveloped RNA virus, perhaps 50 nm in diameter, that sometimes infects consumers of unpasteurized milk and milk products in Central and Eastern Europe.

c. Echovirus

Echovirus 4, a member of the enterovirus group like the polioviruses and the hepatitis A virus, was implicated in a single recorded outbreak in 1976; 80 people who had eaten coleslaw at a picnic in Pennsylvania developed severe headaches, fever, and some other symptoms.

B. Human Viruses That Have Been Detected in Foods by Laboratory Testing

Viruses detected in foods by laboratories include various enteroviruses and reo-viruses extracted principally from shellfish and inoculated into cell cultures. The Norwalk virus has been detected, on a single occasion, when a shellfish extract was tested by immunoelectron microscopy; this was perhaps the only instance in which virus was detected in a food in conjunction with an outbreak of foodborne disease.

C.   "Viruses" Not Primarily of Human Origin That Occur in Foods

1.   Zoonoses

Zoonoses are diseases transmitted from animals to other animals or to humans, but rarely from human to human.

a.   Tick-borne encephalitis

Tick-borne encephalitis has already been mentioned. The virus is shed in the milk of goats, cattle, and perhaps sheep that have been infected as a result of tick bites. The problem seems to be confined to Central and Eastern Europe.

b.   Ornithosis

Ornithosis is a chlamydial disease of poultry (in the United States, turkeys are most often involved) that is transmitted by the respiratory route to those who handle or kill infected birds. At least one person is known to have acquired the infection by eviscerating infected ducks at home.

c.   Q fever

Q fever is a rickettsial disease of cattle and sheep. It is most often transmitted to herdsmen and veterinarians by the respiratory route. However, the agent is shed in the milk of infected cattle and may be transmitted to those who drink the milk unpasteurized. This rickettsia is one of the most heat-resistant agents known to be transmitted via milk and is the basis of the present specifications for low-temperature, long-time pasteurization.

2.   Agents of animal disease not generally transmissible to humans

These can have enormous economic importance. The viruses that cause foot-and-mouth disease in hooved animals are most important in this connection, but the viruses of rinderpest of cattle, Newcastle disease of poultry, hog cholera, swine vesicular disease, and African swine fever are also of concern. All of these have led to costly embargoes of meat and animal products in international commerce. Although vaccines against some of these viruses have been developed, quarantine continues to be the most effective means of preventing the diseases they cause.

3.   Oncogenic viruses

Oncogenic viruses are agents that cause tumors or cancer. None of those associated with foods is known to be infectious for humans.

a.   Avian leukosis virus

Avian leukosis virus is a retrovirus that causes tumors in chickens. It is present in poultry carcasses and in eggs.

b. Bovine leukosis virus

Bovine leukosis virus causes tumors in cattle. The virus occurs latently in lympho-cytes in cattle carcasses and in milk.

c. Polyoma virus

Polyoma virus causes an assortment of tumors in rodents and is shed in the urine of these animals. It has been detected in stored grain that was subject to rodent incursions.

VI. Contamination of Foods

A. Primary Contamination

Primary contamination takes place in the raw material stage, before the event of harvest or slaughter. Examples are meat and other products from infected animals, vegetables contaminated in the field by sewage irrigation or fertilization with human wastes, and shellfish growing in contaminated waters.

B. Secondary Contamination

Secondary contamination takes place during processing, storage, distribution, or final preparation of foods.

1. Indirect contamination

Indirect contamination may occur if polluted water carries viruses to food or to food-contact surfaces. Vectors such as insects or rodents might also carry viruses to foods, but no outbreak of foodborne viral disease recorded in the United States has yet been attributed to this source.

2. Direct contamination

Direct contamination by a food handler is the most common way in which viruses have reached foods in outbreaks recorded in the United States. The infected food handler may or may not have been overtly ill, but was obviously well enough to continue working with food. The infecting virus must have been shed actively (which is not necessarily true throughout the entire course of an infection), usually in feces. If feces are essentially the sole means by which a given virus is shed, the presence of that virus in food seems to indicate that some significant breach of proper food handling practice has occurred.

On a more positive note, it should be mentioned that, on average, only about 2 of the approximately 1000 food handlers reported annually to the CDC as victims of hepatitis A are implicated as sources of contamination that has led to outbreaks. At least as many food-associated outbreaks are traced to amateurs handling food while infected. Of course, the source of the virus in many recorded outbreaks cannot be identified; since a great many infections with the hepatitis A virus are inapparent, it may be that food handlers, paid or not, are the sources in these instances as well. The hepatitis A virus may be shed for 10–14 days before and for perhaps a week after onset of illness. Therefore, the virus is shed without warning for considerable periods (and, as it happens, at higher levels) in the feces of those who are not yet overtly ill. In the case of the Norwalk-like viruses, the relative incident of inapparent infections has yet to be determined. However, shedding of the virus by overtly ill persons seems usually to be limited to the symptomatic period, though at least two exceptions that led to outbreaks of foodborne disease have been reported. Inasmuch as a person who is infected with an intestinal virus may not be overtly ill at the time that he or she handles food, proper sanitation and safe food handling practices are the essence of what can be done to prevent virus contamination from this source.

VII. Inactivation in Foods

Although virus contamination of foods should certainly be prevented whenever possible, it is also clear that not all virus that finds its way into foods remains infectious until the food is eaten. Loss of virus infectivity is properly called "inactivation" rather than death. It should also be noted that viruses cannot under any circumstances multiply in foods. Therefore, a virus that contaminates a food can only persist there or be inactivated before the food is eaten. No more virus will ever be present than was introduced when the contamination occurred.

A. Virus Stability

Persistence is generally inverse to temperature. That is, virus persists in refrigerated or frozen foods but is rapidly inactivated at cooking temperatures. Components of the immediate environment (both the body product in which the virus was shed from its previous host and the constituents of the contaminated food) are likely to exert an effect. The temperature stability of viruses that may be transmitted via foods is roughly comparable to that of vegetative bacterial cells of some of the more durable species. However, no virus is infinitely stable at room temperature or below. "Attrition" is one term that may be applied to the loss of viral infectivity that occurs with time, in the absence of any specific antiviral agent.

B. Physical Inactivation

Physical inactivation of foodborne viruses may occur through the agency of heat, drying, or electromagnetic radiation.

1. Heating

Heating is a common part of food preservation and preparation. A great variety of viruses added experimentally to milk were inactivated within 30 minutes at temperatures of 55°C or less. There are at least some conflicting reports that the viruses of foot-and-mouth disease, and perhaps the hepatitis A and Norwalk viruses, will withstand more heat than this. One problem in comparing such experimental results is that the first study cited used quantitative methods to measure virus persistence, whereas the other findings have been based on qualitative procedures. Although residual viral infectivity is simply that, it seems clear that these two experimental approaches are not measuring quite the same thing. It might be noted that heat affects primarily the nucleic acid of viruses under some circumstances and the coat protein under others.

2. Drying

Drying also inactivates some viruses. Air drying of viruses on surfaces of food or surfaces with which food comes in contact is likely to reduce viral titers extensively. Approximately 99% inactivation of experimentally added virus has also been recorded during freeze-drying of food.

3. Irradiation

"Irradiation" refers to electromagnetic energy impacting on viruses. Ultraviolet rays, from sunlight or from a germicidal lamp, are quite effective against viruses. However, this is true only if the virus is on a surface exposed directly to the irradiation, since ultraviolet rays travel in straight lines and do not penetrate, and only if the intensity of the radiation is fairly high, which may not be true with a germicidal lamp that has been in use for some time. Ionizing radiation, such as gamma rays from cobalt-60, is capable of penetrating into foods and inactivating viruses, although viruses present rather small targets and are therefore fairly resistant. The dose for 90% inactivation of several different viruses was found in one study to be near 4.3 kGy (0.43 Mrad). Visible light affects only virus particles that have been treated chemically so that they incorporate a photosensitizing agent. Microwaves will inactivate viruses; it is not yet known whether this inactivation results from electromagnetic effects, the oscillation of water molecules, or simply the heat that these produce.

C. Chemical Inactivation

Chemical inactivation, obviously, results from a reaction between a viral particle and an extraneous chemical substance. The rates of at least some of these reactions are greatly increased with increasing temperatures. Disinfectants are active against viruses in water and on surfaces of foods or on surfaces with which foods come in contact. Useful disinfectants are generally strong oxidizing agents—ozone in water and chlorine (and probably other halogens) in any of the contexts mentioned. Chlorine acts most rapidly when in the form of undissociated hypochlorous acid and most slowly when applied as "combined chlorine," such as chloramine. Phenolic and quaternary ammonium disinfectants tend to be much less active against viruses than against bacteria.

Viruses that are within a food, rather than on its surface, are not accessible to disinfectant action. However, at least some are apparently subject to inactivation by sodium bisulfite and perhaps other food additives. Intrinsic constituents of food evidently affect the rate at which viruses are inactivated as a function of temperature. Fat and protein appear to exert a protective effect, whereas acidity leads to greater lability of the virus.

D. Biological Reactions

Biological reactions of viruses transmissible through foods also have to be considered. First, it seems likely that a substantial proportion of virus shed late in the course of an intestinal infection will be combined with coproantibody (antibody, principally of the IgA class, that occurs in feces); this may complicate detection of the virus but probably does not prevent infection if the coproantibody-neutralized virus is ingested with food. Second, viruses are slowly degradable by the action of bacteria in some water environments. However, neither bacteria added to foods as starter cultures nor spoilage bacteria seem to exert a significant antiviral effect. Therefore, it appears that the biological reactions that act against viruses in other contexts are not particularly significant in foods.

E. Conclusions Regarding Inactivation

In "stable" foods (heated and sealed, or dry), the food *may* outlast the virus, though storage of the food should probably not be regarded as a means of preventing virus transmission by this route. In perishable foods (those having a short shelf life or which are stored chilled or frozen), viral infectivity is likely to persist for at least as long as the food is fit to eat.

VIII. Detection in Foods

Some viruses in foods can be detected by laboratory methods. This affords a desirable alternative to waiting for consumer illnesses to signal that contamination has occurred.

A. The Most Important Foodborne Viruses

Hepatitis A virus and the Norwalk-like viruses are seldom detectable in foods because they do not cause perceptible infections in laboratory host systems.

1. Replication in cell cultures

Replication in cell cultures evidently does not occur at all with the viruses of the Norwalk group. The hepatitis A virus can replicate in cell cultures, but replication proceeds very slowly and does not cause any overt effect upon the cells. Adaptation of field strains of the virus to infect cell cultures may take several weeks, and it appears that some field strains do not adapt at all.

2. Serologic methods

Serologic methods now used to detect the hepatitis A virus and the Norwalk-like viruses in patients' stools and (with rare success) food and water samples include enzyme immunoassay, radioimmunoassay, and immunoelectron microscopy. In each instance, the virus is detected on the basis of the antigenicity of its protein coat rather than the infectivity of the particle. Given that each viral particle weighs only a little over 10^{-17} g, not all of which is protein, none of these serologic procedures is likely to be sensitive enough to detect small numbers of particles. Nevertheless, serologic testing may be the only means available to detect these viruses.

An advantage of serologic testing is that many methods produce results within hours, or not later than the following day, whereas infectivity tests in cell cultures may take several days to weeks to complete. A disadvantage is that the tests can only detect viruses against which antisera have already been prepared and then usually can seek only one type of virus at a time. "Broad spectrum" tests using combinations of antibodies, or antibodies to antigens shared by more than one type of virus, are under development.

3. Nucleic acid probes

Nucleic acid "probes," done with segments of DNA complementary to the RNA of the virus, offer an alternative means by which viruses may eventually be detected. Again, sensitivity will be limited by the extremely small size of the individual viral particles, any one of which is potentially (though not probably) capable of causing an infection. Amplification procedures await testing. Related viruses may share extensive sequences in their RNA. This offers another potential means of broad spectrum testing but may be a problem if a monospecific test is desired.

4. Sample preparation

Sample preparation inevitably presents some problems, regardless of whether the virus to be detected is in feces, food, or water and no matter which of the test methods is to be used. Problem substances in the sample may include solids, bacteria and other microbial contaminants, and excess water. Solids are generally removed by physical methods such as centrifugation, filtration, or precipitation. Bacterial contaminants may be dealt with by physical methods, chemical treatments, or addition of antibiotics. Excess water may be removed from the sample suspension by ultrafiltration, or the virus may be separated from the majority of the water by ultracentrifugation or by differential solubility methods; these are often termed "concentration" methods. In each instance, the goal of sample preparation is to produce a suspension that is compatible with the detection method to be used, with little or no loss of virus in the process.

B. Indicators

Indicators of the probable presence of hepatitis A virus and the Norwalk group in foods would be highly desirable. An indicator, in this sense, is an organism or substance that can be detected easily and the presence of which suggests contamination by a pathogen.

1. Bacterial indicators

Bacterial indicators of fecal contamination (coliforms, fecal coliforms, fecal streptococci, and perhaps others) are routinely sought in some foods. Since the majority of foodborne viruses emanate from the human intestine, these tests should be relevant to the presence of viruses. However, it has been found that, for a number of reasons, the presence of bacterial indicators and of viruses in foods usually is poorly correlated.

2. Other human viruses

Human viruses other than the hepatitis A and Norwalk-like agents are detectable in foods on the basis of their infectivity in living host systems such as cell cultures. These human enteric viruses may be the best available indicators of the probable presence of the hepatitis A virus or the Norwalk-like viruses, if the immediate source of the virus is sewage. Because viruses interfere with each other in intestinal infections, a single food handler is unlikely to contaminate a food with both a virus that is detectable in cell cultures and either the hepatitis A virus or one of the Norwalk-like agents. However, the human enteric viruses, when present, can be regarded as significant pathogens themselves.

3. Coliphages

Coliphages (viruses that infect the enteric bacterium *Escherichia coli*) are now being evaluated as indicators of contamination of food by human pathogenic viruses. Some coliphages resemble the hepatitis A virus in size and chemical composition and so may show similar persistence in foods. Because the host bacterium, *Escherichia coli,* is found in the intestines of all warmblooded animals, the presence of coliphages in foods may not be strictly correlated with contamination by enteric viruses of humans.

IX. Summary

Viruses sometimes contaminate foods. Most often, this contamination results from human carelessness.

Even if contamination occurs, the virus may sometimes be inactivated before the food is eaten. Because the virus cannot multiply in food, temperature abuse of food does not enhance virus risk.

Some foodborne viruses can be detected, but testing is slow and uncertain. Better test methods, and perhaps indicator tests that *suggest* the presence of viruses in foods, are badly needed.

In general, the risk of virus transmission via foods is greatest for foods that are handled intimately and not cooked thereafter. Further, most kinds of viruses infectious for humans would be kept out of food if all fecal contamination were prevented.

Bibliography

Bryan, F. L. (1982). "Diseases Transmitted by Foods (a Classification and Summary)," 2nd ed., DHEW Publ. No. (CDC) 83-8237, pp. 17–21. U.S. Gov. Print. Off., Washington, D.C.

Cliver, D. O. (1979). Viral infections. *In* "Food-Borne Infections and Intoxications" (H. Riemann and F. L. Bryan, eds.), 2nd Ed., pp. 299–342. Academic Press, New York.

Cliver, D. O. (1983). "Manual on Food Virology" (VPH/83.46). World Health Organ., Geneva.

Cliver, D. O., and Konowalchuk, J. (1983). Viruses as agents of food-borne diseases. *In* "Economic Microbiology. Vol. 8: Food Microbiology" (A. H. Rose, ed.), pp. 243–263. Academic Press, London.

Cliver, D. O., Ellender, R. D., and Sobsey, M. D. (1984). Foodborne viruses. *In* "Compendium of Methods for the Microbiological Examination of Foods" (M. L. Speck, ed.), 2nd Ed., pp. 508–541. Am. Public Health Assoc., Washington, D.C.

CHAPTER 21

PARASITES

Dean O. Cliver

Foodborne Diseases
Copyright © 1990 by Academic Press, Inc. All rights of reproduction in any form reserved.

I. Introduction

A parasite, for present purposes, is an animal that derives its livelihood entirely from a larger animal that is called the host. Though viruses and many bacteria are parasites in the true sense, they are not to be considered here. All of the agents to be discussed are *obligate* (as opposed to facultative) internal parasites and are *pathogens,* though it should be noted that pathogenic parasites do not cause illness in every host. The names of diseases caused by these agents end in *-iasis* (e.g., giardiasis) or *-osis* (e.g., toxoplasmosis). The selection of parasites for discussion has been based largely on relative threat to human health in the United States, although all of these agents occur in other countries as well, often at higher levels. Foodborne parasites that are not significant in the United States are mentioned only briefly.

Some parasites are shed in feces and cause infections in those who ingest them with food or water. Others are present, during a portion of their life cycle, in food animals. In the latter case, humans are often the "definitive" host—the host in which the adult parasites carry out sexual reproduction and produce eggs that are shed in feces and contaminate the environment. None of the parasites that are transmissible through food or water is capable of multiplication outside the host. Groups, and the species within them, are presented here approximately in order of increasing complexity.

II. Protozoa

Protozoa (plural noun; singular is "protozoon"; adjective is "protozoan," which is sometimes used as a noun, or "protozoal") are one-celled animals. Only three agents will be discussed in detail: an ameba (*Entamoeba histolytica*), a flagellate (*Giardia lamblia*), and a coccidian (*Toxoplasma gondii*). Each of these has at least one active, feeding form that is usually called a "trophozoite" and can reproduce by simple division, as well as a quiescent form in which the agent retains infectivity during periods outside the host, whereby transmission may take place. This stable form is called a cyst in the cases of *E. histolytica* and *G. lamblia* and an oocyst in the case of *T. gondii,* which is the only one of these shown to undergo sexual reproduction as well as simple division.

The three agents differ in the degree to which they invade the host in carrying out their parasitic activities. *Giardia lamblia* is largely confined to the lumen of the intestine, where it adheres to the mucosal surface. *Entamoeba histolytica* penetrates the mucosa and may enter the blood and be transported to other organs. *Toxoplasma gondii* is an intracellular parasite. It multiplies within the intestinal mucosal cells of its definitive host, the cat, and in cells of other parts of the body in cats and the many other warm-blooded species it infects.

A. *Entamoeba histolytica*

Trophozoites of this species are typically 18–30 μm in diameter, though some may be as small as 10–15 μm and others as large as 60 μm, depending on the race of the agent and other factors. There is a single nucleus and usually a single pseudopodium, and the cytoplasm may contain red or white blood cells of the host, or ingested bacteria. Cysts may be 3.5–20 μm in diameter, again depending on the race of the agent, and when mature will contain four nuclei and two blunt-ended "chromatoidal bars."

Entamoeba histolytica has a simple life cycle with no sexual phase. The human host is evidently most important, but dogs, cats, and other mammals are said to be infected. The incidence in the United States has been estimated at 3%, compared with as high as 50% in some tropical areas. Infections are often asymptomatic, especially in the temperate zones.

Ingested cysts excyst in the ileum, and each gives rise to eight trophozoites, which usually establish themselves in the colon and rectum. The local activity of the trophozoites, eroding and penetrating the intestinal wall, may produce amebic dysentery (bloody or mucoid diarrhea). If the trophozoites enter the bloodstream, they may parasitize the liver (rarely, the lung or brain), with grave consequences. During the diarrheal phase, feces are likely to contain trophozoites, whereas the transmissible cysts predominate during the convalescent phase. Levels of cysts range from zero to 6×10^6 per gram of stool. Infections can be treated with medication but are often allowed to run their course; chronic infections and prolonged shedding of cysts are possible.

Measures against transmission are like those for other agents transmitted by the fecal–oral route. Feces should be disposed of appropriately, wastewater treated properly before discharge, and anal–oral sexual contact avoided. Food contamination by infected persons is prevented by proper handwashing after defecation. Treatments with halogen solutions have been devised to decontaminate vegetable surfaces contaminated by sewage irrigation or night soil fertilization, but cooking is probably the only certain way to counteract such contamination and is not applicable to all vegetables. Treatment of drinking water should include an effective filtration step before disinfection, since the cysts are relatively resistant to chlorine.

Balantidium coli is another ameba that is pathogenic for humans and is probably transmitted in the same way as *E. histolytica*. *Balantidium coli* will not be discussed separately because it is relatively rare; its transmission should be prevented by measures effective against *E. histolytica*.

B. *Giardia lamblia*

The trophozoites of this agent present a highly distinctive appearance, having a blunt front end and tapered rear, with twin nuclei and four pairs of flagella. The cell is 8–16 μm × 5–12 μm, convex dorsally, and flat ventrally—the ventral surface serves as a sucker by which the cell attaches itself to host surfaces. The cyst is a spheroid, 9–12 μm in its greater dimension, which contains two to four nuclei, internal flagella, and other structures.

The incidence of *G. lamblia* is now recognized as being high in the United States, where the agent has become the leading cause of waterborne disease, particularly where surface waters serve as sources. Elsewhere in the world, infection rates of 2.4–67.5% have been reported. Before the agent was recognized as a pathogen in the United States, giardiasis was being reported among American tourists returning from visits to the Soviet Union, particularly Leningrad.

Colonization and pathogenesis typically take place in the upper small intestine, where the trophozoites adhere to the mucosal surface and reproduce by simple division. If sufficient numbers are present, they may interfere with intestinal absorption of nutrients, particularly fats and fat-soluble vitamins. The incubation period may range from 5–25 (typically 7–10) days after ingestion of infectious cysts. Acute illness consists of diarrhea, abdominal cramps, fatigue, weight loss, flatulence, anorexia, and nausea and may persist for 2–3 months if untreated. As with *E. histolytica*, trophozoites are likely to predominate in diarrheal stools and cysts in formed feces produced during convalescence.

In addition to humans, beavers were implicated years ago as hosts of *G. lamblia*. Now there is increasing evidence that many other species can harbor this agent and shed the cysts in their feces. Each host supports asexual reproduction of the agent; there is no sexual phase. Although reproduction in the intestine is certainly significant, the likelihood and severity of illness seem to be at least partly dose dependent.

Measures to prevent transmission resemble those for *E. histolytica*, including appropriate disposal of feces, wastewater treatment, and inclusion of a filtration step before chlorination in the preparation of drinking water from surface sources. Vegetables are assumed to be subject to contamination in the field (by night soil fertilization or irrigation with inadequately treated wastewater), and any food may be contaminated in handling by an infected person whose hands were not properly washed after defecation. Cooking kills the cysts in contaminated foods, and boiling will certainly make water safe. Giardiasis is a problem in some institutions and day care centers, where adequate sanitation may be difficult to maintain.

C. *Toxoplasma gondii*

This agent is an intracellular parasite, so it is predictably smaller than those discussed previously. The various active forms (trophozoites, merozoites, tachyzoites, and bradyzoites) are 4–8 μm $\times$ 2–4 μm in size. Up to 3000 bradyzoites, accumulated within a distended host cell, may be encysted as the host develops immunity; such cysts, as large as 0.2 mm in diameter, are not analogous to the cysts formed by *E. histolytica* and *G. lamblia*, though they are potentially infectious if ingested. The more stable form is the oocyst produced in the intestines of the cat. Oocysts are 10–13 μm $\times$ 9–11 μm.

The incidence of infections with *T. gondii* is apparently high; 50% of humans in the United States are said to harbor the agent, though most of these infections are evidently inapparent. Distribution of the agent is worldwide, with a high prevalence in cats (the definitive host) and a significant incidence in other species, including meat animals.

Pathogenesis results from intracellular parasitism and cell death, particularly in the brain, heart, and skeletal muscles. Congenital infections in humans often lead to abortions or stillbirths, as well as malformations and malfunctions that are especially likely to involve the central nervous system. Other than in humans, effects of congenital infections are seen most frequently in sheep.

The life cycle of *T. gondii* in cats often begins with ingestion of an infected rodent or bird. This leads to intracellular infection of the intestinal mucosa, where trophozoites multiply and give rise to merozoites and then to gametes. Sexual union of the gametes produces oocysts, which are shed in feces. The oocysts undergo sporulation and, when mature, contain eight infectious sporozoites. Elsewhere in the cat's body, intracellular infections progress as they do in other species, with rapid multiplication of tachyzoites followed by slow multiplication and encystment of bradyzoites as the host develops immunity. Meat animals, such as sheep, swine, and perhaps cattle, may be infected and produce cysts. The oocysts, cysts, and bradyzoites are all potentially infectious if ingested, but only the oocysts are shed, and only in the feces of cats.

Transmission of toxoplasmosis via meats can be prevented by eating only thoroughly cooked meat. Gardeners working soils to which cats have access should wash their hands thoroughly afterward. Pregnant women should avoid emptying cats' litterboxes, or emptying should be done at least daily so that deposited oocysts do not have an opportunity to sporulate and become infectious. Since cats become infected by ingesting infected animals, cats can be protected by feeding them commercial foods and curtailing their hunting and foraging activities.

III. Roundworms

In addition to the parasitic roundworms, or nematodes, there are many free-living forms. Among the parasitic nematodes, reproduction is exclusively sexual and each individual is either male or female. Depending upon the species, the female may either lay her eggs or hatch them internally so that she gives birth to larvae by ovovivipary. The life cycles of some species take place entirely within a single host, whereas others are complex. The sizes of individuals also vary greatly with species, as the following descriptions will show.

A. *Trichinella spiralis*

The transmissible form of this parasite is a larval cyst, approximately 0.40 mm × 0.25 mm, that occurs in pork muscle. The adult male is 1.5 mm × 0.04 mm and the female 3.5 mm × 0.06 mm. The larvae are intracellular parasites that are 80–120 μm × 5.6 μm at birth but reach sizes of 0.9–1.3 mm × 0.035–0.04 mm when mature and encysting.

The incidence of *Trichinella* infection and of overt trichinosis in humans has declined significantly in the United States with reduced incidence of the agent in swine and successful education of the public to avoid eating raw or rare pork. Surveys of cadavers during the 1940s indicated that approximately 12% of the United States population was infected, and about 400 cases of overt illness were reported per year, including occasional memorable outbreaks. By the 1970s, the incidence of infection was said to have declined to about 2%, and only about 100 cases were being reported per year. In 1982 a single foodborne outbreak comprising 4 cases was reported to the U.S. Centers for Disease Control; however, the total reported incidence of the illness (outside the context of foodborne disease) was 115 cases that year, followed by 30 in 1983, 61 in 1984, and 56 in 1985. Though foodborne disease summaries for years since 1982 were not available at this writing, at least two foodborne outbreaks of trichinosis are known to have occurred during 1985. In one of these, 5 of 19 persons who had consumed meat (reportedly thoroughly cooked) from an infected sow showed typical trichinosis. The vehicle in the second outbreak was Alaskan grizzly bear meat: 9 of 16 persons who ate it were affected. The reported rate of occurrence of *Trichinella* in United States bears exceeds that in United States swine. The agent is also transmitted on occasion in beef that has been adulterated accidentally or intentionally with pork. Elsewhere in the world, the prevalence of trichinosis is low in areas where people cannot afford to eat meat or specifically choose not to eat pork and high in most areas where pork is frequently eaten raw or rare.

Pathogenesis varies with the stage of the infection. The digestive tract is affected when the adult worms are burrowing into the lining of the intestines. Light infections may be inapparent; but larvae burrowing into striated muscles, and sometimes other tissues, often cause periorbital edema, eosinophilia, muscle and joint aches, and fever. High concentrations of cysts in the striated muscles surely result in some inefficiency of contraction—some who have died of trichinosis have harbored over 1000 cysts (occasionally over 5000) per gram of muscle.

The life cycle of the parasite begins when infectious cysts are eaten with the flesh of any meat-eating animal. The capsules of the cysts are digested, and the liberated larvae mature and undergo sexual differentiation. Adults penetrate the mucosa of the intestine to copulate, after which the male reenters the lumen of the intestine and is carried away. The female burrows deeper into the mucosa and produces 1500 larvae by ovovivipary. The newborn larvae are carried via the lymph and blood principally to striated muscles, where they grow and encyst. Severe symptoms are likely if the levels exceed 100 larvae per gram of muscle. The cysts calcify, and the larvae within may remain infectious for 25–30 years. Some infectious larvae are shed in the feces of the host, especially in rats. The host develops an active immunity as a result of the infection and is likely to show significant resistance to later challenges with *T. spiralis*.

The most reliable means to prevent trichinosis is to cook pork and other potentially infected meats thoroughly. Commercially cooked, ready-to-eat meats are probably safe if a temperature of 58°C (137°F) is reached throughout, whereas home cooking temperatures of at least 66°C (150°F) are suggested. Roasting until there is no pink color in the meat, especially around the bones, corresponds to a temperature of 77°C (170°F); this may be more reliable than using a thermometer. Studies have detected some potential problems with microwave cooking, which may not produce uniform distribution of heat. Freezing will also kill *Trichinella* if a temperature not above −15°C (5°F) is maintained for at least 20 days in pieces of pork that are not more than 15 cm (6 inches) thick and for 30 days in thicker pieces. However, the Arctic strains of the agent that occur in bears, walruses, etc., withstand freezing for longer periods. Ionizing radiation is now permitted by the U.S. Food and Drug Administration for *Trichinella* control and may prove important for this purpose in the future. Other control measures that are worthwhile include cooking garbage fed to hogs and avoiding cross-contamination of beef with pork. A serological screening program to detect *Trichinella* infections in swine on farms in the United States is being undertaken as a pilot study.

B. *Ascaris lumbricoides*

This is an exceptionally large agent. Adult males are 15–31 cm × 2–4 mm and females are 20–40 cm × 3–6 mm. The transmissible form is the egg, which is 60–70 μm × 40–50 μm. When the egg has matured outside the host to the point of infectivity, it contains an embryo that is 200–300 μm × 14 μm.

The incidence of infection with this agent is fairly high in North America; 3 million humans are estimated to be infected with the agent. The worldwide human incidence is supposed to exceed 600 million. The proportion of these infections that was acquired via food and water is impossible to determine.

Pathogenesis occurs when migrating larvae hatch from ingested eggs and cause local damage in the intestines. Larvae leaving the bloodstream in the alveoli of the lungs cause small local hemorrhages. If sufficient numbers are present, pneumonia will result. Adults in the intestine sometimes penetrate the lining or wander into the pancreatic or bile ducts; large numbers may cause obstruction. Small numbers are seldom noticed, except in hosts that are hypersensitive.

The life cycle may be said to begin when mature eggs are ingested and hatch in the intestines. The larvae penetrate the intestinal lining and enter the blood and lymph. They are carried to the liver, then to the heart, and finally to the lungs, where they exit the capillaries and grow. They migrate via the bronchi to the pharynx and are coughed up and swallowed. When they return to the small intestine, they grow and reach sexual maturity. During 8 months or less after copulation, the female lays as many as 2.7 million eggs at a rate of up to 200,000 per day. The eggs are voided with the feces and, if deposited on or in moist soil at temperatures of 15.5–35°C, will develop second-stage larvae after perhaps 14 days. These embryonated eggs can remain infectious in soil for months and in some instances for 5 or more years. Infectious eggs in soil have been shown to be capable of infecting via foods grown so as to be subject to contamination.

Prevention begins with careful disposal of human feces. The practice of fertilizing food crops with night soil is particularly hazardous. The embryonated eggs lose infectivity at any temperature above 38°C, and faster at higher temperatures. One hour at 50°C is said to eliminate infectivity completely. The eggs are also somewhat susceptible to drying.

The whipworm, *Trichuris trichiura,* appears to be spread in similar fashion. It is somewhat less prevalent than *Ascaris lumbricoides,* perhaps because *Trichuris* eggs are less stable in the environment outside the host.

C. Anisakids

This group comprises at least *Anisakis simplex* (the herringworm or sealworm) and *Pseudoterranova decipiens* (the codworm or whaleworm), but others are probably important to human health. The threat to human health is associated with active, invasive larvae, often 2 cm or more in length.

Anisakiasis is fairly rare in the United States but is common in countries where raw fish is frequently eaten. This includes such foods as sushi and sashimi in Japan, raw herring in the Netherlands and the Scandinavian countries, and ceviche in the countries on the West Coast of South America. Other examples surely exist.

The mechanism of pathogenesis of these agents is debated. Certainly there is mechanical damage as the larvae penetrate and invade tissues. Additionally, there are "foreign body" reactions that may have allergic, inflammatory, or other bases. It seems likely that larvae tunneling in one's tissues would exert an adverse effect, especially if many larvae are present.

The life cycles of these agents are generally complex, with one or two intermediate hosts, some of which are ocean fish. The definitive hosts of the species that are infectious for man are generally warmblooded marine animals, such as pinnipeds (seals and walruses) for *A. simplex* and cetaceans (porpoises) for *P. decipiens*. Humans are accidental hosts who become infected by eating larva-infested fish with little or no cooking. The larvae are first present in the viscera of the fish but, depending on the species of parasite, varying proportions of the larvae migrate into the muscle. Attempts to show that this happens after the fish is caught have not been particularly successful.

Given present knowledge, prevention must be based principally on "processing for safety." Larvae that may be present in edible tissues can be killed by cooking to an internal temperature of at least 60°C (140°F) or freezing for at least 60 hours (some countries specify 24 hours) at a temperature not above −20°C (−4°F). The latter approach is said to have proven useful in preventing anisakiasis in the Netherlands. Other more specialized processes have also been shown to kill anisakid larvae in fish flesh.

D.   Other Nematodes

Some other nematodes are transmitted via foods in parts of the world outside the United States. Raw or undercooked freshwater fish in much of Asia may serve as vehicles of *Gnathostoma spinigerum* if the waters from which they are taken are subject to contamination with feces of carnivores such as dogs and cats. Rodents are the definitive hosts of *Angiostrongylus* spp., which infect a variety of freshwater animals (amphibians, snails, prawns, etc.) and some terrestrial animals of ancestrally aquatic derivation (snails, slugs, land crabs, and planarians) in Asia, Oceania, and the Caribbean region. Because most of these parasites are of less than visible size as they occur in foods, only thorough cooking of the potential food vehicles can prevent transmission by this route.

IV.   Tapeworms

Agents in the tapeworm or cestode group generally have complex life cycles and a relatively high order of species specificity. Although large numbers of immature forms may occur in intermediate hosts, it is common for the definitive host to harbor a single tapeworm (exceptions to this are certainly known). The tapeworm may reside for many years in the intestines and may be very long, yet the effects on a healthy, well-nourished host are usually imperceptible. Conversely, tapeworm infections can be serious in those who are undernourished or in otherwise impaired health.

Reproduction is ultimately sexual, but all stages are hermaphrodites. An adult, which inhabits the intestines of the definitive host, comprises a head (scolex), a short neck, and the tapelike body (strobila) which gives the tapeworm its name. The head is equipped with apparatus by which it fastens itself to the lining of the host's intestine. The strobila is made up of many segments (proglottides) linked together by some muscle and nerve strands but otherwise largely independent. Each proglottid absorbs nutrients from the content of the host's intestines. A *mature* proglottid contains competent gonads of both genders, which usually interact directly with each other in sexual reproduction. A *gravid* proglottid is laden with fertilized eggs and ready to leave the host's intestine; the proglottid may be shed intact or break and free the eggs to be shed in feces.

A. *Taenia saginata*

This is the beef tapeworm, which occurs in the striated muscles of infected cattle as "cysticerci"—larvae enclosed in cysts of host material that do not exceed 1 cm in their greatest dimension. The adult comprises a scolex 1–2 mm in diameter that is equipped with four suckers by way of attachment apparatus, a neck, and a strobila that ranges in length from 35 mm to 6 m. Mature proglottides are approximately 12 mm broad and somewhat less than this in length. Gravid proglottides are 16–20 mm long by 5–7 mm wide and contain about 100,000 eggs. There may be 1,000 to 2,000 proglottides per strobila. The eggs are 30–40 μm × 20–30 μm.

Taenia saginata is said to be rare presently in the United States. However, there may be infection rates as high as 75% in parts of the world where raw beef is commonly eaten.

The presence of a single adult tapeworm in a well-nourished human host is likely to have little effect, but symptoms involving the digestive tract may be seen. Heavier infections can lead to obstruction of the intestines. Also, the proglottides are contractile, so that sections of the strobila can exit the intestine without the host's participation, which can cause distress and embarrassment.

When an infectious cysticercus is ingested by a human, the inverted head everts and attaches itself to the intestinal lining (what governs the number of these that attach from among the number ingested seems not to be known). The adult that develops may reside in the host's intestines as long as 25–30 years. Gravid proglottides or their eggs are shed intermittently in the feces of the human host; if these feces are disposed of in a way which allows access by cattle or other ruminants, they may be ingested and lead to the formation of cysticerci in this new, intermediate host. The cysticerci form in the connective tissue of the striated muscles and may remain infectious for up to a year and sometimes longer.

Prevention is based on safe disposal of human feces and on careful inspection of bovine carcasses at slaughter. Cysticerci in beef can be killed by cooking the meat to an internal temperature of 57°C (135°F) or freezing for 5 days at −10°C (14°F).

B. *Taenia solium*

This is the pork tapeworm. It resembles *T. saginata* in that humans are its definitive host, but it differs both in that its principal alternative host is the pig and that the eggs are infective for humans as well as for swine. The cysticercus in pork may be 6–18 mm long—10 mm is typical. The scolex of the adult is 1 mm in diameter and is armed with two rows of hooks in addition to four suckers. The strobila ranges in length from 1.8 to 4 m (sometimes 8 m). The mature and gravid proglottides are somewhat smaller than those of *T. saginata,* and the gravid proglottides contain 30,000 to 50,000 eggs 35–42 μm in diameter. It is said that the eggs of *T. solium* and *T. saginata* cannot be distinguished from each other. A strobila may comprise 800–900 proglottides.

Taenia solium is rare in the United States. However, it is said to be common in several areas of the world where pork is often eaten rare or raw. A principal concern is its potential for causing really serious disease (cysticercosis) in humans.

Pathogenesis is often negligible in a well-nourished adult host infected with a single tapeworm. The problems of multiple infection and of undernourished human hosts are as discussed for *T. saginata.* On the other hand, cysticercosis in humans can be severe if organs other than striated muscle (e.g., the eyes, heart, brain, and spinal cord) are involved.

The life cycle of *T. solium* may be considered to begin when the infectious cysticerci are ingested with pork by a human. Heads evert from the cysticerci, and one or more attach to the intestinal lining. An adult tapeworm may persist in the intestines for as long as 25 years, shedding gravid proglottides and infectious eggs. The eggs can give rise to cysticercosis in swine or in humans that ingest them. Some infected persons evidently inoculate themselves with eggs from their feces as a result of poor personal hygiene. Cysticerci in pork are also infectious for humans, but at most each gives rise to only one tapeworm.

Transmission of *T. solium* via pork can be prevented by the same measures as were recommended for *T. saginata* in beef. Irradiation of pork to control *Trichinella spiralis* probably will kill cysticerci of *Taenia solium* as well. However, there is also concern for the feces of infected humans as a threat to human health, both directly from person to person and by way of food.

C. *Diphyllobothrium latum*

This is the most prominent of several tapeworm species acquired from fish. The infectious form of this agent is the plerocercoid, 10–20 mm × 2–3 mm, which occurs in fish muscle. The scolex of the adult measures 2–3 mm × 1 mm and is equipped with two suctorial grooves. The strobila is 3–10 m in length and may comprise more than 3000 proglottides. The eggs are 55–76 μm × 41–56 μm; one million of them may be discharged per day by a single adult.

Diphyllobothrium latum is common in fish in lake regions worldwide and in humans in these areas if they eat fish raw or lightly cooked. Many other warm-blooded, fish-eating species are also affected.

Infections are often inapparent, particularly when a single tapeworm is present in a healthy, well-nourished host. However, heavier infections can cause obstruction of the intestine or diarrhea. *Diphyllobothrium latum* also appears to have a strong affinity for vitamin B_{12} and sometimes causes deficiency in the host.

The life cycle may be considered to begin when one or more infectious plerocercoids in fish muscle are eaten by a human or any of a number of other definitive hosts: seals, bears, foxes, dogs, etc. The tapeworm that forms in the human intestines may live as long as 20 years. If an egg shed in feces reaches water, it produces a free-swimming larva (coracidium), which is eaten by a copepod such as *Cyclops* and develops into a second-stage larva (procercoid). Infected copepods are eaten by fish, which are eaten in turn by larger fish. The larva matures in fish muscle to the plerocercoid stage, which is infectious if eaten by a warmblooded animal. As an alternative to the formation of a tapeworm in the definitive host, larvae may retain the plerocercoid form and infect the host's flesh.

Prevention of diphyllobothriasis in based primarily on thorough cooking of fish. Proper disposal of human feces is certainly to be encouraged, but the agent has so many alternative hosts that there are always likely to be sources of eggs in the aqueous environment.

V.   Flukes

Although relatively rare in the United States, several species of fluke, or trematode, may also be transmitted via foods and cause significant health problems in humans elsewhere in the world. These will be mentioned only in passing here. The list is not intended to be exhaustive.

The intestinal fluke, *Fasciolopsis buski,* is sometimes transmitted via water nuts and vegetables. The sheep liver fluke, *Fasciola hepatica,* may be transmitted to humans by water plants eaten raw. The human liver fluke, *Clonorchis sinensis,* may be transmitted via freshwater fish such as carp, when human wastes are used in aquaculture. Finally, the lung fluke, *Paragonimus westermani,* is sometimes transmitted to humans via freshwater crustaceans such as crabs and crayfish. Safe disposal of human feces and thorough cooking of foods could prevent such infections, but these measures are not always readily available in areas of the world where flukes are a human health problem.

VI.   Summary

A wide variety of parasites, ranging from single-celled animals to tapeworms 10 m long, may be transmitted to humans via food. There are two general modes of transmission. Some parasites are present in human feces and may contaminate drinking water, foods handled by infected persons, or vegetables and fruits grown on soils fertilized with infectious feces (Table I); a few of the parasites shed in feces require a maturation period outside the host before becoming infectious by the

Table I

Major Foodborne Parasites

Food vehicle	Source or mode of contamination	Parasite species	Infectious form
Drinking water	Feces (human)	*Entamoeba histolytica*[a]	Cyst
	Feces (human and animal)	*Giardia lamblia*	Cyst
Foods contaminated in handling	Handling by infected persons (feces)	*Entamoeba histolytica*[a]	Cyst
		Giardia lamblia	Cyst
Vegetables and fruits contaminated in the field	Agent in feces-contaminated soil	*Entamoeba histolytica*[a]	Cyst
		Giardia lamblia	Cyst
		Ascaris lumbricoides[b]	Egg
		Taenia solium	Egg (proglottid)
Meats (raw or rare)	Infected food animal	*Toxoplasma gondii*	Oocyst, bradyzooite (cyst)
		Trichinella spiralis	Cyst
		Taenia saginata	Cysticercus
		Taenia solium	Cysticercus
Fish (raw or rare)	Infected fish (ocean)	Anisakids	Larva
	Infected fish (freshwater)	*Diphyllobothrium latum*	Plerocercoid

[a]Perhaps also *Balantidium coli.*
[b]Perhaps also *Trichuris trichiura.*

peroral route. Alternatively, the infectious form of the parasite may develop in the tissues of a food animal (cattle, swine, fish, etc.) and infect humans who eat the meat.

All foodborne parasites are destroyed by thorough cooking, but this is not always appropriate to the food. Freezing will kill some parasites in foods; however, artificial freezing is unlikely to be available as a means of food preservation in deprived areas of the world, and parasites found in regions where freezing temperatures are common may have adapted to withstand extreme cold. Hygiene and sanitation are of value in controlling most of the agents that are shed in feces, although cultural and economic factors may limit what can be done to prevent fecal contamination. In affluent nations such as the United States, foodborne parasites are encountered principally in pockets of crowding and poverty and among those who choose to eat animal flesh without thorough cooking.

Bibliography

Ash, L. R., and Orihel, T. C. (1984). "Atlas of Human Parasitology," 2nd Ed. Am. Soc. Clin. Pathologists Press, Chicago, Illinois.

Ash, L. R., and Orihel, T. C. (1987). "Parasites: A Guide to Laboratory Procedures and Identification." Am. Soc. Clin. Pathologists Press, Chicago, Illinois.

Benenson, A. S., ed. (1985). "Control of Communicable Diseases in Man," 14th Ed. Am. Public Health Assoc. Washington, D.C.

Brown, H. W. (1975). "Basic Clinical Parasitology," 4th Ed. Appleton, New York.

Cheng, T. C. (1986). "General Parasitology," 2nd Ed. Academic Press, Orlando, Florida.

Healy, G. R., and Juranek, D. (1979). *In* "Food-Borne Infections and Intoxications" (H. Riemann and F. L. Bryan, eds.), 2nd Ed., p. 343. Academic Press, New York.

PART IV

ILLNESSES LINKED TO FOODS

CHAPTER 22

DIET AND CANCER

Michael W. Pariza

I. Introduction

Most of this textbook is devoted to the microbiological aspects of food safety. This is appropriate in that many experts, including those within the Food and Drug Administration, consider pathogenic microorganisms and their toxins to be the most important of the potential sources of harm associated with food.

Microbiological issues are usually straightforward: foods that contain dangerous microorganisms or their toxins at levels that can cause illness should not be consumed. One may debate the question of levels of contamination necessary to produce illness, but the conclusion that illness occurs as a result of consuming contaminated foods cannot be disputed.

By contrast, the role of diet in the etiology of cancer is considerably more uncertain. Cancer is an exceedingly complex group of diseases the origins of which are only dimly understood. Diet can influence cancer risk in animals under defined experimental conditions, but the extent to which such data can be extrapolated to free-living humans is unsettled. Epidemiological studies suggest that diet may influence cancer risk in humans, but there is considerable uncertainty about the specific effects of individual dietary factors.

In contemplating these matters one ought to keep in mind that diet and nutrition are really part of an individual's lifestyle. Experimental and epidemiologic evidence indicate that lifestyle *as a whole,* in combination with individual genetic and physiologic factors, act together to determine cancer risk.

II. Two-Stage Model for Carcinogenesis

Carcinogenesis is the process whereby a normal cell is transformed into a cancer cell. It consists of two discrete stages: *initiation* and *promotion* (or more completely, tumor promotion).

During initiation, a normal cell is altered to become a latent cancer cell. Presumably this occurs because of chemical reactions between cellular constituents (particularly DNA) and a carcinogenic agent. For most chemical carcinogens, these reactions involve the ultimate carcinogenic metabolite(s) rather than the parent compounds.

Although an initiated cell is a latent cancer cell, it will not necessarily grow into a malignant tumor. To become the focus of a tumor it is necessary for an initiated cell to pass through the stage of tumor promotion. During this stage altered genes are activated and expressed. The cell begins to exhibit the phenotype of a cancer cell, ultimately developing the capacity to grow autonomously.

The two-stage model provides a useful mechanism for developing hypotheses on the possible effects of exogenous agents (like diet) on carcinogenesis. For example, dietary factors may initiate or promote carcinogenesis. Alternatively they may inhibit initiation or promotion. There are also examples of dietary factors that initiate or promote carcinogenesis under one set of experimental conditions, but inhibit initiation or promotion under other conditions.

III.   Metabolism of Carcinogenic Chemicals

Agents that cause cancer are called *carcinogens,* and they may be chemical, biological (certain viruses), or physical (ionizing radiation) in nature. While all three can contaminate food, most concern is directed at carcinogenic chemicals.

Most carcinogenic chemicals are inert and will not react with biological molecules under conditions that might occur within cells. However DNA, RNA, and protein isolated from the tissues of animals exposed to such carcinogens contain residues of the carcinogenic chemicals which are so closely associated that they cannot be removed with organic solvents. This observation was first made by Drs. James A. and Elizabeth C. Miller at the University of Wisconsin and led to the discovery that the metabolites of the carcinogens, not the parent compounds, reacted with cellular macromolecules.

The metabolites of carcinogenic chemicals that bind covalently to cellular macromolecules, irrespective of the parent compound, are all characterized as strongly electrophilic and highly reactive. The most reactive metabolites, referred to as *ultimate carcinogens,* are extremely short lived and difficult to isolate. Therefore, the structure of ultimate carcinogenic metabolites usually has to be inferred by working backward from reaction products.

Cellular enzymes, particularly the cytochrome P-450s, are involved in the generation of ultimate carcinogenic metabolites. Many other (noncarcinogenic) metabolites may also be formed, which are regarded as detoxification products. The concentration, substrate specificity, and metabolic products of cytochrome P-450s may vary widely among different tissues from the same animal or among similar tissues (e.g., liver) from animals of different species or strains. Certain soluble enzymes are also involved in carcinogen metabolism and may also vary among tissues, strains, and species of animal. Differences in cytochrome P-450 and the soluble enzymes are responsible in part for differences in tissue, strain, and species susceptibility to various carcinogens.

The metabolism of carcinogens to chemically active forms is referred to as *metabolic activation.* A relatively small number of carcinogens in the environment are already chemically reactive and can directly bind to nucleophilic sites on biological molecules. These are referred to as *direct-acting* carcinogens because they can produce cancer by direct contact without metabolic activation.

Carcinogens vary greatly in potency, depending on chemical class and structure. The potency of a carcinogen depends in part on its metabolism by cellular enzymes. Cells also have other defenses (in addition to enzymatic detoxification) against the adverse effects of carcinogens. For example, ultimate carcinogenic metabolites may be inactivated by reaction with protective nucleophiles like glutathione or ascorbic acid, or they may react with nonessential nucleophilic sites of cell proteins. There are also enzymatic mechanisms for repairing DNA that has been damaged by a carcinogen.

The reaction of ultimate carcinogenic metabolites with cellular macromolecules is a triggering mechanism for the initiation of carcinogenesis. Such interactions lead to the generation of defects in DNA, and mutations in genes that regulate the expression of oncogenes may be of particular importance. (Oncogenes are genes that are causally associated with the transformation of a normal cell into a cancer cell. It is believed that their activation and subsequent expression triggers cell transformation.)

IV. Testing for Carcinogens

Testing chemicals for carcinogenic activity in animals represents a considerable national effort in terms of both time and money. Various short-term tests have been devised (testing for mutagenic activity in bacteria or mammalian cells). While useful in some cases as predictors, short-term tests cannot replace whole-animal assays.

A major problem with current testing efforts rests not on the tests themselves but rather on proper and appropriate interpretation of the data, particularly for regulatory purposes. The Delaney Clause of the U.S. Food, Drug, and Cosmetics Act specifies that a chemical found to induce cancer in animals cannot be added to food. No allowance is made for the conditions of testing or for possible mitigating effects.

The wisdom of the Delaney Clause has been passionately debated by those seeking to amend it to permit some flexibility in regulation and those wishing to leave it as it is or even to broaden its scope. This is not an issue that science can solve. It is a societal/political issue. However, as examples in the following section will serve to illustrate, the scientific data on this matter are not as clear-cut as we might wish.

V. Carcinogens in Food

In recent years numerous articles have appeared in the popular press expressing alarm over carcinogens in food. Concern usually centers around man-made substances, particularly food additives and pesticide residues. However, few scientists share this view. Most experts have concluded that *if* there is a carcinogenic hazard associated with the United States food supply, it is the naturally occurring, not the synthetic, chemicals that should be the focus of attention.

One such expert, Dr. Bruce Ames of the University of California–Berkeley, has estimated that our intake of naturally occurring toxicants (including mutagens and carcinogens) exceeds the intake of synthetic toxicants by a factor of 10,000. This does not necessarily mean that the daily dietary intake of naturally occurring toxicants in the United States is too high, but rather that exposure to synthetic toxicants through food is very low.

Carcinogens can enter the human food chain from a number of sources.

A. Metabolites of Living Organisms

1. Higher plants

There are numerous examples of higher plants producing toxicants, including carcinogens and mutagens. For example, carcinogens are found among the constituents of some spices.

Safrole is found at relatively high concentrations in oil of sassafras (prepared from sassafras roots). It was once used as a flavoring ingredient in root beer, but was banned in the 1960s following the discovery that it was carcinogenic for mice (safrole is also fairly toxic). Many spices in common use (e.g., black pepper, cinnamon, sweet basil) contain minor or trace levels of safrole.

Estragole and *methyleugenol* are structurally similar to safrole. Estragole is a major constituent of tarragon and sweet basil and is also found in anise. Methyleugenol is present in sweet bay, cloves, and lemongrass. Both estragole and methyleugenol are carcinogenic for mice.

In a major study on the carcinogenicity of safrole, estragole, and methyleugenol, and related substances published in 1983 the Millers and their colleagues concluded: "Since these chemicals occur naturally and as food additives at no more than low ppm [parts per million, or ppm] levels in the total food intake, they appear to make, at most, only a very minor contribution to the burden of exogenous carcinogenic agents to which humans are exposed." This conclusion would appear to reflect the view predominating among experts knowledgeable in this area.

2. Higher fungi and molds

Edible mushrooms (*Agaricus bisporus*) contain trace levels of certain carcinogenic hydrazines. Reportedly, mice fed relatively large quantities of raw mushrooms will in time develop cancer. However, given the chemical reactivity of the hydrazines, they can only be detected in living, not processed, mushrooms.

Carcinogens are also produced by some molds. The most prominent example is aflatoxin B_1, the most potent known carcinogen for the rat liver. Interestingly, aflatoxin B_1 is about 1000 times less carcinogenic for the mouse. This is because the mouse is much more efficient at detoxifying aflatoxin B_1 than is the rat. It is not known if aflatoxin B_1 is carcinogenic for humans. Epidemiologic studies have established only a weak association between aflatoxin B_1 ingestion and the development of liver cancer in humans.

3. Yeast

It is an axiom of food microbiology that yeasts do not produce foodborne toxins. However, during yeast fermentations small amounts of the carcinogen *urethan* may be produced. It is thought that yeasts do not synthesize urethan but rather that urethan forms as the result of a reaction between carbamyl phosphate and ethanol.

Trace levels of urethan (a few parts per billion, or ppb) have been reported in some beers, and in some wines and liquors the levels may be higher (up to a few hundred ppb).

The cancer risk from these low levels of urethan in alcoholic beverages is not known but is probably quite small given that the substance is only a moderately potent carcinogen in rodents.

4. Bacteria

In contrast to molds and higher plants, there are few examples of carcinogens produced by bacteria. For bacteria commonly found in food in the United States, the only clear example is the dicarbonyl compound methylglyoxal, which is closely related to diacetyl. Methylglyoxal is a weak, direct-acting carcinogen that has been shown to produce tumors in mice when injected (the tumors appeared only at the site of injection, where the concentration of the carcinogen was highest). Methylglyoxal has not been shown to produce cancer when ingested. In fact a mammalian enzyme, glyoxalase, converts methylglyoxal to lactate, and since mammalian cells do not produce methylglyoxal it is likely that glyoxalase evolved in mammalian systems solely to make possible the conversion of a potential toxicant into a useful metabolite.

Even though bacteria do not produce carcinogens that are likely to be hazardous to humans, they are active in the conversion of nitrate to nitrite in foods and in the gastrointestinal tract. This consideration is of potential importance given that nitrite can react with amines to produce carcinogenic nitrosamines. However, data from epidemiologic studies indicate that the possible link between nitrate/nitrite ingestion and cancer risk in humans is at present inconclusive.

B. Formation in Food by Nonenzymatic Chemical Reactions

Carcinogens can also enter the food supply as a result of heat processing or cooking. One example concerns polycyclic aromatic hydrocarbons (PAH), particularly benzo(a)pyrene. The PAH can contaminate foods (particularly fatty foods such as meats) as a result of cooking over an open flame. The PAH are not produced because of the cooking per se, but rather form when fat from the food drips into the hot coals and is incinerated. The resulting smoke, containing PAH, can then adsorb to the food.

Heterocyclic amines, some of which are carcinogenic, are another class of chemicals that may be found in cooked food. These substances form as a result of reactions involving proteins, amino acids, or other nitrogen-containing food constituents and hence are associated with proteinaceous foods. Carcinogenic heterocyclic amines may form at relatively high cooking temperatures ($>500°C$) due to the pyrolysis of proteins or amino acids. They may also form at lower cooking temperatures because of reactions involving creatine and other meat constituents.

In considering the possible health implications of carcinogenic PAH and heterocyclic amines in cooked foods, it is important to realize that the levels found in foods typically consumed in the United States (e.g., fried hamburgers, charcoal-broiled steaks) are very low (a few ppb).

C.   Man-Made Contaminants or Intentional Food Additives

Although the popular media tend to dwell on this source of potential food contamination, it is regarded by virtually all experts as the least significant of the
potential food-associated carcinogenic hazards. The FDA closely monitors foods for
pesticide contamination. In general only traces (ppb levels) of pesticides and man-
made contaminants are detected, and fewer than 5% of the samples tested contain
even these low levels.

Of the total food additive use in the United States, 93% is accounted for by three
substances: sucrose (47%), high-fructose corn syrup and other corn sweeteners
(40%), and sodium chloride (6%). Under the usual conditions of consumption in the
United States, these food additives are not associated with cancer.

Much concern is directed toward synthetic food colors. However, the daily
intake of synthetic colors is very low and the approved colors have been or are being
rigorously tested for carcinogenicity. Some of the colors have been found to exhibit
weak carcinogenic activity when fed at very high levels to rodents. The significance
of such observations is unknown, but literal application of the Delaney Clause
requires the banning of food additives found to be carcinogenic under any set of
conditions, however extreme.

VI.   Modulation of Carcinogenesis by Dietary Factors

The term *modulation* refers to the enhancement or inhibition of carcinogenesis.
Many dietary factors can modulate the process by acting at the initiation and/or
promotion stages.

A.   Nonnutritive Factors

There are numerous nonnutritive factors in food that can modulate carcinogenesis.
For our purposes here three examples will suffice.

1.   Butylated hydroxytoluene (BHT)

If the synthetic antioxidant BHT is fed before or with a carcinogen, fewer tumors
than expected will develop. In this case BHT acts as a tumor inhibitor. By contrast,
if rats are fed 2-acetylaminofluorene (a liver carcinogen) at relatively low levels
(0.02% of diet) for just 2 weeks, to initiate carcinogenesis, and then switched to a
carcinogen-free diet containing BHT, they will develop more liver tumors than
expected. In this case BHT acts as a liver tumor promoter. Hence, the same substance, BHT, can either inhibit or enhance carcinogenesis depending on experimental design.

2.   2,3,7,8-Tetrachlorodibenzo[*p*]dioxin

2,3,7,8-Tetrachlorodibenzo[*p*]dioxin (TCDD) is an environmental contaminant
which may be present at very low levels in drinking water and fish from some areas

of the United States. Dr. Henry Pitot and his colleagues at the University of Wisconsin have found that at relatively low dietary doses TCDD will inhibit tumor promotion in rat liver, whereas at higher levels it will serve as a tumor promoter for the same tissue.

3. Indole-3-carbinol

Indole-3-carbinol occurs naturally in edible cruciferous vegetables (broccoli, brussels sprouts, cabbage, cauliflower). It inhibits carcinogen-induced carcinogenesis in several animal models by acting in part to increase enzymatic detoxification pathways. However, Dr. George Baily and his colleagues at the Oregon State University have found that, when fed to trout following exposure to aflatoxin B_1, indole-3-carbinol increased the incidence of liver cancers.

These examples serve to emphasize that carcinogenesis in animals is extremely complex, a conclusion that greatly complicates the task of legally regulating exposure to dietary carcinogens and modulating agents in a rational manner. For example, is it wise to ban a substance that inhibits cancer at relatively low dietary levels (which people are apt to encounter) because it induces or enhances cancer in animals when fed at excessively high levels (above what humans would reasonably consume)? Might such a policy actually be self-defeating? These are not hypothetical questions, but rather ones that are regularly encountered by those charged with maintaining the safety of the food supply.

B. Nutrients

There is no good evidence that any substance commonly regarded as a nutrient can initiate carcinogenesis. However, many nutrients can modulate carcinogenesis and the effect (positive or negative) may depend on experimental design.

1. Vitamins, minerals, and fiber

For example, there is evidence that ascorbic acid (vitamin C) inhibits tumor promotion when applied directly to mouse skin prior to application of a mouse skin tumor promoter. On the other hand, high dietary levels of ascorbic acid (5% of the diet), fed after exposure to a carcinogen that initiates bladder carcinogenesis in rats, has been found to promote tumor development at that site. Vitamins A and E have also been shown to inhibit carcinogenesis under some conditions of test and to enhance carcinogenesis under other conditions, as has dietary fiber. The realization that the outcome (inhibition or enhancement of carcinogenesis) depends on experimental protocol is one of the reasons that dietary recommendations for the reduction of cancer remain a controversial subject.

Mineral intake may also influence carcinogenesis. Selenium inhibits carcinogenesis in several animal model systems, but there is evidence that one form of the mineral may be carcinogenic in animals. There is evidence from clinical studies indicating that dietary calcium may inhibit colon cancer in humans, particularly in people at high risk for the disease because of genetic predisposition. Unlike some of the substances discussed earlier, there are not yet data suggesting that calcium might also enhance cancer.

2. The calorie effect

The amount of fat relative to carbohydrate or protein in the diet may also affect carcinogenesis. The primary aspect of this effect appears to relate to caloric consumption. Specific effects of individual fatty acids, sugars, or amino acids appear to be secondary.

Over 50 years ago it was discovered that calorie restriction had an extraordinary inhibitory effect on tumor promotion. Since it was related to calorie reduction it was designated the "calorie effect." In the 1940s the calorie effect was one of the main subjects of cancer research investigation. To this day moderate calorie restriction remains one of the most impressive means known to reduce cancer risk and increase lifespan for rodents. Recent studies have shown that most of the effect of high-fat diets in apparently enhancing carcinogenesis is due to a reversed manifestation of the calorie effect (i.e., the effect of increased calorie intake or increased calorie utilization rather than to a specific effect of fat per se).

The mechanism of inhibition is not completely understood but it appears related to changes in hormonal balance. Hormones thought to be particularly important are the glucocorticosteroids and prolactin. Glucocorticosteroids, which are elevated during fasting, have been shown to inhibit tumor promotion. Prolactin (a protein closely related to growth hormone) can serve to promote mammary carcinogenesis in rats. It is decreased in the blood of rats subjected to moderate calorie restriction on a continued basis.

In humans there is epidemiologic evidence that cancer risk at some sites may be elevated by calorie intake in excess of physiological need. There are also epidemiologic correlations between increased physical activity and reduced cancer risk at some sites, notably breast cancer in women and colon cancer in men.

VII.   Cancer Mortality in the United States

When considering the impact of cancer mortality on American society, two points should be borne in mind. First, death from cancer is *increasing* in the United States. This is caused primarily by the fact that people are living longer, and death from heart disease and stroke are declining. Hence, more people are living long enough to develop cancer.

However, there is also another less gloomy side to this issue. Since cancer is basically a disease of old age it is important to ask how *age-adjusted* death from cancer has changed in the United States in recent years. If we control for the fact that the United States population is aging, is there still an increase in cancer death? The answer to this question is *no*. Age-adjusted cancer mortality in the United States is *not increasing*. In other words, while individual risk of contracting cancer increases with each birthday, at any given age one is no more likely than ever before to die of cancer.

The American Cancer Society publishes annual statistics on changes in the age-adjusted death rates from cancer in the United States between 1930 and the present.

During this time span of almost 60 years some types of cancer *declined* dramatically. A notable example is stomach cancer, which was the most common cause of cancer mortality in 1930. Since then stomach cancer has rapidly declined and today it is very rare in the United States (by way of comparison, stomach cancer mortality is eight times higher in Japan). The reason for the decline in stomach cancer in the United States is not known, but it is believed to be related to improvements in diet and increased availability of a wide variety of foods. Another form of cancer which has declined greatly during this time is uterine cancer among women in the United States.

In contrast to stomach and uterine cancer, lung cancer mortality was relatively rare in the United States in the 1930s but has steadily risen since then. Lung cancer became the leading cause of cancer death among men in the mid-1950s and among women in the mid-1980s.

Death rates from other major forms of cancer, such as breast and colon cancer, have not changed much during the past 60 years. Hence, with the exception of lung cancer (particularly among women) we are not in the midst of a cancer epidemic.

VIII. How Much Cancer Can We Realistically Expect to Prevent by Dietary Means?

In a major paper published in 1981, Sir Richard Doll and Richard Peto (two of the world's most eminent epidemiologists) estimated that as much as 35% of the cancer in the United States might be related to the diet. If this is true, then diet would be the primary factor in cancer incidence since tobacco use was given only a 30% "share" while all other possible factors (e.g., industrial chemical pollution) were, individually, given 10% or less. Since this figure has been widely quoted without qualification in the lay press and elsewhere, it may be instructive to consider what the two epidemiologists had to say about their own estimate.

In the text of the paper (Doll and Peto, 1981, p. 1258), the authors warn, "It must be emphasized that the figure chosen is highly speculative and chiefly refers to factors which are not yet reliably identified." Moreover, in the abstract Doll and Peto state, "By far the largest reliably known percentage is the 30 percent of current U.S. cancer deaths that are due to tobacco, although it is possible that some nutritional factor(s) may eventually be found to be of comparable importance."

Others have also been quite circumspect in their estimate of possible benefit (decreased cancer) to be derived from dietary changes. For example, the very last sentence in the report of the U.S. National Research Council's Diet, Nutrition, and Cancer Committee stated: "The data are not sufficient to quantitate the contribution of diet to the overall cancer risk or to determine the percent reduction in risk that might be achieved by dietary modification."

Bibliography

Ames, B. N. (1983). Dietary carcinogens and anticarcinogens. *Science* **221**, 1256–1264.
Ames, B. N., Magaw, R., and Gold, L. S. (1987). Ranking possible carcinogenic hazards. *Science* **236**, 271–280.

Doll, R., and Peto, R. (1981). The causes of cancer: Quantitative estimates of avoidable risks of cancer in the United States today. *J. Natl. Cancer Inst.* **66,** 1191–1308.

Miller, E. C., Swanson, A. B., Phillips, D. H., Fletcher, L. T., Liem, A., and Miller, J. A. (1983). Structure–activity studies of the carcinogenicities in the mouse and rat of some naturally occurring and synthetic alkenylbenzene derivatives related to safrole and estragole. *Cancer Res.* **43,** 1124–1134.

National Research Council, Committee on Diet, Nutrition, and Cancer, Assembly of Life Sciences (1982). "Diet, Nutrition, and Cancer." Natl. Acad. Press, Washington, D.C.

National Research Council, Division of Biological Sciences, Food and Nutrition Board (1980). "Toward Healthful Diets." Nat. Acad. Press, Washington, D.C.

Pariza, M. W. (1984). A perspective on diet, nutrition, and cancer. *J. Am. Med. Assoc.* **251,** 1455–1458.

Pariza, M. W. (1988). Dietary fat and cancer risk: Evidence and research needs. *Ann. Rev. Nutr.* **8,** 167–183.

Pariza, M. W., and Simopoulos, A. P., eds. (1987). Calories and energy expenditure in carcinogenesis. *Am. J. Clin. Nutr.* **45,** Suppl., 149–372.

CHAPTER 23

DIET AND CHRONIC DISEASES AND DISORDERS

Alfred E. Harper

I. Introduction

Chronic and degenerative diseases are the leading causes of death in the United States and other rich, technologically advanced nations. Cardiovascular diseases (CVD)—heart disease (HD) and cerebrovascular disease (stroke)—and malignant neoplasms (cancer) account for about 65% of all deaths in the United States. Chronic disorders and diseases such as diabetes, osteoporosis, and hypertension, although they account for a much smaller proportion of deaths, contribute greatly to the incidence of disability, particularly among elderly people.

Many health officials and organizations assert that these chronic diseases and disorders are epidemic in our population and that this is attributable to the present Western diet. This viewpoint has been so widely accepted that health organizations, Congressional committees, and government agencies in the United States and many other countries have proposed modification—sometimes drastic modification—of the national diet as a means of reducing the incidence of these ailments. Claims that the present United States diet is hazardous to health have been questioned vigorously by many scientists and physicians who are skeptical of simplistic explanations for high death rates from chronic and degenerative diseases. It is certainly a strange type of epidemic that can account for more than two-thirds of the mortality in a population but which, according to the U.S. Surgeon General, has been accompanied by declining death rates at all ages, increased longevity, and a steadily rising proportion of elderly people in the population. These differing views raise questions about the validity of the assumptions on which claims of deteriorating health are based and emphasize the need for critical evaluation of current knowledge of relationships between diet and disease.

The basic question to be addressed in this chapter and its companion (Chapter 22) is: How adequate is the evidence that dietary trends during this century have contributed to high mortality from chronic and degenerative diseases? Discussion of this question will raise others, such as:

- □ What is the explanation for rising mortality from major diseases with declining total mortality?
- □ Have the changes in death rates from various diseases actually occurred in parallel with changes in the composition of the food supply?
- □ How much do the life expectancies of populations with different diets and environments differ?
- □ Are the increasing crude death rates from chronic and degenerative diseases associated more strongly with an aging population than with various environmental factors?

Besides these questions, many issues that are beyond the scope of this chapter deserve consideration. Is it possible to lengthen the human life span through nutritional manipulations? Can the physiological deterioration that occurs with aging be retarded by diet modification? What would be the impact of drastic dietary modifications, even those now being proposed, on agriculture and the food industry generally? What would the impact be if the assumptions about diet–disease relationships currently being put forward are wrong? What will be the social, economic, and political impacts of further increases in the numbers of people who are no longer in the work force? What will be the impact on the health care system if the increasing proportion of elderly in the population has immense medical needs for prosthetic devices, organ transplants, expensive drugs, and surgery? Finally, what are the social, economic, and political implications of the increases in life expectancy that have already occurred and which, without any lengthening of the human life span, are predicted to continue? This issue will have to be faced, even if birth rates are curtailed, unless the world's population is reduced drastically by some devastating catastrophe such as a highly lethal viral pandemic or a nuclear holocaust.

II. Trends in Diet, Health, and Disease since 1900

With the continuous expansion of knowledge of science and technology that has occurred during this century, industrialization progressed, the standard of living rose, knowledge of nutrition expanded, the importance of sanitation was recognized, and medical care and housing improved. These developments led to changes in the nutrient composition of the food supply and in the health status of the population.

A. Trends in the Food Supply and Diet

The trends that have occurred in the United States food supply are trends that occur in countries throughout the world as either national or personal income rises. They have been summarized for some 85 countries by the Food and Agriculture Organization of the United States. When income is low, diets consist mainly of plant products—cereal grains and root crops; these are low in fat and high in carbohydrate—only 10–15% of the energy (calories) they provide is from fat and about 75% is from carbohydrates, largely from starch. As income rises, the proportions of animal products, fats and oils, and sugar in the diet rise and the proportion of plant products falls. This type of transition has occurred generally in industrialized countries. In the United States, Canada, Australia, New Zealand, and Western European countries, the proportion of energy from fat is now about 40%. In Japan, where the trend is more recent, it is only about 25%. The increase in fat consumption has been accompanied by a decline in the proportion of energy from starch, a rise in the proportion from sugar, and replacement of plant proteins by proteins from animal sources. Foods of animal origin now provide about 70% of the total protein in United States diets.

Comparisons of the nutrient content of the United States food supply over the years since 1910 have shown that increases have occurred in the content of most essential nutrients and in the quality of the protein. The nutritive value of the food supply has thus improved. There is much debate, however, over the health significance of the decline in starch consumption and the rise in fat consumption, mainly from increased use of separated vegetable oils.

B.   Trends in Health Status—Demographic Transition

A general assessment of the state of health of a population can be obtained from measurements of various indicators of health status. Those used most commonly include infant mortality, mortality from various diseases, the incidence of nutritional deficiency diseases, growth rates of children, death rates at various ages, and life expectancy. At the beginning of this century the state of health in the United States, and in most of the highly industrialized nations, resembled very much that of the poorer, less industrialized nations today. The transition that has occurred in health status in the United States during this century has been impressive.

During the period between 1900 and 1920, infant mortality exceeded 100/1000 live births; less than 40% of infants born could be expected to reach 65 years of age (Fig. 1); infectious diseases, especially gastrointestinal and bronchial diseases, were major causes of death; nutritional deficiency diseases were common; and life expectancy was less than 50 years (Fig. 2).

Mortality from infectious diseases that were major causes of death in the early 1900s declined steadily as sanitation, nutrition, and medical care improved so that, by the 1940s, these diseases had become minor causes of death. Infant mortality declined steadily until at present it is about 10% of what it was between 1910 and 1920. Nutritional deficiency diseases have been virtually eliminated through improvement of the food supply and fortification of specific foods with certain critical nutrients, for example, salt with iodine to prevent goiter; milk with vitamin D to prevent rickets; cereal grain products with iron and the water-soluble vitamins, thiamin, riboflavin, and niacin, to prevent deficiencies of these essential nutrients. The heights of children have increased steadily until it is thought that most are now approaching their genetic potential for growth and development. Trends in mortality at all ages have been downward so that close to 80% of infants born in the 1980s can be expected to survive for at least 65 years (Fig. 1). Life expectancy at birth has increased to 75 years, 72 years for males and 79 years for females (Fig. 2).

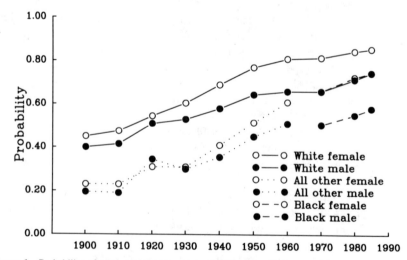

Figure 1   Probability of newborn infants surviving to 65 years of age according to race and sex. From the National Center for Health Statistics. Health United States, 1987.

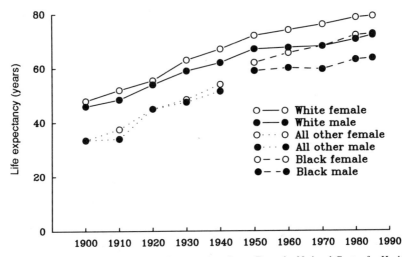

Figure 2 Life expectancy at birth according to race and sex. From the National Center for Health Statistics. Health United States, 1987.

These trends are indicative of remarkable improvements in health. They should not, however, be allowed to obscure the blots on the record. In at least 13 countries, infant mortality is lower than it is in the United States, in large measure because of the high mortality among black infants. Also, a higher proportion of young children in poverty are found in national health surveys to be lower in height for age than would be predicted (Fig. 3). Low height for age in young children is a classical

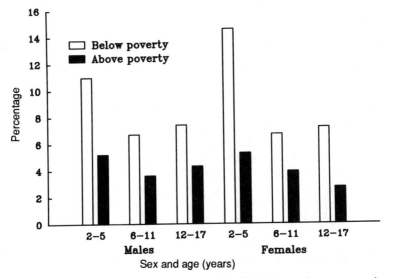

Figure 3 Percentage of children below the 5th percentile of height for age by sex, age, and poverty status, 1976–1980. From the National Health and Nutrition Examination Survey (1986). DHHS Publication No. (PHS) 86-1255.

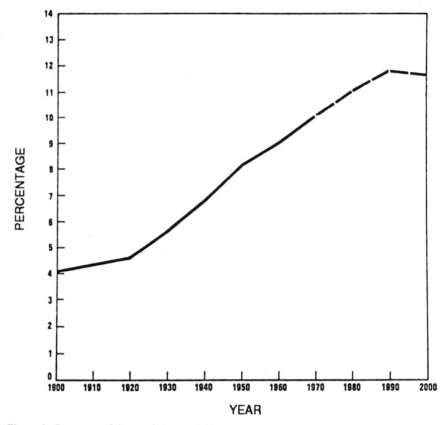

Figure 4 Percentage of the population aged 65 years and older. From the National Center for Health Statistics (1977). USDHEW Publication No. 77-1096.

indicator of inadequate nutrition for some period of time during development. Problems of this type, when they occur in poor countries, are attributed to socio-economic inequities. Health benefits are not shared equally across the population even in highly industrialized nations such as the United States.

The end result of the overall improvement in health has been a demographic transition. The proportion of people 65 years of age or older in the population has increased from about 4% in the early 1900s to about 12% at the present time (Fig. 4). The proportion of young people has declined owing to a decline in birth rate. The Surgeon General, after reviewing this information a few years ago concluded, "The health of the American people has never been better." Despite this, there have been some other trends, especially overweight, that have created concern about whether the state of health is as good as it might be.

C. Body Weight and Obesity

The changes that have occurred in the food supply have been accompanied by increasing mechanization in the workplace and the home and a decreased need for physical activity even in jobs that traditionally have involved heavy labor. With an

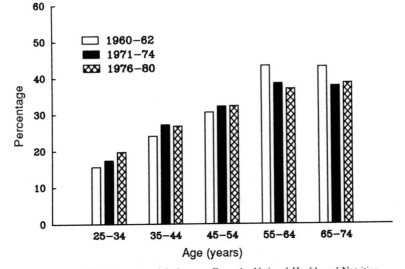

Figure 5 Percentage of females overweight by age. From the National Health and Nutrition Examination Survey (1986). DHHS Publication No. (PHS) 86-1255.

abundant supply of food that is appetizing, nutritious, and relatively inexpensive, a substantial proportion of the population consumes, assimilates, and stores an amount of energy in excess of the amount expended. In the United States, 20–30% of men and 25–40% of women—the percentage increasing with increasing age over 25 years—are considered overweight (Fig. 5). The percentages have changed little

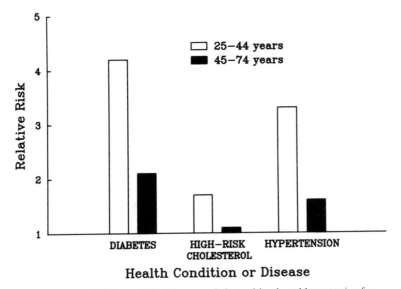

Figure 6 Relative risk of diabetes, high-risk serum cholesterol level, and hypertension for overweight persons (relative to non-overweight persons) by age, 1976–1980. From the National Health and Nutrition Examination Survey (1986). DHHS Publication No. (PHS) 86-1255.

over the past 20 years. In age groups above 25 years, 5–10% are judged to be severely overweight. Excessive body weight is a health risk, particularly if it occurs at an early age (Fig. 6). Risk increases steadily with increasing body weight in excess of what is considered desirable weight. The risk of developing diabetes, hypertension, gall bladder disease, and endometrial cancer increases as body weight increases. Since diabetes and hypertension are risk factors for heart disease, excessive body weight is also a risk factor for coronary heart disease (CHD). Severe overweight was reported in a recent study to be a risk factor for CHD independently of its contribution to hypertension and diabetes.

The term "risk factor" is a term used by epidemiologists, usually as if its meaning were obvious, but this is not so. A risk factor is not necessarily a cause of a disease; it is a factor associated with an increased incidence of the disease. The causes of chronic and degenerative diseases are complex; few have been identified. However, associations between characteristics of individuals and the environment and mortality from such diseases have been examined in large populations. If certain personal characteristics, for example, overweight, or certain environmental factors, for example, a diet high in salt, are found to be associated with a higher incidence of a particular disease than is observed when those characteristics are absent, these are called risk factors. They are based on probabilities that apply to large populations; for example, if, in a large population, mortality from a disease is 4/1000 among the people with certain risk factors but only 2/1000 among those without risk factors, the probability of the disease occurring in those with the risk factors has doubled. Note well, this increase in risk is usually reported as an increase of 100%; in actuality, it is an increase from 2/1000 to 4/1000. The increased risk cannot be assumed to apply equally to every individual, however. The incidence of diabetes is higher among severely overweight people than among those who are lean, but whether the overweight people develop diabetes depends very largely upon whether they are genetically susceptible to the disease. Also, lean individuals may be susceptible to the disease but whether or not they develop it depends very largely upon whether they become severely overweight. Development of most of the chronic and degenerative diseases is influenced greatly by genetic–environmental interactions and, as these diseases are multifactorial (have multiple causes), on many other interactions as well.

It is important to realize that underweight is also undesirable. The relationship between mortality and body weight is J shaped, indicating that mortality increases with increasing deviation in either direction from appropriate body weight. In some studies among the elderly, however, the most desirable body weight for continued longevity was found to be that currently considered as moderately overweight. The risk for health from being overweight appears to depend upon age and genetic susceptibility to the diseases associated with aging.

D. Patterns of Disease—Epidemiologic Transition

The decline in mortality from infectious diseases, brought about by improved sanitation, immunization, advances in medical care, and the greatly improved state of health of Americans during this century, has been accompanied by changes in the major causes of death (Fig. 7). This has been referred to as an epidemiologic

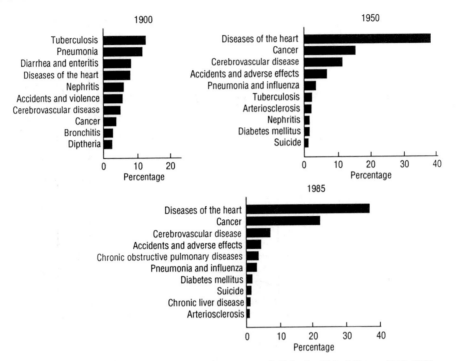

Figure 7 The 10 leading causes of death as a percentage of all deaths, United States, 1900, 1950, 1985. From the National Center for Health Statistics. Health United States, 1987.

transition. Life expectancy lengthens and the proportion of people living to older ages increases when diseases that take a heavy toll of the very young are controlled. As this occurs, chronic and degenerative diseases and disorders that are associated with aging become the major causes of death. This has been occurring throughout all of the industrialized nations despite their different environments and diets. The proportions of deaths from different diseases, however, vary considerable from country to country. The proportion of deaths from malignant neoplasms is similar in Japan and the United States, 25 and 22%, respectively; but for deaths from stroke, the percentages are 19 and 8%, and from heart disease, 20 and 37%, respectively.

In examining trends in mortality from different chronic and degenerative diseases, changes in both the proportion of total deaths and crude death rates can be deceptive. The demographic transition has resulted in an increasing proportion of elderly who are susceptible to such diseases and a decreasing proportion of younger people in the population who are not. In the early 1900s, for example, when only 4% of the population was 65 years of age or older, CVD (heart disease and stroke) accounted for only 15% of total deaths; now, when 12% of the population is in the older age group, CVD account for 45% of all deaths (Fig. 7). The percentages have changed but the proportions are similar.

A similar problem is encountered when comparing time-trends in crude death rates. The crude death rate from total CVD was between 350 and 375 per 100,000 people between 1910 and 1920; and it rose to slightly over 500/100,000 between 1950 and 1960, then it began to level off. Subsequently it has declined slowly but is

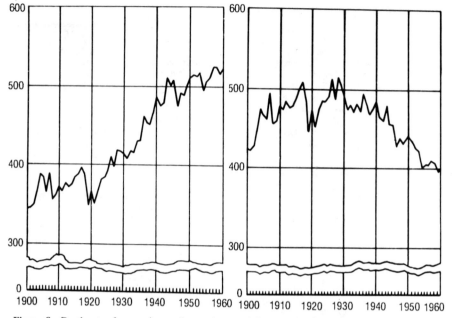

Figure 8 Death rates from major cardiovascular–renal diseases; Death-registration states, 1900–1932, and United States, 1933–1960. Rates are per 100,000 population. *Left:* Crude death rates. *Right:* Age-adjusted death rates. From National Center for Health Statistics, 1968.

still above rates for the early part of the century. The rising death rates and proportion of deaths from CVD have been associated with the increasing proportion of elderly people in the population. It is therefore necessary, if these trends are to be placed in perspective, to compare the rates after an adjustment has been made to take into account changes in the relative proportions of the population in different age groups. This has been done throughout the century by the National Center for Health Statistics.

When these age-adjusted trends for death rates from total CVD, heart disease, and stroke are examined, they are seen to be different from those for crude death rates. The age-adjusted death rate from total CVD was between 450 and 500 per 100,000 people until about 1940 but had declined to 400 by 1960 (Fig. 8, right), whereas the crude death rate was rising throughout this period (Fig. 8, left). The age-adjusted death rate from CVD has continued to decline until it is now about 250 (Fig. 9; diseases of the heart plus cardiovascular diseases). When death rates for CVD for different age groups of men are examined it becomes clear why the crude death rate rises in the total population if the proportion of elderly people increases. Death rate from CVD increases with increasing age, from 37/100,000 at ages 35–44 years to 445/100,000 at ages 54–64 years and to 2750/100,000 at ages 75–84 years. Note the similarity of the slopes of the curves in Fig. 4 and the left panel of Fig. 8. This prompts the question: Have we had an epidemic of chronic and degenerative diseases or is the assumed epidemic merely a reflection of the increased proportion of elderly people in the population? In evaluating statements about associations between diet and chronic and degenerative diseases, it is important to consider the effects of demographic transitions on death rates from various diseases

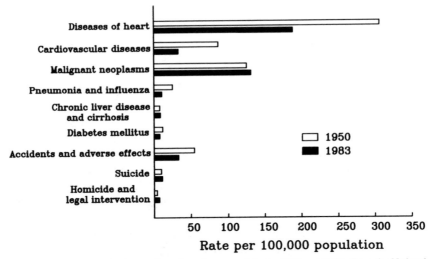

Figure 9 Age-adjusted death rates for selected causes of death, 1950 and 1983. From the National Vital Statistics System (1986). DHHS Publication No. (PHS) 86-1255.

and to distinguish clearly between crude death rates and age-adjusted death rates which take into account changes in the age distribution within the population.

E. Changing Emphasis in Dietary Recommendations

Dietary recommendations made during the 19th century and the early part of the 20th century were mainly responses to disasters. Recommendations for appropriate intakes of energy sources (calories) and protein (the nutritional importance of vitamins and most minerals was not discovered until the early 1900s) were proposed during periods when economic crises, social dislocation, and wars caused severe food shortages. The recommendations were parts of programs designed to preserve the working capacity of the labor force and to relieve the debilitation and disease that resulted from deprivation and starvation. Infectious diseases were the major causes of death. Malnutrition and undernutrition were common. Life expectancy was less than 50 years (Fig. 2).

Since then, knowledge of the causes of nutritional and infectious diseases and of how to treat such illnesses successfully has increased immensely. Application of this knowledge has been spurred by changing concepts of society's responsibility for maintaining the public's health. The purpose of dietary recommendations was expanded after World War I, particularly during the period of the Great Depression (1930–1935). The new direction was to provide not just information needed to improve survival during disasters, but knowledge about the food supply that would contribute toward achievement of genetic potential for growth and development of infants and preservation of health of the entire population.

During this time the nutritional essentiality of many minor components of foods—vitamins and trace minerals—was recognized. These discoveries made possible the treatment and prevention of dietary deficiency diseases. Subsequently recommendations for appropriate intakes of essential nutrients—Recommended Dietary Allowances (RDA)—were proposed by several national and international organizations.

The RDA provided the basis for formulation of an easily understood set of dietary recommendations—a food guide—by the U.S. Department of Agriculture directed toward assuring the nutritional health of the population. Knowledge of food composition and of needs for essential nutrients was used to group foods into four categories according to their content of the different essential nutrients. Then the number of servings needed daily from each food group to meet the nutritional needs of different age groups was estimated. The recommendation for adults was to consume each day two servings of dairy products, two of meats and legumes, four of cereal grain products, and four of fruits and vegetables. After this approach to diet selection was adopted and a few staple foods were fortified with specific nutrients that appeared to be low in the food supply, nutritional deficiency diseases ceased to be public health problems. Despite these efforts, 2–5% of people have low intakes of one or more nutrients and somewhat more than 5% of young women, and as high as 10% of those in poverty, have low iron stores.

As the importance of nutritional deficiency diseases declined and effective methods for preventing or treating many infectious diseases were developed, chronic and degenerative diseases became the major medical problems of highly industrialized societies (Fig. 7; 1950 versus 1900). Observations, particularly epidemiologic observations, indicated that the incidence of these diseases differed among the populations of different countries and that there were associations between the types of diets consumed in different countries and mortality from these diseases. This gave rise to the idea that diseases and disorders such as heart disease and hypertension, and more recently cancer and osteoporosis, might be public health or environmental rather than medical problems. The suggestion was made that such diseases might be prevented if the diets of the highly industrialized nations were modified to resemble those of nations, often the less industrially developed nations, where the incidence of such diseases was low. As a result, dietary guidelines for prevention of these diseases have proliferated as if mortality from chronic and degenerative diseases were the only meaningful measure of the state of health of the population.

This change in both the purpose and the concept of dietary guidelines raises many more questions. Is knowledge of associations between diet and disease adequate to ensure that recommendations of this type will be effective in preventing diseases that are associated with aging and have a strong genetic component? Do such recommendations, like those for obtaining an adequate diet, apply to the entire population or only to segments of it? Are such guidelines based on a realistic assessment of the present state of health? Before intimating that such recommendations will prevent these diseases, should there not be incontrovertible scientific evidence of both their effectiveness and their safety, and possibly even of their cost effectiveness?

III. Cardiovascular Diseases and Diet

Ischemic or coronary heart disease is the single disease responsible for most deaths (37%) in the United States (Fig. 7; 1985). Most CHD results from atherosclerosis, a disease process in which material rich in lipid accumulates in the walls of arteries. These accumulations or plaques thicken the arterial wall, narrowing the internal diameter of the vessel. This reduces the rate of flow of blood to the heart and, particularly during periods of increased physical activity, may cause angina pectoris, painful sensations in the chest. Further reduction in the flow of blood through these narrowed vessels, owing to spasms of the artery or the formation of blood clots, is the major cause of heart attacks.

The underlying causes of CHD are not understood but individuals with the genetic disorder familial hypercholesteremia who develop CHD early in life have greatly elevated concentrations of cholesterol in blood owing to a genetic defect in the system for degrading cholesterol. Their livers lack or contain only a small number of the receptors needed for removal of cholesterol-laden low-density lipoproteins (LDL) from the blood. The nature of the process that results in formation of plaque in the arteries is not understood, but once it has been initiated through damage to the arterial wall, a high blood concentration of cholesterol evidently accelerates it.

A.   Risk Factors for Heart Disease

Results of epidemiological studies—studies of associations between mortality from different diseases in large populations and characteristics of the environment and the people—revealed in the early 1950s that both blood cholesterol concentrations and death rates from CHD tended to be high in populations consuming diets high in lipids, particularly in saturated fatty acids and cholesterol. Associations between dietary intake of lipids, blood lipid concentrations, and arterial lesions have also been observed in clinical studies and investigations on experimental animals. The hypothesis that consumption of a diet high in saturated fats and cholesterol elevates blood lipid and LDL levels which in turn increases the progression of atherosclerosis and results in development of CHD arose from studies of this type. Such studies also revealed associations between the incidence of CHD and many other characteristics of both individuals and their environments. These characteristics are risk factors for CHD.

We should recall here that such risk factors are not necessarily causes of the disease. They are factors associated with an increased incidence of the disease. They are identified by comparing mortality from CHD with the occurrence of a particular characteristic in the population. From such comparisons among different populations estimates are made of the probability that a population with a particular characteristic will have an increased incidence of CHD. Thus, identification of risk factors cannot establish whether an individual will develop CHD, only what the probability is compared with that for others who do not have those characteristics. Also, the absence of risk factors does not guarantee that the disease will not occur. Among the many risk factors for CHD are male sex, age, family history (genetics), hypertension, hypercholesteremia, cigarette smoking, diabetes, low physical activity, and high consumption of fat and cholesterol. Lists of 30 or more risk factors for CHD are not uncommon and some physicians and scientists have compiled much longer lists.

Since serum cholesterol concentration can be influenced by the type and amount of fat in the diet, diet modification has been advocated as an effective means not only of treating but of delaying or reducing the incidence (frequently the term used is "prevention") of CHD. With such a large number of risk factors for the disease, it is difficult to assess the significance of any one factor alone; however, relationships between dietary fat and cholesterol intake and serum cholesterol level have been examined extensively in animal experiments and clinical trials, and many studies have been done in an effort to demonstrate the value of diet modifications and drug treatments which lower blood cholesterol level as a measure for "preventing" CHD. Evaluation of the results of these measures can provide some perspective on the influence of diet on susceptibility to CHD.

B.   Diet, Serum Cholesterol, and Heart Disease

In clinical studies of men with serum cholesterol concentrations in the normal range and consuming diets in which 40% of the calories were from fat, increasing the proportion of saturated fatty acids raised serum cholesterol concentration whereas increasing the proportion of polyunsaturated fatty acids lowered it. The effect of a change in the saturated fatty acid content is about twice as great as the effect of an equivalent change in polyunsaturated fatty acid content. Increasing dietary cholesterol intake over the range of 0–600 mg/day also increases serum cholesterol concentration, but within the usual range of cholesterol intakes of about 300–600 mg/day, the effects are small; they are influenced by the type of fat consumed and vary greatly among individuals. Also, 600–1500 mg of cholesterol is synthesized by the body daily and, if cholesterol intake changes, the body tends to compensate by adjusting the amount synthesized. Dietary cholesterol is one of the less important dietary variables affecting serum cholesterol level. In trials of this type, done under carefully controlled conditions with subjects consuming rigidly defined diets, serum cholesterol concentration can be lowered 15–30%. In large-scale trials with free-living subjects, the reduction is seldom greater than 10% and is commonly between 5 and 10%—partly owing to high individual variability in the response to diet and partly undoubtedly to the inability of most people to adhere to rigid dietary restrictions.

Based on the knowledge that elevated serum cholesterol concentration is a risk factor for CHD and that diet modification and several drugs will lower serum cholesterol, 20 or more intervention trials have been conducted with large numbers of men whose serum cholesterol concentration was high enough to place them at high risk for developing CHD. The objective was to determine if treating them with diets or drugs (or both) to lower serum cholesterol concentration would reduce CHD mortality. The results of these trials have not been consistent. The conclusion from an analysis of 19 such trials lasting 5–10 years and involving 36,000 individuals was that, overall, the numbers of coronary infarcts (heart attacks) and deaths were reduced in association with reduced serum cholesterol concentrations. Total mortality in the treated and untreated populations, however, was not significantly different. It seems, then, that lowering serum cholesterol concentration can lower the incidence of CHD in a population considered to be at high risk from greatly elevated serum cholesterol levels without lowering overall mortality. Success with dietary treatment has been much less than with drug treatment, but results from the major

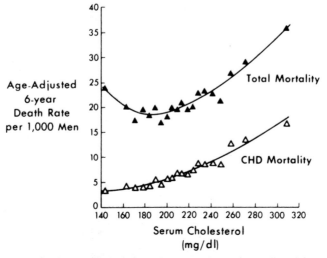

Figure 10 Relationship between serum cholesterol concentration and age-adjusted 6-year CHD and total mortality among 361,662 men, aged 35–57 years, screened for the Multiple Risk Factor Intervention Trial. From M. J. Martin, S. B. Hulley, W. S. Browner, L. H. Kuller, and D. Wentworth (1986). *Lancet* **II,** 934.

successful drug study with high-risk subjects have been used to support dietary recommendations for the entire population.

In connection with the results of these trials, a plot of the relationship between serum cholesterol concentration and both CHD and total mortality for some 360,000 men aged 35–37 years (Fig. 10) is instructive. Although CHD mortality increased progressively with increasing serum cholesterol concentrations above about 190 mg/dl, total mortality among those with concentrations between 160 and 225 mg/dl was essentially the same and rose very little as the concentration increased to 250 mg/dl. Also, death rates of men aged 35–74 years from CHD in France is one-third that in the United States, life expectancy of French men is the same as that of American men (Table I). These observations lead to the conclusion that the incidence of CHD is influenced by environment, including diet. Both sets of observations, however, suggest that modifications of the risk factors, such as diet, to reduce the incidence of CHD in those susceptible to it affects others adversely. When recommendations for adoption of diet modification for the entire population are being promoted, this poses a dilemma. What is the appropriate approach?

C. Dietary Approaches to Control of Heart Disease

There are strong differences of opinion over whether CHD is primarily a public health problem or a medical problem. Ardent advocates of the public health approach recommend that everyone over the age of 2 years reduce consumption of total fat, saturated fat, and cholesterol to reduce the probability of developing CHD. An equally qualified group of physicians and scientists consider that such a recommendation is not appropriate. They consider that healthy children require intervention only if they have a family history of CHD and evidence of high-risk serum

Table I

Age-Adjusted Mortality from Heart Disease among Men
Aged 35–74 Years in Selected Countries and Life Expectancy
at Birth and Age 65 Years (1975)[a]

Country	Age-adjusted mortality from heart disease (deaths/100,000)	Life expectancy	
		At birth (years)	At age 65 (years)
Norway	581	72	14
Netherlands	506	71	14
Japan	115	71	13
United States	793	69	14
Italy	309	69	13
France	205	69	13

[a]Adapted from A. E. Harper (1987). *Am. J. Clin. Nutr.* **45**, 1102.

cholesterol levels and that the majority of healthy adults require dietary intervention only if their serum total cholesterol exceeds 240 mg/dl.

The proportion of people at high risk of CHD is difficult to establish. The serum total cholesterol levels of three-quarters of the men in the United States and most women under 45 years of age do not place them at high risk of CHD. Although CHD is the major cause of death in the United States, two-thirds of all deaths are from causes other than CHD. One-third of those who die from CHD are over the age of 80. A high proportion of those who die at ages below 55 years suffer from genetic defects of lipid metabolism which are not highly responsive to diet. In fact, 50–60% of heart attacks before age 55, according to a study done in Utah, occur among only 2–5% of families. Also, the average age of death from CHD is as high as or higher than the average age of death generally. Only about 50% of the risk for CHD can be accounted for by known risk factors; of the known risk factors, diet is only one of several, and less important than either hypertension or cigarette smoking. Even though high intakes of saturated fats may increase the rate of progression of the disease in those who are predisposed toward developing it, it would seem improbable that diet is a major cause of CHD.

Family history and blood lipid analyses are essential for identifying individuals with a genetic predisposition for CHD. Methods for evaluating blood lipid abnormalities have been improving steadily. Plasma total cholesterol concentration is an indicator of limited value. Cholesterol is carried in the blood mainly in the LDL fraction but a portion is present in a high-density lipoprotein (HDL) fraction. HDL carries cholesterol back to the liver for degradation. A high HDL level reduces risk of CHD even if blood cholesterol is elevated. The total cholesterol : HDL cholesterol ratio is a better indicator of risk than either plasma total cholesterol or LDL concentrations alone. Even with high total cholesterol, risk is low if this ratio is four or less. Also, it is now becoming possible to measure concentrations of the specific apoproteins associated with different lipoproteins and soon it should be possible, using the techniques of molecular biology, to characterize lipoprotein profiles in detail. With these tools, prediction of susceptibility to CHD will improve greatly and it will become possible to devise specific treatment programs for reducing risk of CHD for individuals with different genetic problems.

For those at high risk, CHD is not a public health problem. It requires comprehensive, continuing medical care with retesting at regular intervals. General dietary recommendations are not adequate for those at high risk and create an unjustifiable sense of complacency when they are followed. They are unnecessary for most of the population and pressure to follow them creates apprehension among those not at risk. Overzealous application of general dietary recommendations for prevention of this disease has resulted in withholding of food from children by parents to the point where they have been hospitalized for failure to grow.

Further, the age-adjusted death rate from CHD has been declining steadily in the United States for many years (Figs. 8 and 9). Efforts to relate this trend to changes in risk factors, including changes in dietary patterns, have been unsuccessful. The influence of improved medical care on CHD mortality has received little attention and is often brushed aside. In one comparison of a large population of patients with CHD admitted to hospital in the early 1970s with another admitted in the early 1980s, the improvement in survival during the decade was great enough to account for 40% or more of the decline in death rate from this disease. Another factor that deserves attention but which has not been evaluated is that 65% of CHD patients performed "heavy" occupational work in the 1950s compared with only 5% now. Thus, the likelihood of excessive physical exertion which can precipitate a heart attack is much less now.

In efforts to reduce the death rate from this disease there would seem to be no viable alternative to increasing efforts to identify those at high risk and treat them comprehensively and vigorously. As for general dietary guidance, advice to consume a nutritionally adequate diet from a wide variety of foods and to do so in moderation so that body weight is maintained within the desirable range would seem both logical and adequate. If these guidelines are followed, fat intake should not be inordinately high and caloric intake would not be excessive.

IV. Hypertension and Diet

Hypertension is defined as persistent high arterial blood pressure. High blood pressure is the major risk factor for stroke and is associated with increased risk for cardiovascular–renal diseases generally and for CHD in particular. Blood pressure is usually measured over the brachial artery in the upper arm. The highest pressure (systolic) occurs during contraction of the ventricles of the heart and normally ranges between 100 and 140 mm of mercury. The lowest pressure (diastolic) occurs during relaxation of the ventricles and usually ranges between 60 and 90 mm of mercury. Blood pressure levels within a large population follow a normal or Gaussian distribution pattern with no clear line of demarcation between normal and high blood pressure. The high end of the range is considered on an operational basis to represent hypertension. The lowest mortality among young adults is associated with diastolic blood pressure of less than 70 and systolic blood pressure of less than 130 mm of mercury. Values above these are associated with increased risk of developing diseases such as stroke and CHD. Hypertension is usually defined as diastolic blood pressure greater than 90 or systolic blood pressure greater than 150 mm of mercury with major emphasis being placed on the diastolic pressure.

A. Incidence and Nature of Hypertension

When this definition is used, about 25% of adult Americans over 30 years of age are classified, on the basis of their initial blood-pressure reading, as being hypertensive. In a large study, however, one-third of the individuals initially classified as hypertensive were found subsequently to have diastolic blood pressure readings below 90 mm of mercury. Blood pressure can vary greatly from moment to moment for many reasons. Therefore, several blood pressure readings are needed in order to identify hypertensive individuals. Also, as the degree of risk associated with elevated blood pressure increases gradually with increasing diastolic or systolic pressure, an element of judgment is involved in selecting the line of demarcation between the high end of the normal range and blood pressure that is considered indicative of hypertension. The criteria used to define hypertension are not always consistent and estimates of the incidence of hypertension among Americans range from 10 to 20%. In addition, the risk to health from hypertension is influenced by the presence of other risk factors for cardiovascular diseases. The degree of risk from a given elevation of blood pressure does not, therefore, apply uniformly across a population but will vary greatly from individual to individual.

The cause of elevated blood pressure can be established in less than 5% of individuals classified as hypertensive and, in these, it is usually secondary to other diseases such as renal or endocrine diseases. The remainder are said to have "primary" or "essential" hypertension; about 75% of them have "mild" hypertension, that is, diastolic blood pressures falling between 90 and 104 mm of mercury.

The mechanisms controlling arterial blood pressure are complex and include a variety of neural and endocrine systems. Since most individuals with hypertension are from families with a history of the disease, the underlying cause is most likely an inherited defect in one or more of the systems that control blood pressure. The occurrence of hypertension in susceptible individuals is influenced by various environmental factors, among them dietary factors such as the amounts of energy (calories), sodium, potassium, calcium, and polyunsaturated fatty acids consumed. Animal studies support this view. Strains of rats that are genetically susceptible to hypertension have been selected and blood pressure in these animals can be influenced by diet.

Since the underlying cause of most hypertension is not known, treatment and preventive measures are directed toward control of the signs of the disorder—the elevated blood pressure. Many effective antihypertensive medications have been developed and these are used widely to reduce blood pressure. In clinical trials, individuals whose diastolic pressure exceeds 105 mm of mercury have been found to benefit from medication. There are, however, many side effects of antihypertensive medication. As a result, there is a question as to whether treatment of individuals with "mild" hypertension, blood pressure between 90 and 105 mm of mercury, with medication does not carry more risk than the limited elevation of blood pressure. In the Multiple Risk Factor Intervention Trial (MRFIT), more deaths occurred among men with diastolic pressures between 90 and 94 mm of mercury who were treated intensively with medications than among those who were not. Therefore, despite the effectiveness of antihypertensive medications, increasing attention has been given to the possibility of controlling hypertension by dietary modification.

B.   Dietary Factors

Since the early part of this century, after restriction of sodium chloride intake was found to reduce the blood pressure of many hypertensive individuals, control of salt intake has been the dominant approach to dietary treatment and prevention of this disorder. This approach was reinforced by epidemiologic observations made subsequently, showing that high blood pressure occurred only rarely among isolated, nonacculturated populations with sodium intakes below 60 mEq, equivalent to the amount provided by 3.5 g of sodium chloride, daily. Since then, it has become evident that some 10–20% of people are genetically susceptible to hypertension and that those who are genetically resistant show no elevation of blood pressure while consuming 12 g or more of salt daily. Investigations of diet and blood pressure relations have revealed that body weight and several dietary factors besides sodium influence blood pressure in both humans and animals who are genetically susceptible to the disorder. Thus, hypertension is a multifactorial disorder; it does not result simply from excessive sodium intake.

In addition, the anion accompanying sodium is reported to influence the blood-pressure response to altered sodium intake. In a recent study in which several sodium salts were tested for their ability to increase blood pressure in hypertensive men, only sodium chloride was found to produce an elevation. The effectiveness of salt restriction alone as a means of preventing and controlling hypertension has come into question as knowledge of diet and blood-pressure relations has expanded. The low-salt diets of nonacculturated populations are now recognized as being high-potassium diets or diets with a high potassium-to-sodium ratio. Both epidemiologic and clinical studies have provided evidence, not always consistent, that increased potassium intake or an increase in the potassium/sodium ratio of the diet is associated with lowering of blood pressure and, in one epidemiologic study, with reduced mortality from stroke.

Results of epidemiologic studies have also suggested that elevated blood pressure is associated with low calcium intake. Increased calcium intake has been reported to lower high blood pressure in some animal studies and clinical trials but results have not been consistent. A response to calcium would appear to depend on the relative intakes of calcium and sodium. Knowledge of these apparent interactions among sodium, potassium, calcium, and chloride is still too fragmentary to permit firm conclusions about the appropriate use of nutrients other than sodium in treatment and prevention of hypertension. The information presently available does, however, emphasize the complexity of the problem.

Excessive body weight is associated with a high incidence of hypertension (Fig. 6) and weight reduction is accompanied by a fall in blood pressure in most severely overweight, hypertensive individuals. A decline in blood pressure accompanying weight reduction is observed even when sodium intake is not restricted. Control of caloric intake to maintain appropriate body weight provides a safe method for reducing the incidence of hypertension in many overweight persons even though the basis for the relationship between body weight and blood pressure has not been established.

Besides the potential roles of body weight and mono- and divalent ions in dietary control of blood pressure, investigations in both animals and human subjects have shown that blood pressure can be influenced by the linoleic acid content of the diet. The beneficial effects were observed when intakes of sodium, potassium, calcium, and calories were maintained constant, and are thought to involve the role of linoleic acid as a precursor of certain prostaglandins that can affect blood pressure.

C.   Public Health Approaches to Control of Hypertension

It should be evident from this cursory survey of diet–blood pressure relations that simple dietary proposals for prevention of a disorder as complex as hypertension are unlikely to be effective. Restriction of salt intake by the entire population has, nevertheless, been advocated vigorously by many health organizations and some government agencies as a public health measure for prevention of hypertension. Assumptions underlying such proposals are that the entire population is susceptible to essential hypertension from high salt intake; hypertension is a single disorder; moderate salt restriction will prevent elevated blood pressure in the entire population; salt restriction will control blood pressure in those susceptible to severe hypertension; and that, even if the policy is not effective, it will do no harm.

Depending upon the stringency of the definition of hypertension, only 10–20% of the population will develop the disorder. Variability in susceptibility to hypertension from high salt intakes and variability in blood-pressure responses to salt restriction among those who have hypertension argue against hypertension being a single disorder which is uniformly responsive to salt restriction.

As for the potential of moderate salt restriction to control blood pressure in hypertensive individuals, experience in clinical studies has demonstrated that not more than half of those who have hypertension respond to salt restriction. Usually, for those who do respond, restriction must be much greater than the 5-g limit for salt intake advocated in public policy proposals. It seems most unlikely that moderate restriction of salt intake would benefit severely hypertensive individuals.

The argument that, even if salt restriction will not be beneficial, at least it will do no harm, is specious as a basis for public policy. Objective scientific evidence of both benefit and safety should be the only criteria for instituting public health programs. General recommendations for simplistic solutions to health problems divert attention from the unique problems of the most severely affected individuals and create a sense of complacency when comprehensive medical attention may be needed. They also divert attention from the complexity of the problem, and from the importance of developing new methods for treatment and prevention by gaining basic understanding of the underlying causes of the disorder. They lead to categorization of foods as "good" or "bad" based solely on their content of a single nutrient rather than on the basis of their total nutritional value. This makes selection of an appropriately balanced diet difficult, a hazard particularly for the young and the elderly.

Sodium restriction is an important part of comprehensive therapy for hypertensive individuals. For many the restriction must be below the equivalent of 3.5 g of salt daily. Some with mild hypertension may be helped by moderate restriction and for some the requirement for medication may be reduced by salt restriction. The variability among hypertensives in responsiveness to salt, medication, and weight control makes hypertension primarily a medical rather than a public health problem.

The most important public health approach for control of hypertension is to identify those who have the disorder and to treat them comprehensively. Awareness of the importance of having blood-pressure measurements taken has been created and has already contributed to control of the disorder. According to the most recent Surgeon General's Report, the proportion of hypertensive persons who have their high blood pressure under control more than doubled between the early 1970s and 1980. Even more important will be to develop improved methods and programs for identifying at an early age those who will develop the disease later in life.

V. Diabetes, Obesity, and Diet

Diabetes mellitus is a chronic disorder resulting from defective glucose metabolism owing to either impaired ability of the pancreas to produce insulin or reduced sensitivity of tissues to insulin. About 1% of adults under 45 years of age in the United States are diabetic, but more than 10% percent of those over 55 have diabetes (Fig. 11). Diabetes is the seventh leading cause of death but is a major

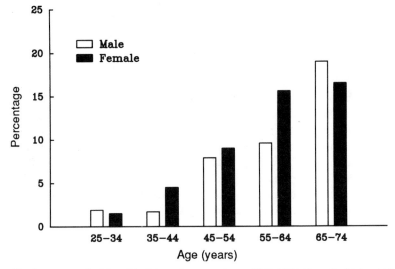

Figure 11 Percentage of adults with diabetes by sex and age, 1976–1980. From the National Health and Nutrition Examination Survey (1986). DHHS Publication No. (PHS) 86-1255.

cause of disability because one-third of diabetics suffer some limitation of activity. It is the leading cause of blindness in adults in the United States, accounts for about half the amputations of the lower limbs or digits and about 25% of kidney failure, and is a major risk factor for cardiovascular disease. When complications from this disease are taken into account, it is ranked third as a cause of death.

A. The Nature of Diabetes

There are two major forms of diabetes. Insulin-dependent diabetes (type I or juvenile-onset diabetes), which makes up about 10% of cases, usually develops during childhood. It accounts for only about 1% of diabetics over age 45. It results from destruction of the β cells of the pancreatic islets which produce insulin. The etiology of insulin-dependent diabetes is complex. There is evidence for genetic susceptibility, but expression of the disease appears to depend on the impact of environmental factors, primarily viral infections and possibly some chemical agents. Daily injections of insulin are required to control the disease, and food, usually with some limitations on the amounts of simple sugars it contains, must be ingested at regular intervals.

There is no evidence that diet is a factor contributing to the development of type I diabetes nor that the disease is preventable.

The other form of diabetes, noninsulin-dependent (type II or adult-onset) diabetes, is also a disease of complex etiology. It has a strong genetic component, but in a high proportion of individuals expression of the genetic susceptibility occurs only after age 40, and usually later, and mainly after the susceptible individual has accumulated an excessive amount of body fat (Fig. 12). Impairment of glucose metabolism, seen as elevated blood glucose (hyperglycemia) and urinary excretion of glucose (glucosuria), occurs even though type II diabetics may have normal, or even elevated, blood concentrations of insulin. The defect in glucose metabolism results from reduced sensitivity of tissues, particularly muscle and liver, to insulin, but the underlying biochemical defects appear not to be the same in all cases. Also, in some type II diabetics, insulin secretion is delayed or inadequate.

The strong association of this disease with excessive body weight—some experts estimate that 80% of type II diabetes is associated with obesity—suggests that it should be considered as a public health problem which can be largely prevented, despite its strong genetic component, by appropriate public health measures.

There has been controversy in the past over whether type II diabetes might be induced by the type of diet consumed, particularly by a high-sucrose diet. There is no convincing evidence that it is caused by diet. It is, however, a disease in which nutritional status is a predisposing factor. Excessive body fat accumulation, the major adverse effect of lowered energy expenditure and the ready availability of an appetizing food supply in industrialized nations, as has been mentioned, greatly increases the risk of developing this disease in those who are genetically susceptible.

B. Obesity and Diabetes

Overweight is excessive body weight for height; it is an indicator of excessive body fat. Degree of overweight is assessed most simply by calculating the "body mass

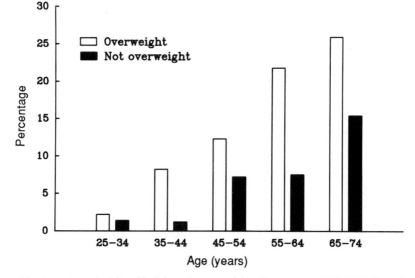

Figure 12   Percentage of adults with diabetes by overweight status and age, 1976–1980. From the National Health and Nutrition Examination Survey (1986). DHHS Publication No. (PHS) 86-1255.

index" (weight in kilograms divided by height squared in meters; W/H^2). Body mass index (BMI) in the range of 20 to 24.9 is considered normal; obesity is defined as BMI more than 20% above this. Within a large population, death rates rise steadily with increasing BMI above 25, more for men than for women and more for those who become overweight at an early age than for those who become overweight later in life (Fig. 6). In fact, some studies indicate that a moderate increase in body weight in old age is beneficial. Excessive body weight, nonetheless, particularly in the range considered to represent obesity, is associated not only with increased risk of developing diabetes mellitus type II but also, as was mentioned earlier, with increased risk of hypertension, hyperlipidemia, gall bladder disease, and cardiovascular disease (Fig. 6).

The incidence of excessive body weight in the industrialized nations is high. In the United States, 26% of men and 30–35% of women over age 25 are classified as overweight (Fig. 5) and somewhat over 5% of men and somewhat over 10% of women are considered to be severely overweight, or obese. Excessive body weight results from expending less energy than is obtained from the food consumed. The ability to store fat is important for survival and becomes increasingly so when energy expenditure is high, food is not abundant, it is available only sporadically, and the ability to store uneaten food is limited. Overweight seems not to have been a problem generally in societies before the advent of industrialization. When the environment changes so that energy expenditure is low and food is abundant, the ability to store fat, with no upper limit other than that at some point immobility occurs, can become detrimental for a large proportion of people.

It would seem evident from observations on the high rate of failure in efforts at weight reduction that the body has evolved a system that stores energy highly efficiently but mobilizes energy reserves readily only under conditions of severe deprivation. Why this is so, and why it is a serious problem for about a quarter of the population but not for the rest, has been the subject of intensive investigation. As with many chronic disorders, evidence is now available to indicate that susceptibility to obesity has a strong genetic component. Among the possible mechanisms which may contribute to accumulation of excessive body weight are defective control of food consumption, highly efficient use of energy by the body, metabolic defects in fat metabolism, and endocrine disturbances. There is equally good evidence that other factors influence body weight. Among these are the amount of physical activity, social and psychological attitudes toward food, and early feeding patterns.

The increased risk of type II diabetes among severely overweight individuals (Fig. 12) suggests that a solution for the problem of overweight would go far toward providing a solution for the high incidence of diabetes. Unfortunately, this theoretically simple solution has proven almost impossibly difficult in practice. Simple dietary advice to limit or restrict food intake, as is advocated in public health programs not only for the overweight but also for diabetics, hypertensives, and those at high risk for heart disease, has not been successful, as is evident from the limited change in the proportion of overweight individuals during the past two decades (Fig. 5).

Like diabetes, excessive body weight is a chronic problem. People who lose weight tend to gain it back. Most of those who are severely overweight need continuous counseling in order to achieve substantial weight reduction. They usually need programs designed to encourage both limitation of food consumption and increased physical activity. Motivation is critical, and for maintenance of lowered body weight once it is achieved, changes in style of life—in patterns of eating and physical activity—are required. Although type II diabetes and obesity appear to be disorders amenable to a general public health approach, it has become clear that means of achieving the degree of body weight control needed to reduce their incidence are highly complex. The need for individual or group counseling and guidance would seem to preclude any simple public health solution for them.

VI. Osteoporosis and Diet

Osteoporosis is defined as a decrease in bone mass and strength which leads to increased susceptibility to fractures. It probably begins between 35 and 45 years of age, when the rate of bone formation declines below the rate of bone breakdown, and progresses gradually and imperceptibly with increasing age until bones become porous and brittle. Eventually the bone is weakened to the point where minor slips and falls cause fractures, particularly of the wrist, spine, and hip. It is not considered to be a disease but is a disorder or syndrome in which the reserves of the tissue, in this case the bone, are not sufficient to withstand minor stresses or trauma. Osteoporosis is a major medical problem in the United States. It is more frequent and more severe in women than in men and in whites than in blacks. At some time after the menopause, about 25% of white women will develop osteoporosis which is severe enough to lead to fractures.

A.   The Nature of Osteoporosis

Loss of bone with increasing age is not an abnormal phenomenon. Peak bone mass occurs at about age 35. Thereafter bone mass declines. This occurs in both men and women and in all populations that have been studied, regardless of diet, activity, and way of life. Also, it is not a modern phenomenon; it has been reported in bones recovered from archaeological sites. The incidence of bone loss severe enough to cause fractures will obviously be higher in modern industrialized societies in which life expectancy is long than in societies, past or present, with shorter life expectancies. What is striking, however, is the great variability in bone loss among individuals and the variability in susceptibility to fractures among persons with similar degrees of bone loss. This has led to extensive studies of associations between various environmental and personal characteristics and the occurrence of osteoporosis.

Age-related bone loss is more rapid in women than in men and in whites than in blacks, as might be inferred from comparing the incidence of osteoporosis among these groups. The more rapid bone loss in women is associated strongly with decreased production of the female sex hormone, estrogen, after the menopause, but rate of bone loss and development of osteoporosis appear to be influenced by many factors besides age and sex. Among these factors, usually identified as risk factors, are low physical activity, small body size, smoking, alcoholism, excessive use of glucocorticoids or thyroid hormones, chronic kidney or liver disease, low calcium intake, and high intakes of dietary constituents such as protein that may increase calcium loss. Despite evidence of associations between many of these factors and the incidence of osteoporosis, information about them has not made it possible to predict accurately the occurrence of the disorder. Clinical observations suggest strongly that osteoporosis is heterogeneous in nature and that it has multiple causes, that is, it is multifactorial. The accumulated observations also suggest just as strongly that differences in susceptibility are attributable to still unidentified factors such as impairment of regulatory systems that control bone formation and resorption (breakdown) owing either to genetic differences or to pathophysiologic factors. Clearly, the underlying causes of severe expression of this disorder have not been established.

B.   Diet and Osteoporosis

Dietary modification as a method of treatment and prevention of osteoporosis has received great attention in recent years. Major emphasis has been given to calcium intake and factors that affect calcium utilization in the body. Calcium is an essential element. It is essential for bone formation. The adult body contains 1–1.2 kg of calcium and 99% of it is in the bones. Calcium deficiency results in mobilization of calcium from bone, and vitamin D deficiency, which impairs calcium absorption, leads to rickets. Inadequate calcium intake or absorption in adults causes osteomalacia, a disorder in which there is low mineral (calcium) content of bone, whereas in osteoporosis, overall bone mass declines but the composition of what remains is normal. Despite this difference, undoubtedly because the essential role of calcium in bone structure and development is well established and many women are reported to consume inadequate amounts of calcium, the hypothesis that inadequate calcium intake is a critical factor in the development of osteoporosis has become a dominant theme in public health approaches to control of this disorder.

Extensive epidemiologic studies in which radiologic and absorptiometric measurements of bone density have been made in populations with vastly different calcium intakes have failed to reveal significant differences in the rate of bone loss or in the density of the bone in relation to calcium intake. Results of studies of effects of calcium supplements on calcium balance, and on the rate of bone loss by postmenopausal women, have not been consistent and have led to controversy over the role of increased calcium intake in both prevention and treatment of osteoporosis. Despite some observations of improved calcium balance and modest decreases in loss of calcium from the compact bone of the arm, evidence that increased calcium intake reduces loss of bone from the spine is unconvincing except in women who have unusually low calcium intakes and may be suffering from both osteomalacia and osteoporosis.

Estrogen treatment appears to offer the greatest promise in preventing bone loss in postmenopausal women; there is some evidence that the effective dose is lower if calcium intake is increased at the same time. Interestingly, obese women have a relatively low fracture rate, which is thought to be attributable to the formation of estrogens in adipose tissue.

Factors that affect calcium absorption and retention have also received attention as possible contributors to the development of osteoporosis. A high protein intake can increase urinary calcium loss but in an appropriately balanced diet seems to have little effect. There is some evidence that the rate of conversion of vitamin D to the active form needed for calcium absorption in the body may decline with age but evidence that this is a significant effect is limited. Inactivity, such as prolonged bed rest, increases calcium loss but the trend is reversed when activity is resumed. A moderate degree of activity is therefore recommended to reduce this possible cause of bone loss.

An adequate calcium intake during the growing years is critical for achieving maximum bone mass at maturity. Most scientists and physicians recommend this as the best way of ensuring that total bone mass will remain high despite the continuing bone loss that occurs during aging. There is no disagreement over the need to meet calcium requirements in order to ensure normal growth and development of bone, but the extent to which this protects against osteoporosis has been questioned.

As with chronic and degenerative diseases generally and many disorders associated with aging, osteoporosis is a complex health problem for which there is not a simple solution. Despite the recommendation of the Consensus Conference on Osteoporosis sponsored by the National Institutes of Health, for calcium intakes of 1–1.5 g/day for postmenopausal women to reduce the likelihood of osteoporosis, objective evidence supporting such a recommendation is lacking. There is no evidence that the incidence of the disorder is unusually high in populations that consume half these amounts of calcium. The current recommendation of 800 mg/day for adults would seem to be ample and, to ensure health, it would seem much more important to develop ways of increasing calcium intakes of the large proportion of women, more than 50%, who consume less than 500 mg/day, rather than to encourage the use of large supplements to prevent a disorder that seems to bear little relation to nutrition.

VII. Nutrition and Public Health

A nutritious diet is essential for health. Food guides were designed to enable people with limited knowledge of nutrition to select a healthful diet which would meet the RDA for essential nutrients. The public health objective was to ensure that each individual in the population would achieve his/her genetic potential for growth and development, work performance, and resistance to disease. The objective was not to prevent chronic and degenerative diseases, only to prevent nutritional deficiencies which cause a highly unique group of diseases. The high degree of success in achieving this was discussed in Section I, and some of the changes that have occurred in dietary guidance more recently have been mentioned in the subsequent sections on specific diseases. These changes represent a shift in public health policies and programs toward the use of diet as a preventive measure for diseases that are multifactorial and for which specific dietary causes have not been established. This brings us back to some of the questions that were raised in Section I concerning the adequacy of nutrition knowledge used to support this shift and the appropriateness of a public health policy directed more toward medical rather than general public health problems. This new direction has created controversy. It merits attention.

A. Public Health Approaches to Disease Prevention

The objective of public health programs is to reduce morbidity and mortality by preventing rather than curing diseases and disorders that may affect the entire population or large segments of it. At least three approaches have been used highly successfully to accomplish this.

For infectious diseases and dietary deficiency diseases, to which the entire population is potentially susceptible, programs have been directed toward institution of measures that will protect the entire population. When specific vaccines have become available, programs for vaccination of as much of the population as is feasible have proven highly effective. Elimination of smallpox and the near elimination of poliomyelitis are two most successful programs. For dietary deficiency diseases, education about the essentials of a nutritionally adequate diet and fortification of the food supply with essential nutrients likely to be consumed in inadequate amounts, for example, niacin, thiamine, iron, vitamin D, and iodine, have virtually eliminated deficiencies of essential nutrients as public health problems in the United States. Fluoridation of water supplies, despite political and emotional resistance to it which has prevented some communities from instituting this measure, has not eliminated but has immensely reduced the incidence of dental caries (tooth decay).

A second approach has been used to control water and foodborne infections and prevent hazards from potentially toxic substances. This has been to identify the sources of infectious organisms and undesirable chemical compounds that might enter food and water supplies and to take measures to prevent contamination from them. Protection of water supplies against contamination with sewage and other sources of hazardous waste, requirements for following sanitary procedures, and safety measures in food production, manufacturing, and food-service facilities all represent applications of this approach. Control of cholera and typhoid fever, botulism, and many foodborne diseases was accomplished by these methods. They have also been used successfully to reduce or prevent chemical contamination of the food supply with, for example, heavy metals. Success in using this approach requires constant vigilance, continuous health surveys, and enforcement of regulations.

A third approach has been used in dealing with certain diseases and disorders that are basically medical problems, problems that, even though they may affect a substantial part of the population, require measures directed toward the individual. Tuberculosis is an example of a disease of this type. The public health approach has been used to identify, initially through X-ray examinations and subsequently through tuberculin tests made available to large segments of the population, individuals who have the disease or have been exposed to it. Then, by treatment of those identified, spread of the disease has been controlled.

This type of approach is currently being used in efforts to control certain diseases and disorders that affect only segments of the population but which are not contagious. Education programs designed to encourage people to visit centers where they can have blood-pressure measurements made free of charge are being used to identify individuals with elevated blood pressure. Those found to have this disorder are advised to undergo further tests and, if it seems desirable, treatment. The programs have not been emphasized as forcefully as the tuberculosis prevention programs, perhaps partly because individuals with hypertension pose no threat to the rest of the population and partly because of the competition for resources from education programs emphasizing control of this disorder through restriction of salt consumption. Blood-pressure awareness programs, nonetheless, perhaps in large measure because of the active interest of insurance companies in having such information, have been highly successful in creating consciousness of the risks from high blood pressure and in increasing greatly the number of people undergoing some type of treatment for it.

This approach to the control of diseases that are not contagious and which do not affect the population at large but only segments of it is a recent direction in public health. Is represents an effort to protect the individual, not the population. It is directed toward reducing the probability of disability and early death and, thereby, hopefully, the cost of medical care. The objective is to identify those with the disease or disorder, or those who are likely to develop it, and encourage them to obtain treatment or to follow guidelines that are thought to be preventative. Application of this approach to health problems of individuals can be viewed as a public health education program designed to shift the responsibility for health care from government agencies back to the individual. It therefore becomes important to look at the differences between the major medical problems for which a public health approach is now being proposed and traditional public health problems.

B. Chronic and Degenerative Diseases and Disorders and Public Health

Promotion of dietary guidelines for the entire population is currently being advocated as a public health measure for control of the most prevalent chronic diseases and disorders—heart disease, stroke, cancer, hypertension, diabetes, obesity, and osteoporosis. This approach resembles that used to control infectious diseases and dietary deficiency diseases which have well-defined causes and to which the entire population is susceptible, and from which the entire population can be protected.

The chronic and degenerative diseases and disorders, in contrast, do not have well-defined and readily-identifiable causes. They are generally accepted as having multiple causes. Each is thought to be heterogeneous in nature. For the most part they are treated successfully only with medications or surgery.

It is not possible, therefore, to focus public health—prevention—programs for these diseases on eliminating specific causes or on adoption of specific preventive measures, only on probable causes—risk factors—of which there are many. Individual variability in susceptibility to chronic and degenerative diseases and disorders is great and, even with current knowledge of risk factors, predictions as to who will and will not develop them are far from accurate. Results of the many prevention trials conducted to determine the effectiveness of controlling risk factors have been disappointing.

The chronic and degenerative diseases and disorders that have been studied most intensively are known to have a strong genetic component, with a large part of the population being resistant to them and succumbing only at a late age. Another small part of the population develops one or another of these diseases early in life and there is little evidence that such cases are preventable. Chronic and degenerative diseases are associated strongly with aging, a time in life when physiological functions have begun to deteriorate and the ability to adapt and respond to stresses has declined. There is evidence for a strong genetic–environmental interaction in the development of most of these diseases. For the proportion of the population that is highly susceptible to them, as has been emphasized in the discussions of hypertension and diabetes, development of these diseases appears to depend upon exposure to environmental conditions that do not adversely affect the majority of the population. These are diseases or disorders for which effective control will depend upon having specific and sensitive methods for identifying susceptible individuals early in life and encouraging those who are identified to follow a comprehensive program for reducing their risk.

C. Approaches to Control of Chronic and Degenerative Diseases and Disorders

Intense controversy exists about the approach that should be used in efforts to control chronic and degenerative diseases and disorders. There is no disagreement about these being major medical problems, about the merit of attempting to control risk factors when the causes of these diseases are not known, and about increased importance of such control for individuals who are identified as being at highest risk. The controversy centers around the merit of dealing with diseases of this type by the classical public health approach of mass intervention, with the entire population as the target, as compared with the merit of a selective approach of identifying high-risk individuals as the target population and providing them with comprehensive health care programs. The most vocal school of thought, which includes many health organizations and agencies, favors mass diet modification for the entire population; the American Heart Association recommends that this begin at age 2 years. Major assumptions underlying this approach are that knowledge of diet–disease relationships is adequate to provide confidence in the effectiveness of such a program; although all may not benefit from it, those who are most at risk will; it will not be harmful to those who do not need it; it is too difficult and expensive to identify high-risk groups and target them with comprehensive programs; individual variability in susceptibility to the disease, and in responsiveness to reduction of potential risks, is not great enough to curtail seriously the effectiveness of a program of mass diet modification.

The reasons for supporting the approach of developing comprehensive programs for high-risk individuals are that this approach has been successful in dealing with diabetes and hypertension; those who are most susceptible to this group of diseases are least likely to benefit from a mass education program because they require individual attention; a high proportion of the population is not at high risk, therefore they should not be subjected to a prophylactic approach which, when it is not or cannot be followed, creates apprehension unnecessarily; knowledge of the effectiveness of dietary measures in reducing susceptibility to these diseases is inadequate; individual variability in responsiveness to diet is too great to instill confidence that the mass diet-modification approach will be effective; intervention trials have not provided convincing evidence of decreased total mortality; dietary differences among the industrialized populations are not associated with significant differences in longevity; methods for identifying individuals at risk have been improving steadily, therefore efforts should be directed toward those who are most likely to benefit; the mass diet approach makes disease prevention the main focus of nutrition programs and shifts attention away from the critical nutritional needs for growth, development, and reproduction, and the needs of the elderly.

Quite apart from these considerations, little has been done to assess the feasibility of modifying diets generally to meet guidelines of the American Heart Association and the American Cancer Institute. The U.S. Department of Agriculture recently examined the probable effects on the diets of women if guidelines for reducing fat intake to 30% of calories, saturated fat to 10% of calories, and cholesterol to 300 mg/day, and increasing fiber intake to 20 g/day were followed, while keeping sodium intake at 3300 mg/day (8.4 g of salt, well above the recommendation for controlling hypertension), and meeting the recommended dietary allowances of the National Research Council. The conclusion of the study was that it would require increases in lowfat milk consumption of 2-fold; lean meats, 1.7-fold; legumes, 1.4-fold; cereal products, 3.5-fold; vegetables, 3.5-fold; and almost complete elimination from the diet of cheeses, luncheon meats, desserts, snacks, potatoes, and separated fats. The report of the study included a comment: A recommendation for a change in a single nutrient must be assessed in terms of its potential effect on the total diet. Practicality is an essential condition. Is the recommendation likely to be achieved through informed food choices?

It is certainly appropriate that government agencies should provide the entire population with sound nutritional advice for maintaining health. It is difficult to accept that this advice should consist largely of prescriptions that have not been adequately tested for prevention of chronic disorders and diseases mainly among middle-aged males, while recommendations that can be made on a sound scientific basis for ensuring that growth and development of the young will not be impaired are neglected. Prescriptions for disease prevention do not include consideration of basic nutritional needs; hence, foods, regardless of their nutritive value, tend to be classified as "good" or "bad" on the basis of their utility in ameliorating the effects of metabolic limitations, usually of hereditary, not dietary, origin. Characterizing foods in this way undermines the basic principles of nutrition education, encourages the use of foods as medications, and distracts attention from the special needs of the groups—infants, adolescents, the pregnant, and the elderly—who are most at risk of nutritional inadequacy.

In dealing with chronic disorders and diseases effectively we need to know more about the genetic diversity of the population and how to distinguish among environmental effects, genetic effects, and effects of senescence. We need better and simpler ways of distinguishing between individuals who are truly at risk of developing these health problems and those who are not, and of portraying their relative risks accurately and meaningfully. We also need to recognize the limits of effectiveness of dietary manipulation in correcting and preventing disorders that are not caused by dietary inadequacies.

Bibliography

Harper, A. E. (1987). Evolution of recommended dietary allowances—new directions? *Annu. Rev. Nutr.* **7,** 509–537.

McCannon, D. A., and Kotchen, T. A., eds. (1983). Nutrition and blood pressure control. *Ann. Intern. Med.* **98,** 699–890.

National Center for Health Statistics (1988). "Health United States, 1987 (also 1986 and 1985)," DHHS Publ. No. (PHS) 88-1232, Public Health Service. U.S. Gov. Print. Off., Washington, D.C.

Nordin, B. E. C., ed. (1988). "Calcium in Biology." Springer-Verlag, New York (esp. pp. 209–240, 447–471, for osteoporosis).

Shils, M. E., and Young, V. R., eds. (1988). Diet and nutrition in the treatment and prevention of disease. *In* "Modern Nutrition in Health and Disease," 7th Ed., pp. 1069–1482. Lea & Febiger, Philadelphia, Pennsylvania.

Simopoulos, A. P., ed. (1987). Diet and health: Scientific concepts and principles. *Am. J. Clin. Nutr.* **45,** Suppl., 1015–1414.

USDHHS and USDA (1986). "Nutrition Monitoring in the United States," DHHS Publ. No. (PHS) 86-1255, Public Health Service. U.S. Gov. Print. Off., Washington, D.C.

PART V

PREVENTION

CHAPTER 24

ORGANIZING A SAFE FOOD SUPPLY SYSTEM

Dean O. Cliver

I. What Is "Safe"?

Food safety is a concern in every developed nation, yet any scientifically advanced society must face the fact that absolute safety is unattainable. Great gains in food safety may be achieved initially at modest cost, but further gains become increasingly expensive, and no amount of money will buy complete safety. The general goal must be to make eating safer than most other activities, without raising the price of food so much that substantial numbers of people cannot afford to eat.

A. Risks in the United States

Several common causes of death, or "risks to life," in the United States are shown in Table I. These were compiled for 1975 but apparently have not changed very much since. The entry for inhalation and ingestion of food, which does not include food poisoning, is of particular interest: 2200 people evidently choked to death on food, whereas only 10 people are known to have died of food poisoning during 1975. Total food poisoning deaths have not yet been reported for 1985, but the "inhalation and ingestion" toll declined to 1663, perhaps through more use of the Heimlich maneuver. Granted there were probably more than 10 unreported deaths due to food poisoning during 1975, but the fact remains that the hazards of eating in the United States are, rather than the infections and intoxications classified as "food poisoning," more mechanical in nature (by analogy, "waterborne disease" is much less common than drowning). For young adults in the United States the most prevalent causes of death are accidents and suicide. The safety of the United States food supply is no accident. The goal of this chapter is to consider what is being done right (so it doesn't get away) and what might be done even better without excessive cost.

Table I
Selected Risks to Life in the United States[a]

Cause of death	Deaths per year	Deaths per year per 100,000 people
Heart disease	716,200	336
Cancer	365,700	173
Stroke	194,000	91.9
Auto accidents	45,900	21.8
Suicide	27,100	12.8
Homicide	21,300	10.1
Inhalation and inges- tion of food[b]	2,200	1.04
Lightning	120	0.06
Food poisoning	10	0.005

[a]Based on 1975 data from the National Center for Health Statistics and Center for Disease Control, U.S. Department of Health, Education and Welfare.
[b]Does not include food poisoning.

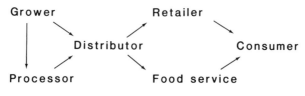

Figure 1   The human food network.

B.   The Human Food Network

A simplified diagram of the human food network appears in Fig. 1. The ultimate source of food is the "grower" (sometimes called "producer"), who might in fact be a farmer, a rancher, or a fisherman. The "processor" converts raw materials into final, edible products or preserves foods to prolong their useful life. Some perishable foods go directly to distribution without processing—these are less available during winters in northern zones, except to those who can pay to have their food transported rapidly from the tropics. "Distributors" move food from place to place and often store food until it is needed. Food in distribution reaches the consumer by way of "retailers" (e.g., grocery stores) and "food service" establishments such as restaurants. The "consumer" is whoever ultimately eats the food. Each of these individuals has an important role to play in making and keeping food safe.

C.   How Does Safe Food "Happen"?

Production and marketing of food involve many interactions. If the food is to be *safe*, further interactions are required. Responsibility for food safety is shared by industry, government, and consumers. The role of each will be considered in the sections that follow.

II.   Industry's Role in Food Safety

The food industry comprises both individual companies and trade associations. Some trade associations have made important contributions to food safety, but responsibility for the safety of any given product lies with the individual company.

A.   Functions of the Food Industry

Growers' production of raw food material entails relatively few safety concerns, although the proper use of pesticides, herbicides, and fertilizers have been emphasized in earlier chapters. Distributors' and retailers' activities are not *intended* to modify the food, so their work should entail relatively little risk. Food processors and food service establishments manipulate foods most extensively, so theirs are the functions with the greatest potential to cause hazards. The epidemiologic record shows that food poisoning is more often associated with food service than with food processing. This is true at least partly because food is more intimately exposed to those who do final preparation in food service than to those who work in processing. Earlier chapters have shown that many agents of foodborne disease are introduced into foods by handlers.

B. Motivations to Food Safety

Both individual workers and corporations must be performing a useful service, since they are being rewarded for their efforts—and they expend effort because they expect to be rewarded. As with so many other activities, the reward (profit) motive is what drives the system. For a number of reasons, safe food is likely to prove more profitable than unsafe food.

Humanitarian considerations are certainly important. It is most unlikely that those working in the food industry would intentionally cause consumer illnesses. The good will of customers, associated with specific corporate names or brands, is a very important asset; therefore, companies know they must strive to produce consistently safe products to protect their good names. There is also a "regulatory hazard" to be considered—companies that handle food unsafely are likely to come to the attention of the regulatory agencies that will be discussed in a following section. In all, the production of safe food is a matter of enlightened self-interest to the food industry in the United States. Specific food products, and at times entire companies, have disappeared because of incidents involving hazards to consumers.

C. Programs for Food Safety

Until approximately 1966, the United States food industry's efforts for safe food were based principally on good intentions—methods in use tended to be based on technical tradition more than on scientific knowledge of microbiologic hazards associated with foods. Although a good deal of information concerning the causes of foodborne disease already existed, industry tended to treat such knowledge as theoretical. Then, a series of events involving human illness from foods in interstate commerce led to a substantial increase in funding for the U.S. Food and Drug Administration (FDA) and permitted that organization to take a more aggressive approach to regulating food safety than previously. There were recalls and seizures of foods by the FDA and some states and a great deal of publicity adverse to the food industry.

These events got industry's attention and produced a great many jobs for microbiologists. Now trained microbiologists form an important part of quality assurance groups, at least in the larger food companies. Microbiology now plays a significant role in research and development of most new food products and in routine surveillance of foods during processing. In recent years, the "Hazard Analysis/Critical Control Points" (HACCP) approach to quality assurance has helped guarantee that microbiological analyses make a maximum contribution to the safety and stability of foods.

Microbiological quality control is being used in several ways (cf. Chapter 3). Purchase specifications are used by processors to stipulate to their suppliers of raw materials the absence of certain hazardous organisms or to impose limits on levels of organisms that may cause stability problems in the product. Continuing micro-biological surveillance is also applied to raw materials as received at the plant, the environment within the plant, food during processing, and the final product.

Industry associations have made substantial contributions to food safety, despite competitive pressures between food companies that tend to inhibit cooperation. Some industry associations perform research on industry-wide problems, conduct industry surveys, and serve as advisors to their member companies and to government. The National Canners' Association (now National Food Processors' Association) established its own laboratories and developed industry-wide standards for safe heat treatment of canned foods. The Flavor and Extract Manufacturers' Association was mentioned in Chapter 10 as maintaining a list of flavors and extracts that are generally recognized as safe. Other organizations, such as the Institute of Food Technologists and the International Association of Milk, Food and Environmental Sanitarians conduct national and local meetings and publish journals that present current information on food safety. The National Restaurant Association produces training materials to encourage safe food service. Many more examples could be listed if space permitted.

Both individual food companies and some industry associations fund research on food safety. Much of this research is conducted at universities, but other nonprofit and profit-making organizations do some of the work. As will be mentioned in a following section, important food safety research is also conducted in government laboratories and in university and other laboratories with government support.

D. Events beyond Processors' Control

No matter how diligent a processor may be in producing safe food, some events are beyond the processor's control. For example, much of the storage and distribution of foods is conducted by corporations other than those that do processing. This may prevent an undesirable degree of vertical integration, but it also puts many safe, centrally processed products into the hands of several organizations, not all of which are equally dedicated to food safety. Failures to refrigerate some sensitive foods continuously during distribution, for example, have led to outbreaks of disease. Great care must also be taken that conveyances for food have been cleaned properly after their previous use, especially if that use was for something other than food.

Retailers begin where the distributors' function ends, and retailers, too, have many opportunities to abuse food. Refrigerated and frozen foods may be unloaded behind a store and stay there for hours before being placed at a proper temperature. Other foods may be stored or displayed in ways that permit incursions of insects or rodents. Refrigerated display cases may be overloaded, so that some of the product is outside the cold zone. Cans may be handled so roughly that their seams are compromised. This is not to suggest that retailers deliberately abuse food; however, food retailing is a very competitive business, and some seemingly innocent attempts at cost cutting may lead to unsafe conditions. Also, retailers' knowledge of food safety may be only as complete as a city or state health department inspector makes it. Despite the known problems just listed, it is established practice in some segments of the food industry for the food processor to indemnify the retailer against any claim that may result from the retailer's negligence.

Finally, there is the consumer. The consumer's role in food safety will be discussed at length later in this chapter. It should simply be noted here that no set of instructions on a food package is absolutely foolproof and that there is little more the processor can do to prevent some of the extremely ingenious ways in which consumers abuse food.

III. Government's Role in Food Safety

One of the most important functions of government is to insure public safety. By analogy to the police that protect the public against other kinds of hazards, there are agencies at each level of government that are responsible for various aspects of food safety. The discussion that follows will focus on government activities in the United States because these are most familiar to the author. Clearly, there are many other ways to organize government activities in food safety, and many other governments undoubtedly accomplish the task as well.

A. Federal Agencies

The domain of federal agencies is principally foods in interstate commerce, but there are several instances of federal activity involving foods in intrastate commerce, either by invitation or default of the state in question. Although agencies of the United States government are to be emphasized here, it should at least be mentioned that national organizations such as the American Public Health Association and the Association of Official Analytical Chemists make important contributions to food safety by screening and publishing methods (especially microbiological methods) for testing foods.

1. Food and Drug Administration

The FDA is a unit of the U.S. Department of Health and Human Services and is directed by a commissioner. It has jurisdiction over all foods traveling in interstate commerce (including imports) except meat and poultry. The FDA operates under the authority of the federal Food, Drug, and Cosmetic Act, as amended, which prohibits the sale of adulterated or misbranded food. For purposes of the law, food is adulterated if it contains any poisonous or deleterious substance that could be injurious to health, contains any filthy or putrid substance or is otherwise unfit to eat, or has been prepared under unsanitary conditions whereby it might have been contaminated. Enforcement is conducted by a field force, comprising perhaps 3000 inspectors, that is organized into regions and districts. The inspectors make unannounced inspections of food processing facilities on an irregular basis. They make notes of their observations and collect samples for analysis by FDA laboratories. If they detect problems, they can get a court injunction, have the product seized, or "suggest" that the product be recalled from distribution. The FDA regulatory approach is based partly on promulgation of codes of Good Manufacturing Practice—"GMPs." In addition to food processing and distribution, the FDA regulates eating establishments on common carriers, federal property, and interstate highways. The agency conducts research in its own laboratories, funds some research at universities and other organizations, and drafts model ordinances and codes (e.g., the Pasteurized Milk Ordinance) for possible adoption by state and local governments.

2. Department of Agriculture

The U.S. Department of Agriculture (USDA) has jurisdiction over meat and poultry in interstate commerce, and in intrastate commerce in about half the states. It also has quarantine responsibility for meats, vegetables, and fruits being imported into the United States. Its authority derives from the federal Meat and Poultry Inspection Acts. Inspection activity is based in the Food Safety and Inspection Service (FSIS), whereas international quarantine is conducted by the Animal and Plant Health Inspection Service (APHIS). FSIS operations are based on continuous, in-plant ("resident") inspection. About 9000 inspectors are engaged in this work, and one or more of them is expected to be present during all operating hours in larger meat and poultry slaughter and processing plants. The inspectors make their judgments on the basis of what they see, with limited assistance from reference laboratories testing samples taken in the plant. Any time that operations are judged not to be safe and sanitary, the inspector can shut down the line or the entire plant until the situation is corrected. APHIS inspectors operate at points of entry into the United States (ports, airports, etc.) to prevent introduction of exotic insect pests and agents of plant and animal disease. The USDA also conducts an extensive research program in support of its regulatory activities.

3. Other federal activities

a. Centers for Disease Control
The Centers for Disease Control (CDC) in Atlanta have no regulatory responsibility, but they investigate disease outbreaks, including those in which food may have served as a vehicle, and compile statistics regarding the incidence of diseases in the United States. They have also, until fairly recently, issued year-end summaries of foodborne and waterborne illness in the United States. Although such activities appear to be in eclipse at present, one can hope that they will be restored eventually, so that the CDC can resume its former influence over which aspects of food safety are emphasized in inspection and research.

b. Environmental Protection Agency
The Environmental Protection Agency (EPA) sets standards for the microbiologic and chemical purity of drinking water in the United States. Since water used in food plants must be of potable quality, this puts the EPA indirectly into the regulation of food plants. Additionally, the EPA is responsible for the registration of pesticides, including those that may be used in conjunction with foods.

c. National Marine Fisheries Service
The National Marine Fisheries Service (NMFS) of the National Oceanic and Atmospheric Administration, U.S. Department of Commerce, operates a voluntary inspection service for domestic fisheries and seafood. There appears to be growing interest in making this inspection mandatory.

d. Bureau of Alcohol, Tobacco, and Firearms

This bureau of the U.S. Department of the Treasury regulates the production and distribution of alcoholic beverages in the United States.

B. State Agencies

The domain of state agencies is food produced and distributed within their own political and geographic boundaries, although some states' programs range even wider. At present, a state can pass laws or regulations that are more stringent than those of the federal government and apply them even to foods that are traveling in interstate commerce.

1. Departments of health

Departments of health often are responsible for inspection of restaurants and milk processing establishments, except where such activities are conducted by city or county agencies.

2. Departments of agriculture

Departments of agriculture may carry, at the state level, responsibilities comparable to those of the FDA and USDA combined. They can, if their state chooses to have them do so, inspect processing and distribution of all foods within the state, including those that will be sold outside the state and including meat and poultry. If the state does not undertake inspection of meat and poultry with a rigor comparable to that of the USDA, the latter agency is required by federal law to take over inspection even of meat and poultry destined for intrastate consumption.

3. Cooperation with federal agencies

Cooperation is established, where possible, so that the state can carry out inspections when the FDA or USDA is not present.

C. Local Agencies

These include agencies of county and municipal governments, which function largely within their own political jurisdictions, except in some instances where milk is concerned. Cities (e.g., Chicago) have at times taken jurisdiction over their entire "milkshed," conducting inspections all the way to the farm.

Cities or counties may choose to supervise food service establishments and retail stores within their political boundaries. Many counties and most larger cities have their own inspectors and laboratories to conduct inspection and testing and perhaps to investigate outbreaks of foodborne disease. Interactions with state agencies depend on the local political climate. Relationships range from cordial and cooperative to strained.

D. International Agencies

Several international organizations concern themselves with various aspects of food safety. Cooperative efforts by many countries are made to bring order in the chaotic field of international commerce in food. None of these groups has lawmaking power, so their actions are *advisory* to national governments, more or less as the model ordinances drafted by the FDA are advisory to state governments.

1.   United Nations agencies

Some United Nations agencies carry out food safety activities on behalf of their member nations, which are usually also members of the UN.

a.   World Health Organization

The World Health Organization (WHO) conducts many activities in the area of food safety. In addition to staff functions, it convenes "expert committees" to consider topics such as food microbiology and hygiene and food additives.

b.   Food and Agricultural Organization

The Food and Agricultural Organization (FAO) is concerned with the production and preservation of food worldwide. It interacts with the WHO in the areas of wholesomeness and safety and is the sponsor of Codex Alimentarius activities.

c.   Codex Alimentarius

This program of the FAO directly produces advisory documents on regulatory issues. The Committee on Food Hygiene of the Codex addresses most safety and wholesomeness questions.

2.   International Commission on Microbiological Specifications for Foods

The International Commission on Microbiological Specifications for Foods (ICMSF) is a subsidiary of the International Union of Microbiological Societies. Groups of microbiologists with expertise in various aspects of food spoilage and safety have convened and written books that are rapidly becoming standard references in their field.

IV.   Consumers' Role in Food Safety

In several ways, it appears that the consumer is his or her own worst enemy. That is, much of the contamination and temperature abuse that leads to foodborne disease is perpetrated by consumers—for reasons of ignorance or indifference. It might be noted that the term "consumer" may apply not only to the person who eats the food, but also to the purchaser or to the very same persons in other roles as taxpayers and voters. The message of the section that follows is that those who prepare and eat their food at home must accept responsibility for their safety, almost as if they had grown and harvested the food themselves.

A. Basic Self-Protection

Consumers need to recognize that certain types of food contamination should be assumed (cf. Section II,D of Chapter 3). For example, vegetables grown in or on the soil are likely to contain spores of *Clostridium botulinum* (cf. Chapter 6). The spores themselves are not injurious, but any raw vegetable and any fruit that grows close to the soil should be assumed to contain these spores and be treated accordingly. Furthermore, the American cuisine assumes that *Trichinella spiralis* is present in any given piece of pork (so that thorough cooking is practiced even though the current incidence in slaughter swine in the United States is only 0.1%). Similarly, one should expect *Salmonella* and *Campylobacter* to be present in raw poultry and other animal products as purchased, even though in this instance the probability is somewhat less than 50%. Consumers need to be aware of these assumed sources of contamination to minimize opportunities for cross-contamination with or growth of pathogens in foods in the home. The sole alternative would be sterilization of all foods before sale, which would result in products that few would favor. An important outbreak of listeriosis from coleslaw made from raw cabbage (fertilized with manure from *Listeria*-infected sheep; cf. Chapter 18) is a case in point—cole slaw from cooked cabbage is likely to be a distinctly less acceptable product.

B. Shopping

Packaged foods offered for sale in the United States typically have a great deal of information printed on their containers. All of those who do their own marketing should develop the habit of reading the information on containers, even if some of the names of ingredients, etc., cause consternation because they are unfamiliar. In addition to qualitative concerns, purchasers should accept the challenge of comparing the cost per pound, ounce, or other unit of measure among competing products or even among packages of the same product. Despite some adverse sentiments in the United States, the inevitable advent of metric units of measurement in food sales will help the consumer with these comparisons.

Qualitative decisions are also very important in shopping. Most American shoppers can exercise ethnic and personal preferences as they wish because typically there is always enough food and one can always select among species, varieties, or brands. People from elsewhere in the world will surely recognize that the choices available to the American consumer are exceptionally broad. Probably, if not certainly, this breadth of choice stems from the competitive nature of the United States food supply system. If any substantial segment of the consuming public wants a product or a version of a product that is not already available, someone (or some organization) will find a way to produce and market it. Though truth in labeling is generally a fundamental principle of United States food law, it is important to note that Standards of Identity apply to many specific foods but do not include the term "natural" (cf. Chapter 4). That is, "natural" and its derivative terms can appear on food packages as descriptors or as parts of brand names with no concern for whether the word has any specific meaning.

In any case, consumers are obliged to select among products in the market on the basis of information on packages; conflicting nutritional advice from manufacturers, government, and the press; and personal preferences that need have no rational basis. Some information is decidedly better than none, but rejection of *misinformation* is a continuing challenge. Perhaps the most important point is that the consumer must weigh information and make decisions. Almost any buyer in the United States can select among many foods and, by doing so, cast a vote that will ultimately affect the selection of products that will be available in the market a year later. This means that it is up to the consumer to set priorities among foods that are offered for sale. For example, protein has been highly glamorized in the United States, yet nutritional research indicates that many Americans' diets exceed requirements for protein to the point of insulting the kidneys. If the consuming public were more aware of this, the proportion of lower-protein foods offered for sale would be likely to increase. Advertising notwithstanding, the food industry in the United States and much of the western world responds to consumer demand.

Nutrition probably is not a preeminent basis for the buying decisions that are made in a food store. Nevertheless, those who read labels on food packages probably also read publications, if only newspapers, that address nutritional topics. The nutritional aspects of safe eating are discussed elsewhere in this book. It should suffice to note here that undernutrition has emerged in the 1980s as a major concern in the United States (affecting 8–9% of the United States population) and that the longstanding problems of obesity and of iron-deficiency anemia in women of childbearing age continue. Vitamin deficiencies certainly occur on occasion, but so do intoxications due to excess vitamin intake. The options available to the more affluent of the United States food buyers are not always exercised wisely. In those countries where fewer options are offered the food buyer, nutritional decisions are made by the government or by economic circumstances.

Aside from decisions about which food purchases to make, the buyer must also take responsibility for safe handling of food from the time it is selected in the store. Many stores are so arranged that some of the most perishable foods are offered for sale nearest the entrance, so that the shopper may spend long periods with highly perishable foods in a cart, out of the refrigerator or freezer, before paying and leaving for home. This problem can be circumvented by selecting the most highly perishable items last before leaving the store, even if it requires some additional walking. The buyer should also note that food may be mishandled by retailers and by other shoppers. One must be alert to the potential for holding foods at improper temperatures, either as the food enters the store or while it is being offered for sale. Shoppers who observe such practices should complain to the management of the store. A shopper who observes repeated violations of safe food retailing practices should bring these to the attention of the responsible branch of government and should change vendors.

Abuse of food by other shoppers is also a concern. Sometimes this results from innocent (or ignorant) unsafe handling of foods that will ultimately be purchased by someone else, but malicious abuse of products has become an increasing problem. The only bright side, if there is any, to this is that packages designed to prevent malicious tampering also tend to preclude thoughtless abuse of food by shoppers other than the ultimate purchaser.

One would hope that a buyer who has shopped at the food store in a properly enlightened way would also arrange other stops so that the purchased food would not be subjected to temperature abuse in the interior or trunk of the car on the way home. Readers who have no cars with which to take their food purchases home may well wonder how this could be problem, but it certainly is. American mobility adds a dimension to the dangers of consumer transportation of food.

C. Food at Home

When food arrives at home it should, obviously, be stored in the refrigerator, the freezer, or on a shelf at room temperature as indicated by the directions on the package. However, it is important to note that the expected temperature of a freezer in the United States is −18°C (0°F) and of a refrigerator, 5°C (not above 40°F). These temperatures should not be taken for granted: occasional verification with a reliable thermometer is important. Beyond this, it is important that foods to be cooked be cooked thoroughly and that hot foods be served hot and cold foods, cold. During preparation and final serving, opportunities for cross-contamination and for temperature abuse should be recognized and avoided. A thawing chicken, for example, must not be allowed to drip onto a salad stored on a lower shelf of the refrigerator, nor should a cutting board used to cut raw meat be allowed to contaminate foods that are being sliced or otherwise prepared for final serving. Although eating carries an inevitable, small element of risk, no one who has read this book or completed a course for which it is used as a text should suffer from self-inflicted food poisoning. Risks in the home can and should be controlled.

Once food is served, it should be appreciated as a nondurable form of art. Only undercooked pork or poultry is probably hazardous enough to warrant rejection at the table, although there are those who would be equally concerned about undercooked or raw fish and seafood, and perhaps even beef. Foods that are not eaten (i.e., leftovers) must be refrigerated promptly; they should not be left to cool at room temperature before being placed in the refrigerator or freezer. Reheating of leftovers should be rapid and thorough; for reasons explained elsewhere in this book, time spent in the danger zone of temperatures must be minimized. Also, several foodborne disease agents (though assuredly not staphylococcal enterotoxin) that may be present in leftovers can be destroyed by thorough reheating. Even in professional hands in a restaurant, safe storage and serving of leftovers are often among the greatest challenges in food safety.

D. Amateurs in the Food Network

Foods are often abused outside the home by persons who are not professional food handlers. For example, group picnics and "potluck" dinners afford many opportunities to cause foodborne disease. Foods for such occasions may be prepared in unwontedly large quantities by persons who lack the skill, the facilities, or both for large-scale food preparation. Scaling up of old, familiar recipes can cause large quantities of food to remain for dangerous periods at inappropriate temperatures. Food service by amateurs may also take place where proper hand-washing and general hygienic facilities are unavailable, inasmuch as government regulation seldom applies to such situations. This has led to several of the more memorable outbreaks of foodborne disease described in this book.

E.   Rights and Responsibilities

In the United States and probably many other countries, there is a principle of "implied warranty"—goods offered for sale should be useful for the purpose for which they are sold. Applied to food, the implied warranty is that foods as sold are nutritious and safe. Other laws in the United States prohibit adulteration and mis-branding. However, it is important that every consumer learn what can and cannot be expected of food in the market. Absolute safety cannot be attained, and safety greater than presently exists can only be achieved, in most instances, at substantially increased cost to the consumer. Specifically, a purchaser of raw vegetables in the United States can reasonably expect that cysts of *Entamoeba histolytica* will not be present, but must also accept the high probability that spores of *Clostridium botulinum* in the food may express themselves and cause disease if inappropriate means of home preservation are employed. In another example, American consumers accept the risk that viable cysts of *Trichinella spiralis* may be present in United States government inspected pork, whereas people in Europe expect their governments' inspections to deal with this agent. A result is that American consumers "assume the worst" and cook pork more thoroughly than is often done in Europe. What can reasonably be expected with respect to *Salmonella* and *Campylobacter* contamination of market poultry and other raw meats is being argued in the political arena in the United States and elsewhere at this writing. It seems important to point out that undernutrition has become a major problem in the United States, and that attempts to "idiot-proof" food which result in a substantial increase in price will be a disservice to those who are already unable to feed themselves adequately.

This brings up the question of how consumers can participate in decisions concerning the safety of their food. They can, of course, communicate with vendors and (where applicable) processors, either by voicing complaints or by spending their money at different places or for different products. If government is expected to take a role, the consumer as a voter and taxpayer can contact elected or appointed officials and state the case. Groups that claim to represent consumers are also widespread. If one chooses to let such a group act as representatives, it is important to take careful heed of what is being said. Many "consumer" groups have been formed not by consumers but by individuals whose principal qualification is charisma. The rhetoric that results may look good in the newspapers but does not necessarily serve the interests of those who merely wish to eat safely and well at reasonable cost. It is clear that Americans spend fewer hours at work earning enough to feed themselves than people anywhere else in the world, and the incidence of foodborne disease in the United States is probably no higher than elsewhere (granted that foodborne disease is poorly reported everywhere), so attempts to improve the situation in the United States must be very carefully considered before being acted upon.

F.   Information Needs and Sources

What seems to be lacking in the United States, and probably in many other developed countries, is reliable information on nutrition and food safety, expressed in terms that a reasonably literate consumer can understand. It is probably not surprising that vendors of foods are reluctant to enunciate hazards associated with their products—in a competitive marketplace, the food that is *perceived* as least hazardous by consumers is likely to sell best. Government funding for food safety research conducted outside of government laboratories generally includes money to publish the results of the investigation in scientific journals but not to publicize the results in media that will reach the consumer. This means that a great deal of research sponsored by government (and ultimately by the taxpaying public) yields results that are not presented to the public in a useful way. It seems to me that the United States government must accept more responsibility for putting the results of nutritional and food safety research into a reasonable perspective and sharing it with the public. The USDA has made a modest beginning in this direction, but a great deal more could be done to develop information for consumer use and to publicize its availability.

Ultimately, only a small proportion of consumers looks to the government for food safety information, perhaps because information has seldom come from that source in the past. This means that the "media" must srve, at least temporarily, as the channel through which food safety information passes to consumers. Given the communications medias' problems with holding an audience for even short periods of time, it is not reasonable to hope for a major emphasis on accuracy. One can only hope that government will in time assume a sufficiently visible role as a source of information that both consumers and the media will look in this direction. Whether the situation in other countries resembles that in the United States is problematical, but it seems clear that valid information about nutrition and food safety is in short supply everywhere. This book is intended to strike a balance between the *very latest* information and that which has already withstood the test of time. These noble aspirations are probably applied to many other sources of information, and all undoubtedly fall short of their potential.

V. Summary

Safe food does not happen by accident. Those in the food business, and government, and those who ultimately prepare and eat the food all share the responsibility for keeping food safe. Food in the United States is relatively inexpensive and safe, but there is certainly room for improvement in informing consumers about how to protect themselves (perhaps from the consequences of their own folly). There are no valid generalizations about how food is kept safe in other countries, but it seems clear that American tourists can go many other places and eat the food (and drink the water) without fear of illness. Clearly, many kinds of institutional arrangements can yield a basically safe food supply. However, it seems clear also that the food industry, the government, and the consumer all play roles in the safety of food in every country. None of the three can abdicate its responsibility and still expect food to remain safe.

Bibliography

U.S. Department of Agriculture (1984). "The Safe Food Book—Your Kitchen Guide," Home Gard. Bull. No. 241. Food Saf. Inspection Serv., FSIS Publ. Off., Rm. 1165-S, USDA, Washington, DC 20250.

U.S. Department of Agriculture (1985–1986). "Safe Food to Go," Home and Gard. Bull., No. 242. Food Saf. Inspection Serv., FSIS Publ. Off., Rm. 1165-S, USDA, Washington, DC 20250.

U.S. Department of Agriculture. "Food News for Consumers." A quarterly news publication available by subscription from the Superintendent of Documents, U.S. Gov. Print. Off., Washington, DC 20402.

U.S. Department of Agriculture Meat and Poultry Hotline (weekdays 10 a.m. to 4 p.m. EDT): 800-535-4555, or write to the Meat and Poultry Hotline, USDA, FSIS, Rm. 1165-S, Washington, DC 20250.

CHAPTER 25

PERENNIAL ISSUES IN FOOD SAFETY

Edwin M. Foster

I. Introduction

A. American Experience through the 19th Century

From its beginnings in colonial times to the American Civil War in the 19th century the United States was basically an agrarian society. Most people produced and preserved their own food supply, which was far different than the one we enjoy today. Drying, salting, and pickling were the main processes of preservation.

The American Civil War gave a boost to the fledgling canning industry, and postwar growth of the cities encouraged development of the meat and dairy industries. No longer could each family have its own garden, cow, pigs, and chickens. The nation was moving rapidly into an urbanized society.

Safety and honesty soon became important issues. In 1869 news writers complained that city people were in constant danger of buying unwholesome meat, that dealers were unscrupulous, and that the people were uneducated. This was only 5 years after Pasteur disproved the theory of spontaneous generation and even before Robert Koch demonstrated that microbes can cause disease.

Milk soon became recognized as a dangerous source of infection. As dairies grew in size, so did the outbreaks of typhoid fever, diphtheria, scarlet fever, tuberculosis, and other infectious diseases that were easily transmitted by milk.

Economic cheating was everywhere. Milk was diluted with water, coffee with charcoal, cocoa with sawdust, olive oil with coconut oil, butter with oleomargarine, honey with sugar, and candy with paraffin. Some operators preserved milk with formaldehyde, meat with sulfurous acid, and butter with borax.

During the last third of the 19th century Americans had plenty to complain about from the standpoint of both safety and economic cheating. The times were right for some kind of regulatory program.

B. Regulation Begins

Throughout the 19th century the food industry was based essentially on the theory of "caveat emptor," let the buyer beware. A few large cities and a handful of states had enacted limited controls on certain types of food sold within their jurisdictions, but there was no regulation whatever at the national level. This situation changed early in the 20th century, when Congress passed the Food and Drugs Act of 1906. This was done largely at the urging of Dr. Harvey W. Wiley, a chemist in the U.S. Department of Agriculture, who had been campaigning for years to outlaw the abuses being imposed on the American people. The Food and Drugs Act covered all food except meat, which was regulated by the Meat Inspection Act of 1906. Both laws had similar provisions, although the Meat Inspection Act included a requirement for resident inspectors and much more rigorous attention during slaughter and processing than did the Food and Drugs Act.

The Food and Drugs Act of 1906 was a relatively short document that simply made it illegal to sell misbranded or adulterated food in interstate commerce. Food was considered adulterated if (1) any substance was added that reduced its quality or strength; (2) any substance was substituted wholly or in part for the article of food; (3) any valuable constituent of the food was removed; (4) the food was treated in a way that concealed damage or inferiority; (5) the food contained any added poisonous or other deleterious ingredient which might render it injurious to health; or (6) it consisted in whole or in part of a filthy, decomposed, or putrid substance, or any portion of an animal unfit for food, or the food was the product of a diseased animal or one that had died otherwise than by slaughter.

There was one serious problem with this law. To take any regulatory action the government had to prove that a given product was adulterated or misbranded. Manufacturers still could do just about anything they wished. If the government elected to claim that a product on the market contained an added adulterant substance, it was incumbent upon the government to prove that the substance was both present and also injurious to health.

We lived with this law for over half a century. Responsibility for proving the safety of food ingredients was not transferred to the manufacturer until the Food Additive Amendment was passed in 1958.

C. Impact of World War II

Meanwhile, World War II in the 1940s brought enormous developments in the chemical industry. All kinds of insecticides, fungicides, herbicides, fertilizers, plastics, and other useful chemicals appeared on the scene. There seemed to be no limit to the ingenuity and resourcefulness of the chemical industry's scientists.

Much the same thing can be said about the developments in food technology. A great deal of effort during the war went into the development of better rations for the troops, who were located all over the world from arctic to tropic climates. These efforts were continued after the war in the development of new foods for the civilian population. New products, new processes, new packaging methods, and new functional ingredients were developed. Many of these new ingredients were synthetic chemicals, such as antioxidants, emulsifiers, sweeteners, and the like.

The net result of these developments was a huge increase in the use of synthetic chemicals in our daily lives. This increase began to worry some people, including members of Congress. There was a growing doubt in the wisdom of adding a large assortment of new chemicals to our foods and to our environment. There was concern about upsetting the balance of nature, and there was growing mistrust of industries that manufactured and used these chemicals.

Finally, in 1950, the U.S. House of Representatives appointed a Select Committee to Investigate the Use of Chemicals in Foods. The chairman was Congressman James J. Delaney of New York. This action was a prelude to passage of the Pesticide Chemical Amendment in 1954 and the Food Additives Amendment in 1958.

The latter amendment was the first major change in the basic food law since it was enacted in 1906. The 1958 Amendment established three categories of food ingredients: (1) substances that were generally recognized as safe (GRAS) on the basis of prior usage or scientific information, (2) regulated food additives, and (3) substances that were banned from use in foods. For the first time the food manufacturer was required to provide acceptable evidence that a food ingredient was safe before he used it rather than have the government prove that it was unsafe after it was on the market.

This action was extended to color additives by a separate amendment adopted in 1960.

The decade of the 1950s saw a growing concern about dissemination of man-made chemicals in our environment and our food supply. One of the most effective events in crystallizing the opposition to pesticides and other chemicals was the publication in 1962 of Rachel Carson's book "Silent Spring." This eloquent plea to turn back the clock and save the robins gave a tremendous boost to the burgeoning environmental movements that were then beginning.

Controversy increased sharply, with particular concern about DDT. This insecticide is reputed to have saved more lives than any other chemical made by humans, yet it was banned in 1970 on the grounds that it caused thin eggshells in fish-eating birds.

Concern and controversy over chemicals added to our foods and to our environment grew rapidly in the 1960s, culminating in an order by President Nixon to reexamine the entire GRAS list of food ingredients. This job took several years and a great deal of money to complete. It revealed nothing of special concern about the safety of food components except to reemphasize something we already knew— there is no way to prove that a chemical is safe. We can feed a material to animals and we can look for evidence of harm that tells us the material is *unsafe* for the particular animal under the particular conditions of test, but that evidence does not prove safety under some other conditions and it does not even prove lack of safety for man under any conditions.

So, with imprecise and uncertain methods coupled with our inability to experiment with humans it should not be surprising that controversy has arisen and grown, especially around anything that appears to incite the development of any kind of cancer or tumor in any organ of any animal species, whether it relates to humans or not.

The result is an environment of ignorance in which the proponents of any idea, no matter how ridiculous or impractical, can make themselves heard and gain headlines in the news media simply because this is a land of free speech and there is no way to prove them wrong.

II. Food Safety Becomes a National Issue

The controversies that developed up to and during the early 1970s led the Food and Drug Administration (FDA) to establish six categories of hazard in the following descending order of risk:

1. Microbiological contamination
2. Nutritional problems
3. Environmental contaminants
4. Naturally occurring toxicants
5. Pesticide residues
6. Food additives

This list provides a convenient basis for discussing the various safety issues that have arisen over the past 25 years. However, it should be supplemented with a "miscellaneous" category covering such items as reaction products formed during cooking.

A. Microbiological Contamination

From the standpoint of solid information there is no question that microbiological hazards are the most common, and probably the most serious, of all foodborne disease hazards. Botulism has been recognized for over two centuries. Both salmonellosis and staphylococcal food poisoning have been known for more than 50 years. Others are still being discovered. Table I lists the long-known pathogenic and toxigenic agents of foodborne disease with the reported incidence of each. It is well recognized that these figures represent only a small fraction of the true number of outbreaks and cases of foodborne illness in the United States. Most outbreaks are never investigated, and many of these are never confirmed with the organism and the food identified. Thus, we are left with estimates based on extrapolations from known figures, but there is a general belief that the American public suffers several million cases of foodborne disease each year.

Controlling and preventing foodborne illness depends a great deal on the nature of the organism. *Bacillus cereus* and *Clostridium perfringens* are widely distributed sporeformers that cause trouble only in certain cooked foods that are subjected to gross temperature abuse. At one time *Clostridium botulinum* was a serious problem for the canning industry, but safe food processes were developed which virtually eliminated botulism from commercially canned foods. The bacterium is still a problem for home canners.

Table I
Confirmed Outbreaks of Foodborne Disease
in the United States

Causal organism	Number of outbreaks[a]	Number of cases[a]
Bacillus cereus	6	127
Clostridium perfringens	21	1108
Clostridium botulinum	13	27
Salmonella spp.	50	2322
Shigella spp.	7	433
Staphylococcus aureus	31	1651
Viruses	8	1196

[a]Figures represent annual averages for the 5 years from 1978 to 1982 as published in "Foodborne Disease Surveillance Annual Summaries." Centers for Disease Control, U.S. Public Health Service, Atlanta, Georgia.

Salmonella organisms are not a serious health problem in processed foods, but they are frequent contaminants of animal products (milk, meat, and eggs). Handling and cooking food properly is presently the only way to deal with these organisms. A great deal of controversy has arisen over the presence of salmonellae in chickens, though it is doubtful that they are any greater health problem in chickens than they are in other animal products.

Staphylococcus aureus is no longer a serious problem with processed foods excepting, occasionally, such fermented items as cheese and dry sausages. The organism can still be a problem with foods that are prepared, contaminated, and then mishandled before consumption. *Shigella* spp. and the enteric viruses originate from human sources and get into food only by the fecal route. This can happen from infected food handlers or through contaminated food (e.g., shellfish) grown in polluted waters.

Several other bacterial species, most of them well-known pathogens of animals, were first recognized as foodborne disease agents during the past 10 years. *Campylobacter jejuni,* for example, is now believed to cause more outbreaks of gastroenteritis than *Salmonella* and *Shigella* combined. *Escherichia coli* is a member of the normal flora of the gastrointestinal tract and long was considered harmless. In recent years, however, several serotypes have been discovered that cause gastroenteritis. One of them, *E. coli* **O**157:**H**7, causes an especially serious type of bloody diarrhea that sometimes spreads to the urinary tract and causes permanent kidney damage.

Yersinia enterocolitica is a widespread animal pathogen that grows well at refrigeration temperatures. It has caused several serious outbreaks of gastroenteritis in recent years. *Listeria monocytogenes,* a cause of lethal nervous disorders in domestic animals, is now known to be able to infect man via the oral route. Sizeable outbreaks with numerous deaths have been traced to contaminated cabbage and a soft, Mexican-type cheese. The organism is widespread in nature and, like *Yersinia,* it can grow at refrigeration temperatures.

The cholera bacillus *Vibrio cholerae* is known to be in our coastal waters. It contaminates our shellfish and crustaceans and causes occasional outbreaks of Asiatic cholera. *Vibrio vulnificus,* a highly invasive bacterium, also is common in shellfish from coastal waters. This organism is especially hazardous to people with liver disease or compromised immune systems. *Aeromonas hydrophila* has only recently been recognized as an agent of foodborne disease. Its full significance is yet to be established.

Nonbacterial hazards in foods include the mycotoxins, or fungal poisons, which develop in cereal grains and peanuts under certain conditions of cultivation. These substances have been recognized for about 30 years, but we have little evidence to date that they are, in fact, a serious threat to public health.

Anyone who is familiar with the evidence is bound to agree with the FDA's conviction that microbial contamination is the most serious of the known hazards to health that can be transmitted to man by food.

B. Nutritional Problems

We have long known that scurvy, rickets, beriberi, pellagra, goiter, and a few other diseases were the result of deficiencies in certain dietary components, primarily vitamins. As a result, most of these deficiency diseases have been eliminated from the United States population. Dietary supplements have become popular with many people and now we hear about problems caused by excessive intake of essential nutrients—selenium, iodine, and vitamins A and D, to name a few. Some of these materials have a surprisingly narrow range between optimum and toxic levels.

Controversy exists over the safety and effectiveness of what amounts to nation-wide experimental dietary manipulation. Experts tell us to (1) consume less sodium to ward off hypertension; (2) eat less saturated fat and cholesterol to reduce the risk of heart attack; (3) eat less unsaturated fat and more fiber to reduce the risk of cancer; and (4) take huge doses of vitamin C to assure good health and well being. Other equally qualified experts give contrary advice. Clearly, we don't understand all we need to know about the relationship between diet and health.

C.   Environmental Contaminants

Growth of the environmental movement during the past 25 years has raised many issues that impinge on food safety. Food can become contaminated with potentially toxic chemicals in various ways. Table II lists 13 materials that have been demonstrated in food at one time or another in recent years and whose safety has been questioned.

There is no doubt about the toxicity of heavy metals; the problem comes in deciding what is a safe intake level. Cadmium and selenium are found at undesirably high levels in localized areas of the soil. Plants grown in those areas accumulate the elements to excess. Lead is widely used in commerce and gets into food from various sources. One source that has come under scrutiny is the solder used for sealing tin cans. The canning industry has greatly reduced exposure to lead from this source. Mercury occurs naturally, but the areas of most concern are the rivers and bays that receive discharge from chemical plants that emit mercury. There have been several outbreaks of mercury poisoning following the consumption of fish and other seafood taken from contaminated waters.

Chlorine and iodine are among the most widely used sanitizing agents in food plants. Chlorine also is the universal disinfectant to assure safe drinking water. However, it is now known that chlorine can react with organic matter to form products that cause cancer in experimental animals. Likewise, excessive intake of iodine can lead to goiter formation. Finding effective replacements for chlorine and iodine as food-plant sanitizing agents will not be easy.

Table II
Some Chemical Contaminants of Concern in Foods

Heavy metals	Halogenated compounds	Others
Cadmium	Chlorine	Antibiotics in
Lead	Iodine	animal feed
Mercury	Polybrominated biphenyls	Asbestos
Selenium	Polychlorinated biphenyls	Diethylstilbestrol
	Trichloroethylene	
	Vinyl chloride	

Vinyl chloride is the building block of polyvinyl chloride, one of our most useful plastic polymers for packaging food. The vinyl chloride monomer is carcinogenic for experimental animals, and at one time traces of the monomer remained in the finished product. Manufacturers now are able to eliminate the monomer. Trichloroethylene is an organic solvent that has been used for removing certain components from food (e.g., decaffeinating coffee). It too is carcinogenic in animals and its use in food has been stopped. Polychlorinated biphenyls (PCBs) once were widely used as heat exchange fluids, but this application was halted following a few episodes of accidental food and feed contamination with PCBs. Polybrominated biphenyls have long been used as fire-retardant chemicals, but this application was stopped after some of the material was accidentally incorporated in dairy cow rations. Many cattle were poisoned, and safety of their milk came under scrutiny.

For at least 30 years low levels of antibiotics have been added to animal feed to stimulate growth and efficiency of feed utilization. The practice has been controversial almost from the beginning. The primary objective is based on the belief that antibiotic-resistant bacteria will develop and contaminate the environment. Proponents of the practice say that no such selective action has occurred thus far and therefore is unlikely to be a problem. The controversy continues.

Asbestos is a widely used filtering medium and can contaminate liquid foods during filtration. This substance can cause lung cancer if inhaled. Its effect on ingestion is not known. Diethylstilbestrol is a synthetic steroid that also has been widely used to stimulate growth of domestic animals. This compound was found to cause cancer in experimental animals and was banned several years ago. The wisdom of the ban is still argued. Dioxins are contaminants of certain pesticides and therefore may get into food if used improperly.

D. Naturally Occurring Toxicants

Over the centuries humans have discovered that certain plants and animals are harmful when eaten. He has learned to survive by avoiding those that are poisonous or by treating them in some way to eliminate the toxicity. Table III lists some of the many toxicants that occur naturally in food. Ames (1983) has published a much longer and more detailed list that pertains only to mutagens and carcinogens.

Table III
Some Toxicants That Occur Naturally in Food

In plants	In animals
Bracken fern	Ciguatoxin
Caffeine	Paralytic shellfish
Cyanide	poison
Gossypol	Tetrodotoxin
Hydrazines	
Pyrrolizidine alkaloids	
Quercetin, other flavonoids	
Quinones	
Safrole, estragole	
Solanine	
Theobromine	

Cyanide is found in lima beans. It is driven off during cooking. Safrole and related compounds are found in many edible plants, including sassafras and black pepper. These compounds are carcinogenic in rodents. Solanine is a strong cholinesterase inhibitor and possible teratogen in potatoes. Formation of this glycoalkaloid is stimulated when the potato is diseased, bruised, or exposed to light. It can reach levels that are lethal to humans. Quercetin and similar flavonoids are widespread in the human diet. As a group they are mutagenic in short-term test systems and quercetin has been found carcinogenic in some test animals. Quinones are very common in the diet. They participate in numerous toxigenic reactions and many are mutagenic. Theobromine is a relative of caffeine and acts in much the same way.

Gossypol is a major toxic component of cottonseed, comprising about 1% of the seed's dry weight. The compound has a variety of toxic actions including carcinogenicity in mice. Plant breeders have developed a "glandless" cottonseed which contains very low levels of gossypol. Hydrazines are present in edible mushrooms. Many of them are carcinogenic in rodents. The pyrrolizidine alkaloids are common in many plant species but are ingested by humans mainly in the form of herbs and herbal teas. These compounds are carcinogenic, mutagenic, and teratogenic in experimental animals. Bracken ferns are eaten as green vegetables in some parts of the world. They are carcinogenic to humans.

Among the animal sources of toxins, ciguatoxin poisoning is a common result of eating certain fish that live on and around reefs in the warm waters of the Caribbean Sea. The original toxin is formed in microscopic life and is passed through the food chain up to the fish that are eaten by humans. Tetrodotoxin is a natural component of the puffer fish, or *Fugu,* as it is known in Japan. The tetrodotoxin is concentrated in the liver, gonads, and certain other internal organs which must be removed before the fish can be safely eaten. Paralytic shellfish poisoning results from the accumulation of toxic dinoflagellates in clams, mussels, and related shellfish during periods of algal "blooms" in shoreline waters. The toxin is a very potent nerve poison that survives cooking. When an algal bloom or "red tide" develops, shellfish harvesting must be stopped until the situation corrects itself. This can take months.

Despite all the concern about man-made chemicals in the environment and in the foods we eat, it is clear that nature herself has provided many more dangers than we like to admit. At the same time, however, nature has provided a measure of protection in the form of anticarcinogens which are believed to have considerable protective effect against cancer. Vitamin E (alpha tocopherol) and beta carotene are antioxidants that help protect the body against cancer. Carotenoids, such as beta carotene, are found in green and yellow vegetables, which are believed on epidemiologic grounds to offer substantial protection against cancer. Selenium, glutathione, and ascorbic acid are other naturally occurring antioxidants that show a protective effect against carcinogens.

E. Pesticide Residues

Many of the wonders of today's productive agriculture can be credited to the use of chemical pesticides developed during and after World War II. A wide variety of insecticides, fungicides, and plant-growth regulators have been made available to the nation's farmers to increase yield and reduce labor. The Environmental Protection Agency regulates the use of pesticides, but the FDA establishes tolerances that must be met for presence of pesticide chemicals in foods. Some of these chemicals are highly toxic to animals, including humans.

Our experience of the past 40 years has revealed very little evidence of danger to consumers from pesticide residues in food. There have been accidents in the use of pesticides that affected the farmer or pest-control operator, but these represented massive exposure while handling or spreading the chemicals. Even so, great controversy has arisen over pesticide usage, especially where environmental considerations are prominent, as is true with the so-called persistent pesticides that decompose slowly in soil.

Eliminating any useful chemical has a price. When DDT was banned in the United States, we changed to the far more dangerous organophosphates, which have been involved in several fatal accidents during application. We also saw tussock moths and spruce budworms decimate forests from Maine to Oregon. We saw malaria return to Sri Lanka and other tropical countries, bringing death to thousands of people after the disease had been virtually eliminated. And we saw an increase in aflatoxin levels in corn grown in certain parts of the country. What benefits did we gain? We were told that the eggs of fish-eating birds might hatch better, and we were promised a highly questionable reduction in our risk of cancer. Were the benefits worth the cost? All persons will have to answer for themselves. It is widely accepted that DDT has saved more lives than any other man-made chemical in history. The World Health Organization has stated that "The safety record of DDT for man is truly remarkable." Yet it is banned in the United States.

Ethylene dibromide (EDB) is another long-used pesticide that was banned in the early 1980s. It was used mainly to control insects in grain during storage but was banned on the grounds that it caused cancer in rodents. Like DDT, this compound has never shown evidence of toxicity or carcinogenicity in humans.

F. Food Additives

Without question, the greatest public concern over food safety is associated with chemicals added to foods. This is the same area that the FDA considers least hazardous of the six categories established originally. Table IV lists some of the

Table IV
Some Food Additives Whose Safety Has Been Questioned
in the United States since 1969

Aspartame	Hydrogenated fats	Saccharin
BHA, BHT	Monosodium glutamate	Salt
Caffeine	Nitrate	Sugar
Carbon black[a]	Nitrite	Synthetic colors
Carrageenan	Phosphate	and flavors
Cobalt salts[a]	FD&C red #2[a]	Sulfite
Cyclamates[a]	FD&C red #3	FD&C violet #1[a]
Diethylpyrocarbonate[a]	FD&C red #40	FD&C yellow #5

[a]Banned in the United States.

food additives whose safety has been publicly questioned since 1969. The reasons for controversy have been varied.

A high salt intake exacerbates hypertension; hence, physicians commonly prescribe low-salt diets for hypertensive patients. It is widely recognized that Americans eat more salt than they need for metabolic use. Therefore, certain government agencies, supported by medical groups, have urged a nationwide reduction in salt consumption. It seems a harmless recommendation, though it could be significant if food manufacturers removed salt from those foods in which it is a primary preservative (mostly ripened cheeses and cured meats).

Sugar has been blamed for numerous effects ranging from dental caries through obesity (and possible cancer) to criminal behavior. Aspartame is a recently developed dipeptide that serves as a low-calorie sweetener. It has been thoroughly studied and the FDA approved its use, yet its safety is still being challenged. Saccharin has been used as a low-calorie sweetener for almost a century but now is believed to cause bladder cancer in rodents. The FDA proposed a ban on saccharin several years ago, but the ban was prevented by a special act of Congress. The matter is still under debate. Cyclamates, another class of low-calorie sweeteners, were banned several years ago on the grounds that they caused bladder cancer in rodents. Additional study has cast doubt on the original evidence of carcinogenicity, but the cyclamates are still banned from use in foods.

A great deal of controversy has involved several food colors in recent years, and some of them have been banned from food use. FD&C red #2 was excluded on the basis of questionable evidence that it caused cancer in rodents. FD&C red #3 has been opposed on the grounds that it adds to the iodine content of the diet, but it is still in use. The safety of FD&C red #40 was questioned on the basis that it might cause leukemia. A few people appear to be sensitive to FD&C yellow #5; hence, special labeling is now required to warn consumers of its presence. FD&C violet #1 and carbon black were banned on evidence that they cause cancer in mice.

Sulfite was once considered GRAS. Early claims that it was mutagenic were refuted, and metabolic studies showed no indication of toxicity in experimental animals. However, recent evidence revealed that a few asthmatic people are exquisitely sensitive to sulfite and undergo severe respiratory distress when exposed. This has led to increased restrictions on use and broader labeling requirements.

Nitrite and/or nitrate are used as curing agents for ham, bacon, and other processed meats. Nitrite reacts with certain amines to form nitrosamines, many of which cause cancer in rodents. These compounds offer a good example of the dilemma we face in electing to ban a useful chemical. In the first place, we could not avoid nitrite if we wanted to. Nitrate is common in vegetables and many water supplies. We manufacture our own nitrite in our salivary glands. Therefore, banning nitrite from use in foods would not end our exposure. Furthermore, nitrite plays a very important role in the preservation of cured meat products, especially through inhibiting growth and toxin formation by *Clostridium botulinum*. The regulatory agencies have taken steps to minimize nitrosamine formation in cured meats (chiefly bacon, where the nitrosamines are formed during cooking), but nitrite is still an important component of cured meat products.

The safety of phosphates has been questioned in the belief that they interfere with calcium metabolism and, therefore, bone structure. Experimental evidence does not support this theory. Phosphates have also been accused of causing misbehavior in children.

Cobalt salts were permitted at one time as foam stabilizers for beer. They were banned after the death of several people who regularly consumed over 3 gallons (ca. 11 liters) of beer per day.

Butylated hydroxyanisole and butylated hydroxytoluene (BHA and BHT) are synthetic antioxidant chemicals that have long been used to prevent rancidity in foods. They offer a special concern because of their conflicting reactions in tests for carcinogenicity. Both BHA and BHT have been shown to cause hyperplasia of the forestomachs of rats under certain conditions of feeding. However, they also help prevent cancer under other test conditions.

Caffeine, a natural component of coffee and tea and a prominent ingredient of many soft drinks, has been accused of causing lumps in the breast, birth defects, and pancreatic cancer. The evidence is far from conclusive. Carrageenan is a widely used thickening agent that is extracted from seaweed. In foods it is used in the natural form, but for certain pharmaceutical preparations it is partly degraded. This degraded form, but not the natural form, has been alleged to cause ulcers of the colon when fed in large amounts to monkeys.

Monosodium glutamate is a widely used flavor-enhancing agent in many processed foods. It has been blamed for causing the so-called "Chinese Restaurant Syndrome," a discomfort that some people experience when they consume Chinese food.

Diethylpyrocarbonate has been used as a preservative in beer and wine to prevent yeast growth in the finished beverage. A major advantage of the compound was its hydrolysis to carbon dioxide and ethanol. Later, however, it was discovered that small amounts of urethane, a potent carcinogen, were formed during hydrolysis. Accordingly, the compound was banned from use in food.

The safety of hydrogenated fats was questioned after evidence was obtained suggesting that consumption of *trans* fatty acids led to atherosclerosis. This evidence was used to discourage consumption of margarine. The evidence was obtained in feeding trials with swine but has not been confirmed by other investigators.

Synthetic colors and flavors have long been under attack, mainly on the grounds that they have no nutritive value and therefore should not be in food. Up to now a more substantive reason has been necessary before they could be banned from the food supply.

G. Miscellaneous

A few issues of food safety have arisen in recent years that did not appear in the FDA's six categories of hazard. These may be classed as products of reactions that occur during preparation and storing of food. An example would be the nitrosamines that sometimes form as reaction products of residual nitrite with amines when bacon is being fried. Another example is the benzo(*a*)pyrene that is formed when meat is grilled over charcoal. The true impact of these substances on human health is unknown.

III.   Summary and Conclusions

It has been pointed out many times that the public's conception of hazard in foods does not agree with that of the FDA. Over the past 15 years, for example, it would appear that the public is more concerned about the safety of additives and chemical contaminants in food and less worried about microbiological and nutritional hazards. This is the exact opposite of the FDA's ranking and merely reflects what the public has been told. This situation is subject to change, of course, as more reliable information becomes available. Large and serious outbreaks of foodborne microbial disease in 1985 made a strong impression on the public's conception of food safety.

One reason for the confusion that has developed around food safety is our lack of clear and unequivocal information about the toxicology of food components on humans. We cannot find out if a particular substance causes cancer in humans by feeding it to humans. The best we can do is feed the material to experimental animals and hope the results can be extrapolated to humans. There is a great deal of uncertainty about the meaning of results obtained in this way, and uncertainty always leads to controversy and conflict. Sometimes the conflict can be reconciled only by political means (e.g., the saccharin situation).

Over and over during the past two decades we have learned not to believe everything we hear about food safety. Far too many irresponsible scientists and pseudoscientists have chosen to sound public warnings about one or another component of the diet that *might* be harmful. Usually the basis for such warning is tenuous, hypothetical, and without relevant scientific support. As an example, several years ago an academic chemist saw a reaction when he added deoxyribonucleic acid (DNA, the basic material of heredity) to a $6 M$ sulfite solution. On this evidence alone he hypothesized and warned the public that sulfite may cause mutations and possibly even cancer; therefore, they should avoid foods that contain sulfite. What he did not know, obviously, is that animal tissues contain the enzyme sulfite oxidase, which rapidly converts sulfite to sulfate for excretion in the urine. In extensive studies with fruit flies there was no evidence of mutagenicity of dietary sulfite at any level below acutely toxic concentrations. Clearly, the public should not panic just because someone says that something might not be safe. We need better evidence than that.

Widespread fear of toxic chemicals in food and concern about depleting the soil's nutrients have given impetus to the "natural" food movement (often referred to as organic farming). Animal manure is a good source of plant nutrients, but it often contains pathogenic microorganisms that can cause foodborne disease. In 1981, for example, we had a large outbreak of listeriosis in North America that was traced to coleslaw. The cabbage was grown on land that was fertilized with animal manure. The manure came from a flock of sheep that had recently suffered from an outbreak of listeriosis.

Bibliography

Ames, B. N. (1983). Dietary carcinogens and anticarcinogens. *Science* **221**, 1256–1264.

INDEX